METHODS IN MOLECULAR BIOLOGY™

Series Editor
John M. Walker
School of Life Sciences
University of Hertfordshire
Hatfield, Hertfordshire, AL10 9AB, UK

For other titles published in this series, go to
www.springer.com/series/7651

Type 2 Diabetes

Methods and Protocols

Edited by

Claire Stocker

Clore Laboratory, University of Buckingham, Hunter Street, Buckingham, UK

Humana Press

Editor
Claire Stocker, Ph.D.
Clore Laboratory
University of Buckingham
Hunter Street
Buckingham
United Kingdom MK18 1EG
claire.stocker@buckingham.ac.uk

ISSN: 1064-3745 e-ISSN: 1940-6029
ISBN: 978-1-934115-15-2 e-ISBN: 978-1-59745-448-3
DOI: 10.1007/978-1-59745-448-3
Springer Dordrecht Heidelberg London New York

Library of Congress Control Number: 2009922609

Printed on acid-free paper

Springer is part of Springer Science+Business Media (www.springer.com)

Preface

Diabetes is now reaching epidemic proportions, and the associated complications of this disease can be life threatening and disabling. Over recent years, both clinical and basic researchers have increased our understanding of the mechanisms involved in the progression of diabetes and the relative roles played by both environmental and genetic factors. For example, it is well known that a lifestyle of inactivity and excessive food intake plays an important part in diabetes risk.

The purpose of this volume is to provide up-to-date explanations of commonly used laboratory protocols used in diabetes research. Specifically, the chapters will cover the commonly described in vivo and in vitro model systems, ultimately leading to an overall view of how cellular dysfunction and degeneration lead to susceptibility and diabetes disease progression.

This book is unique in providing a simple explanation of a particular practical technique or model in a short succinct format, thus allowing research scientists and clinicians quick and easy practical information to address a particular question. There are key practical notes at the end of each chapter, as well as numerous helpful tables and figures.

Claire Stocker
Buckingham, UK

Contents

Contributors

PETRA AUGSTEIN • *Institute of Diabetes "Gerhardt Katsch" Karlsburg e.V., Karlsburg, Germany*

SUSAN BONNER-WEIR • *Section on Islet Transplantation and Cell Biology, Research Division, Joslin Diabetes Center and the Department of Medicine, Harvard Medical School, Boston, MA, USA*

GAY M. CROOKS • *Division of Research Immunology/BMT, Childrens Hospital Los Angeles, Los Angeles, CA, USA*

ELEFTHERIA DIAKOGIANNAKI • *Institute of Biomedical and Clinical Science, Peninsula Medical School, Plymouth, Devon, UK*

DONALD R. DUNBAR • *Centres for Cardiovascular Science and Inflammation Research, Queen's Medical Research Institute, University of Edinburgh, Edinburgh, UK*

SHUNDI GE • *Division of Research Immunology/BMT, Childrens Hospital Los Angeles, Los Angeles, CA, USA*

PETER M. JONES • *Beta Cell Development & Function Group, King's College London, London, UK*

KLAUS H. KAESTNER • *Department of Genetics and Institute for Diabetes, Obesity and Metabolism, University of Pennsylvania School of Medicine, Philadelphia, PA, USA*

JASON K. KIM • *Division of Endocrinology, Metabolism and Diabetes Director, UMass Mouse Phenotyping Center University of Massachusetts Medical School, 381 Plantation Street, Suite 200 Worcester, MA, USA*

NICKY KONSTANTOPOULOS • *Metabolic Research Unit, Deakin University, Geelong, VIC, Australia*

EDWARD H. LEITER • *The Jackson Laboratory, Bar Harbor, ME, USA*

WAN-CHUN LI • *Section of Islet Transplantation and Cell Biology, Joslin Diabetes Center, Boston, MA, USA*

LORELLA MARSELLI • *Section on Islet Transplantation and Cell Biology, Research Division, Joslin Diabetes Center and the Department of Medicine, Harvard Medical School, Boston, MA, USA*

JUAN CARLOS MOLERO-NAVAJAS • *Metabolic Research Unit, Deakin University, Geelong, VIC, Australia*

EDUARD MONTANYA • *Endocrine Unit, University Hospital of Bellvitge, Barcelona, Spain*

Department of Clinical Sciences, University of Barcelona, Barcelona, Spain

Biomedical Research Institute of Bellvitge (IDIBELL), L'Hospitalet de Llobregat, Barcelona, Spain

NOEL G. MORGAN • *Institute of Biomedical and Clinical Science, Peninsula Medical School, Plymouth, Devon, UK*

BEVERLY SARA MÜHLHAUSLER • *Early Origins of Adult Health Research Group, Sansom Research Institute, University of South Australia, Adelaide, SA, Australia*

DANY MULLER • *Beta Cell Development & Function Group, King's College London, London, UK*

ANNA L. NOLAN • *Elixir Pharmaceuticals, Cambridge, MA, USA*

JACQUELINE F. O'DOWD • *Clore Laboratory, University of Buckingham, Buckingham, Buckinghamshire, UK*

SHANTA J. PERSAUD • *Beta Cell Development & Function Group, King's College London, London, UK*

MARK A. RUSSELL • *Institute of Biomedical and Clinical Science, Peninsula Medical School, Plymouth, Devon, UK*

ECKHARD SALZSIEDER • *Institute of Diabetes "Gerhardt Katsch" Karlsburg e.V., Karlsburg, Germany*

DENNIS C. SGROI • *Molecular Pathology Unit, Massachusetts General Hospital, Harvard Medical School, Boston, MA, USA*

NOÈLIA TÉLLEZ • *Biomedical Research Institute of Bellvitge (IDIBELL), L'Hospitalet de Llobregat, Barcelona, Spain*

XIULI WANG • *Division of Research Immunology/BMT, Childrens Hospital Los Angeles, Los Angeles, CA, USA, Division of Cancer Immunotherapeutics and Tumor Immunology, City of Hope National Medical Center, Duarte, CA, USA*

EDWARD T. WARGENT • *Clore Laboratory, University of Buckingham, Buckingham, Buckinghamshire, UK*

GORDON C. WEIR • *Section on Islet Transplantation and Cell Biology, Research Division, Joslin Diabetes Center and the Department of Medicine, Harvard Medical School, Boston, MA, USA*

PETER WHITE • *Director, Biomedical Genomics Core, Research Assistant Professor of Pediatrics, The Research Institute at Nationwide Children's Hospital and The Ohio State University*

Chapter 1

Selecting the "Right" Mouse Model for Metabolic Syndrome and Type 2 Diabetes Research

Edward H. Leiter

Summary

This is not a "Methods" chapter in the traditional sense. Rather, it is an essay designed to help address one of the most frequently asked questions by investigators about to embark on a study requiring an animal model of diabetes - what is the "right" model for the reader's specific research application. Because genetic heterogeneity and the requirement for complex gene-environment interaction characterize the various mouse models of Type 2 diabetes as well as the human disease manifestations, the readers may come to share the author's conclusion that more than one model is required if the investigator is interested in knowing how broadly effective a given compound with putative therapeutic efficacy might be.

Key words: Mouse model, Genetic, Transgenic, Knockout, Monogenic and polygenic

1. Introduction

The Jackson Laboratory (TJL) is the world's largest repository of inbred mouse strains and genetically engineered (by gene targeting or transgenesis) or otherwise genetically manipulated mouse stocks useful for biomedical research. Included among these holdings is a large and ever-expanding subset used to analyze the etiology, pathophysiology, and therapy of Type 2 diabetes (T2D). The types of models available, and a resource manual describing them, may be accessed at http://jaxmice.jax.org/models/diabetes_obesity.html. One of the most commonly asked questions is: "Given a list with a large number of choices, what is the best mouse model available for T2D research applications?" The model(s) recommended very likely will differ according to the type of application. This chapter will discuss issues relevant

C. Stocker (ed.), *Type 2 Diabetes,* Methods in Molecular Biology, vol. 560
DOI 10.1007/978-1-59745-448-3_1, © Humana Press, a part of Springer Science+Business Media, LLC 2009

to helping an investigator new to the field of animal diabetes research make well-informed choices.

2. Why There Is No "Best" Model

T2D is widely recognized to be among the most complex, genetically heterogeneous disease conditions of humans, with both heredity and environment generally contributing to disease pathogenesis. Accordingly, there is unlikely to be a single "best" model for a genetically heterogeneous set of conditions collectively known as T2D. T2D may be broadly described as a loss of glucose homeostasis generally attributable to either a subnormal pancreatic insulin secretory response to glucose stimulation, or to development of insulin resistance (the latter generally associated with obesity), or both. Both impaired fasting glucose (IFG) and impaired glucose tolerance (IGT) are intermediate states in the transition from normal glucose tolerance (NGT) through IGT to T2D and have been termed as "prediabetes." The term "Metabolic Syndrome" is sometimes applied to a collection of prediabetic phenotypes conferring increased risk for T2D and associated cardiovascular disease; notably IGT, insulin resistance associated with central obesity, dyslipidemia, and hypertension. Important genus-specific metabolic differences resulting from 65 million years of divergent evolution to fill different niches dictate that rodents "model" rather than exactly reflect a given form of T2D in humans.

Development of diabetic complications represents one example: mouse T2D models generally are resistant to development of the complications common in humans (e.g., diabetic neuropathy, nephropathy, and retinopathy) and when they occur, do not reflect all the features seen in human tissues *(1)*. Although metabolic pathways are remarkably similar in humans and mice, there are notable differences - for example, mice do not express genes thought to be important for development of diabetic complications in humans such as aldose reductase and cholesterol ester transport protein. Moreover, although humans and mice share most of the same transcription factors, there are significant genus-specific differences in the targets with which they bind *(2)*. Finally, humans are not inbred such that heterozygosity at many loci is the norm, whereas all the characterized mouse T2D models are highly inbred and thus homozygous across their autosomes. One consequence of this homozygosity is that different inbred mouse strains have fixed homozygosity for different mutations that render them particularly useful for certain applications. The resources that help the investigator identify what inbred strains are genetically "sensitized" for specific applications will be discussed in a later section.

3. Outbred Versus Inbred Mice

Outbred mice, as exemplified by ICR Swiss mice (marketed as CD-1™ by Charles River Laboratories, Waltham, MA) model for a randomly breeding human population both in terms of their genetic heterogeneity and the fact that they harbor a large number of (segregating) genetic loci capable of conferring susceptibility to either autoimmune, T cell-mediated Type 1 diabetes (T1D), or to IGT and T2D. Although outbred mice are suitable for general toxicity studies because they are less expensive and model the diverse genomes present in humans, this genetic inhomogeneity makes them problematic for obesity/diabesity research. **Fig. 1** depicts the remarkable spread in outbred 10-12-month-old CD-1 female body weights (between 30 and 55 g) and correlative variation in serum leptin concentrations (between 4 and 40 ng/mL) *(3)*.

Inbred strains put constraints on this phenotypic variation by drastically reducing the effects of genetic heterozygosity. The genetic heterogeneity underlying this phenotypic variation in ICR/CD-1 mice provided the "raw material" for genetic selection not only of a new T1D model (the NOD/Shi mouse), but also T2D models (ALS/Lt), and models of IGT (NSY/Shi and NON/ShiLt). (See *(4)* for summary descriptions of these models.) Both the NSY and NON strains were selected for IGT that worsens with age *(5, 6)*. A recent publication has assessed 43 inbred strains (mice of both sexes fed a high-fat/high-cholesterol diet) for ten subphenotypes associated with the Metabolic Syndrome *(7)*.

The definition of the diversity reflected in the strain-specific responses to diet not only attest to how a given inbred strain inherits different genetic components of the Metabolic Syndrome, but also serves as a valuable resource for identifying strains useful for T2D-related research applications. As an example, this analysis identified males of another Swiss-derived inbred strain, KK/HlJ, as exhibiting multiple metabolic abnormalities associated with the Metabolic Syndrome including obesity and insulin resistance. Data in **Table 1** show metabolic phenotyping for aging males of three Swiss-derived inbred strains with predisposition to IGT and T2D (KK/Hl, NZO/Hl, and NON/LtHl). In all three strains, the sex differences distinguishing the glucose tolerant females from the IGT males are striking.

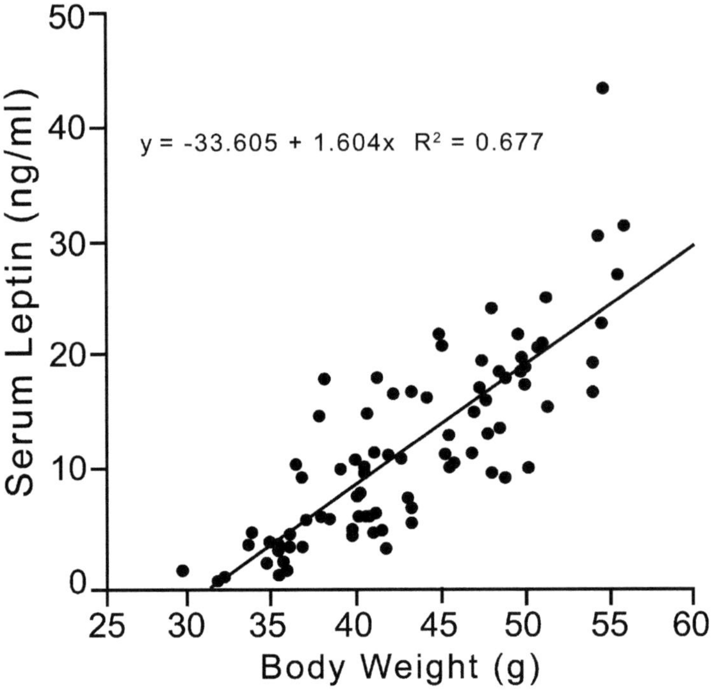

Fig. 1. Aging CD-1 females show a wide spectrum of body weights and serum leptin concentrations. (Reproduced with permission from Pelleymounter et al.[3]).

Table 1
Three inbred strains with components of the metabolic syndrome[a]

Strain sex (*n*)	Body weight (g)	Glucose (mg/dL)	IRI (ng/mL)	Triglycerides (mM)	Cholesterol (mM)
KK/Hl M *(12, 13)*	41.8 ± 0.8	293 ± 24.7	12.1 ± 1.2	7.0 ± 0.7	5.5 ± 0.2
KK/Hl F *(8)*	38.5 ± 2.1	142 ± 6.9	1.7 ± 0.4	4.6 ± 0.3	6.3 ± 0.4
NZO/Hl M *(17, 18)*	59.4 ± 1.4	367 ± 22.3	3.9 ± 0.7	5.2 ± 0.5	7.7 ± 0.3
NZO/Hl F *(8)*	51.2 ± 1.9	128 ± 3.6	0.7 ± 0.1	2.0 ± 0.1	6.1 ± 0.2
NON/LtHl M *(12, 14)*	45.4 ± 0.9	139 ± 5.0	1.0 ± 0.1	5.2 ± 0.5	5.5 ± 0.1
NON/LtHl F *(13)*	36.7 ± 1.0	131 ± 3.6	0.5 ± 0.1	2.9 ± 0.2	4.1 ± 0.4

[a]Data are mean ± SEM at 6 months of age (data collected in collaboration with Dr. Lieselotte Herberg, Diabetes Research Institute, Düsseldorf). All values are for nonfasted mice fed a chow diet containing 5% (w/w) fat. *M* males; *F* females; *IRI* immunoreactive insulin

4. When to Diagnose a Mouse as Diabetic?

Another salient difference between humans and mice is that many inbred mouse strains not considered to have diabetes maintain a higher concentration of glucose in blood than do humans, and some of these "normal" values approach what is considered to be diagnostic for diabetes in humans. The criteria currently offered by the American Diabetes Association for diagnosis of diabetes in humans are nonfasting plasma glucose ≥200 mg/dL; fasting ≥126 mg/dL. Hence, a number of inbred mouse strains considered to exhibit nonfasting glucose homeostasis might be considered borderline diabetic if human criteria for nonfasting glycemia were imposed. As an example, a mean glucose of 195 ± 5 and 223 ± 9 at 8 and 16 weeks, respectively, was recorded in a group of normoglycemic CBA/J males (see Jaxpheno3 data in the Mouse Phenome Database (http://phenome.jax.org/pub-cgi/phenome/mpdcgi?rtn=docs/home).

For a variety of reasons, this author recommends that the diagnostic criterion for clinical diabetes in a mouse be set as a nonfasting glucose concentration in blood ≥250 mg/dL, and preferably a chronic elevation ≥300 mg/dL. In the case of Type 1 diabetic mice, such as the NOD/ShiLtJ mouse at TJL, this higher value for plasma glucose exceeds a renal threshold for glucose spillage into the urine (glycosuria) necessary to have a clear diagnosis of diabetes by urine test reagents such as Diastix™ (Bayer, Elkhart, IN).

5. Impaired Glucose Tolerance Versus Clinical Diabetes

All diabetic mammals will exhibit IGT in a glucose tolerance test (GTT) regardless of whether the bolus is administered orally (OGTT) or intraperitoneally (IPGTT). However, IGT is much more common in humans than is T2D, and there certainly are inbred strains of mice that exhibit IGT without clinical diabetes (usually males). Thus, a distinction should be made between a prediabetic mouse model with IGT, but maintaining nonfasting normoglycemia, and clearly diabetic models showing both IGT and nonfasting hyperglycemia by this definition (≥250 mg/dL).

For humans, the American Diabetes Association lists a fasting blood glucose ≥126 mg/dL or a 2-h glucose ≥ 200 mg/dL after an oral bolus as a diagnostic criterion for diabetes. For most normoglycemic mice, a 16-h food deprivation (generally entailing food deprivation throughout the entire dark period when mice do most of their feeding) drops blood glucose to between 50 and 100 mg/dL (**Fig. 2**, "0" time point). At TJL, we typically observe that T2D mice will exhibit values between 150 and 300 mg/dL after a fast of that duration. When such T2D mice are then injected i.p. with a glucose bolus (1.0-2.5 g glucose in water/kg body weight), the 2-h blood glucose concentration remains well above their already elevated "0 time" baseline. So, again, the human criterion of 200 mg/dL at 2 h in a GTT should be shifted upward to at least 300 mg/dL or higher depending upon the glucose dose administered.

Glucose loading of nondiabetic, insulin-sensitive mice in an IPGTT reaches a maximum between 15 and 30 min, such that the slope of the line between 30 and 120 min allows determination of glucose clearance rate. Glucose tolerance differences are generally expressed either as differences in clearance rates or in "area under the curve," or AUC. One method for AUC calculation has been detailed elsewhere *(8)*. Mice that are either truly diabetic, or nondiabetic but insulin resistant like the obese NZL/Lt females shown in **Fig. 2**, exhibit little to no clearance between the 30 and 120 min time points. These normoglycemic, but severely glucose intolerant NZL females make the point that impaired GTT does not necessarily equate to clinical diabetes (unlike NZL males, NZL females fed standard chow diets maintain fed glucose homeostasis). Another example of a severe IGT syndrome without chronic nonfasting hyperglycemia ≥250 mg/dL is the high-fat diet-induced obesity syndrome (DIO) in C57BL/6J (B6) male mice. In normoglycemic nonobese and insulin-sensitive mice on standard chow diets containing not more than 5% (w/w) fat, the glucose clearance rate is directly related to the glucose-stimulated insulin secretion (GSIS) response of the beta cell mass in the pancreas. In males

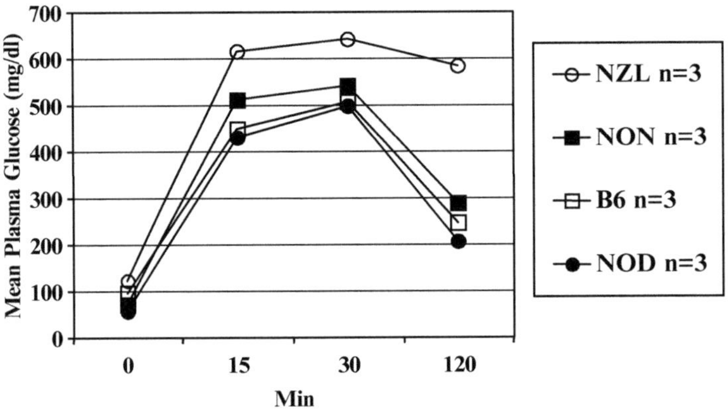

Fig. 2. Severe IGT in obese but normoglycemic NZL/Lt females is contrasted to 2-h plasma glucose (PG) clearance exhibited by young 7-week-old normoglycemic NON/Lt, B6/J, and NOD/Lt males. NZL females received 2.5 g/kg glucose i.p.; NON, B6, and NOD males received 2.0 g/kg. Note that all groups exhibit a "0" time fasting PG within a normal range. Data are mean ± SEM.

of DIO-responsive strains maintained on high-fat diets containing refined carbohydrates, increases in body weight and adiposity are accompanied by increases in both plasma insulin concentrations and islet beta cell mass. However, these physiologic adaptations are blunted by progressive development of insulin resistance as reflected by a severely impaired GTT.

Just as feeding a high-fat/high-cholesterol diet to mice of various inbred strains produces a spectrum of responses, a comparable spectrum of glucose clearances/GSIS responses is observed when males are fed a chow diet with fat content between 4 and 6% (w/w). For example, young, prediabetic NOD males show an excellent glucose clearance, whereas young NON and B6 males exhibit a more protracted clearance (**Figs. 2, 3a**). This difference correlates with a lower GSIS in the latter two strains (**Fig. 3b**). Reduced GSIS has been demonstrated for pancreatic islets in vitro from both NON/ShiLt (compared to NOD/ShiLt) and B6/J (compared to C3H) *(9, 10)*. In B6/J, this phenotype is mapped to a defect in the gene encoding nicotinamide nucleotide transhydrogenase (*Nnt*) *(11)*. In NON, which carries a wildtype *Nnt* allele, the impaired GSIS appears under polygenic control. The *Nn*t mutation provides an excellent illustration of the strain-specific (and random) acquisition of loss-of-function mutations; it has only been found in B6/J; C57BL/6N, a B6 substrain separated from B6/J for more than 50 years, carries the wildtype allele. Potentially, such strain and substrain differences may be critically important for the performance of a given model. The B6/J male is the paradigm for a DIO-sensitive strain; if B6/N males were substituted, deviations in expected plasma insulin changes might be anticipated. However, direct comparisons at TJL showed plasma insulins of B6/NJ males were significantly higher only on a low fat diet, and were comparable to B6/J on a high fat diet.

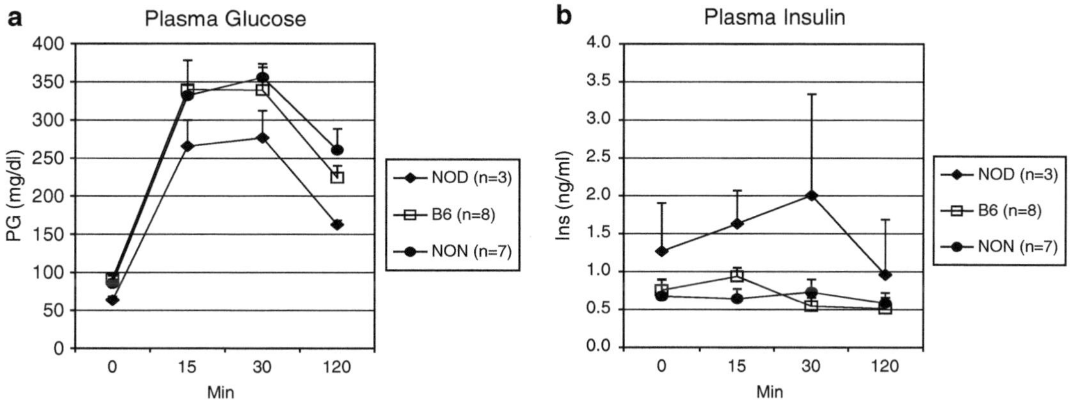

Fig. 3. Glucose clearance following injection i.p. of 1 g glucose/kg (*panel A*) correlates with glucose-stimulated insulin secretory responsiveness (*panel B*). Data are mean ± SEM for groups of 7-9-week-old males.

6. Diabesity in Monogenic Obesity Models Requires Polygenic Interactions

The most widely studied models of obesity-associated T2D ("diabesity") are those with monogenic obesity-producing mutations, notably the "obese" mutation at the leptin locus (Lep^{ob}), the "diabetes" mutation at the leptin receptor locus ($Lepr^{db}$), the "yellow" and "viable yellow" mutations at the agouti locus (A^{y}, A^{vy}), and the "fat" mutation at the carboxypeptidase E locus (Cpe^{fat}). The major phenotypes of the standard Lep^{ob} and $Lepr^{db}$ stocks have recently been reviewed *(12)*; the others are described in a reference manual entitled "Type 2 Diabetes & Obesity" and available upon request from TJL (http://jaxmice.jax.org/library/index.html). There are three important points to consider with regard to these monogenic models. First, although these mutations, when homozygous (Lep^{ob}, $Lepr^{db}$, and Cpe^{fat}) or heterozygous (A^{y}, A^{vy}), are completely penetrant for morbid obesity, development of T2D is contingent on what appear to be a large number of interactive modifier genes (quantitative trait loci, or QTL) in the inbred strain background *(13-15)*. This is demonstrated in dramatic fashion by the earlier finding that both Lep^{ob} and $Lepr^{db}$ homozygosity on the B6/J background produced a transient hyperglycemia that was compensated by sustained hyperinsulinemia and beta cell hyperplasia. In contrast, on the related C57BLKS/J (BKS) strain background, initial hyperinsulinemia produced by either mutation was not sustained, producing a progressively more severe hyperglycemia associated with progressive loss of beta cell mass *(16)*. It is noteworthy that BKS represents a recombinant congenic strain sharing approximately 88% genomic identity with B6 *(17)*. These modifier loci are uncovered by outcross of a mouse of a diabesity susceptible strain to a mouse from a diabesity resistant strain. The results of such studies are often complex, in the sense that the resistant strain can contribute "transgressive" diabesity-predisposing loci when removed from the resistant donor genome. An example is *Sorcs1*, a B6-derived diabetogenic QTL on Chr. 19 contributing to the diabetogenic action of the Lep^{ob} mutation in a segregating stock *(18)*. Another modifier was discovered when a leptin receptor gene mutation ($Lepr^{db3J}$) was introgressed into the FVB/NJ background. In contrast to the abrogation of hyperinsulinemia associated with loss of beta cells observed in BKS-$Lepr^{db}$ mice, development of a marked hyperinsulinemia and beta cell hyperplasia was sustained despite a chronic, severe hyperglycemia. An FVB genetic modifier promoting this beta cell resistance was mapped to Chromosome 5 *(19)*.

7. Choosing the "Right" Model

The selection will be determined by the specific research application and the inbred strain background deemed to be appropriately "sensitized" to develop the targeted phenotype. Much of the current interest in the monogenic obesity mutant mice revolves around their usefulness in drug testing. Among the most often-utilized and widely accepted models for pharmacologic testing have been the B6-*Lep*^{ob}/*Lep*^{ob} and BKS-*Lepr*^{db}/*Lepr*^{db} mice. If investigators pay strict attention to control of the physical environment in which the mice are studied, the obesity/diabesity phenotypes are very reproducible such that therapeutic effects of drugs can be readily assessed with relatively small groups of sex-matched mice. These models generally respond very well to efficacious drugs administered by gavage. In addition to phenotypic predictability, a major advantage of these models is the availability of a nonobese wildtype control (generally a segregant from the same cross producing the homozygous mutants). Such controls are invaluable for analyzing differences in gene expression in tissues and cells from obese versus nonobese segregants. The investigator should give special consideration to testing models that span different etiologic mechanisms. For example, testing responses of B6- *Lep*^{ob}/*Lep*^{ob} and BKS- *Lepr*^{db}/*Lepr*^{db} mice, and for that matter, Zucker Diabetic Fatty (*Lepr*^{fa}) rats are, in fact, looking at treatment of metabolic disturbances produced by defects in the leptin-leptin receptor axis. Although defects in this pathway are central to the two mouse and one rat monogenic obesity syndromes just mentioned, defects of that magnitude in humans are rare.

There are other features of these leptin/leptin receptor mutant mice (and rats) that do not accurately reflect most "garden variety" T2D. In human diabesity, the etiology of the obesity is generally polygenic, not monogenic - with the obese phenotype being more moderate rather than morbid. Moreover, humans with diabetogenic obesity syndromes are not infertile like *Lep*^{ob} and *Lepr*^{db} homozygous mice. Human Type 2 diabetics generally lack the severe juvenile-onset obesity and insulin resistance associated with uncontrolled hyperphagia, hypercorticosteroidism, cold sensitivity, and extremes of plasma leptin and insulin typical of the mouse monogenic obesities. For these reasons, examination of a polygenic as well as a monogenic obesity model is recommended when the general effectiveness of a compound across genotypes is of importance (as it usually is to the pharmaceutical industry and the governmental regulatory agencies approving new drug applications).

8. Polygenic T2D Models

Polygenic mouse models of IGT, obesity, and T2D present a spectrum of different genotypes and susceptibilities, and thus, multiple metabolic targets for drug therapy. Rather than obesity arising from a single mutation, the obese phenotype develops over time in response to a complex interaction between a collection of QTL and the nutritional environment. A summary of certain of these QTLs and the strains associated with them has been published recently *(14)*. NZO/HlLt mice represent a model originally selected for polygenic obesity. The marked obesity developing in this strain results from the interactions between multiple QTL with each other and with the maternal postparturitional nutrient environment *(20)*. When such QTL are examined individually, they may contribute only a small effect to a given phenotypic trait such as fat mass or plasma insulin, but this effect is amplified greatly through epistatic interaction with other QTL to enhance significantly the QTL contribution to the trait *(20)*. All NZO substrains have a metabolic syndrome including hypertension on an elevated fat diet *(21, 22)*. At TJL, development of diabesity in NZO/HlLt is limited to males and represents a threshold phenomenon, dependent both upon rate of weight gain during the peripubertal period *(20)* and carbohydrate content of the diet *(23)*. However, the morbid obesity and the extremely high plasma insulin and leptin concentrations that develop in this strain still remain unrepresentative of the less extreme phenotypes associated with human "garden variety" obesity and T2D.

After extolling the advantages of inbred versus outbred strains, it should be noted that there are multiple examples of "negative heterosis" where combining genomes of two inbred strains, each one without IGT or T2D, produces F1 progeny with IGT or worse *(9)*. This is not surprising given the findings that different components of the Metabolic Syndrome are widely dispersed across various inbred strains *(7, 24)*. Outcrosses between NZO/HlLt and either NON/Lt or ALR/Lt (a model of systemic resistance to free radical damage) produce massive (NZO-type) obesity in the F1 generation *(25)*, reflecting the large number of additive or codominant obesity QTL in the NZO genome. The discovery that (NZO x NON) F1 males more uniformly attained diabetogenic weight gain thresholds and transited from IGT to T2D at 80-90% frequency makes this F1 hybrid a valuable polygenic model of diabesity in its own right. However, the morbid obesity and hyperphagia, as well as extremely high serum concentrations of insulin and leptin, did not differentiate this model from the monogenic models, despite their reproductive competence and functional genes encoding leptin and its receptor. These deficiencies were circumvented by selective introgression of certain of these NZO obesity/diabesity QTL onto the NON/Lt background. The panel of recombinant congenic strains produced by this means exhibited moderate obesity and reflected different levels of T2D stress *(26, 27)*. The most intensively studied of these, NONcNZO10/LtJ, along with another selectively bred polygenic model, the TALLYHO/Jng male mouse *(28, 29)*, serve as paradigms for comparison to the monogenic obesity models.

9. Utilizing Polygenic Models: NONcNZO10/LtJ and TALLYHO/JngJ

The major advantage of these two more recently developed T2D polygenic models over the monogenic obesity models is that the complex mode of inheritance more accurately reflects the more common human obesity/diabesity situation; the less extreme phenotypes are more consistent with human profiles, and the models are very responsive to increased dietary fat. In both new models, fertility is maintained and progression toward adiposity is more protracted and less extreme. Mice are not hyperphagic, and plasma insulin and leptin concentrations are only moderately increased after puberty *(28, 30, 31)*. Euglycemic-hyperinsulinemic clamp analysis demonstrated insulin resistance developing in liver and skeletal muscle of NONcNZO10/LtJ males at 8 weeks of age, prior to development of chronic hyperglycemia *(32)*. Chronically elevated plasma glucose is established from around 12 weeks onward. Initial islet mass increases in both models are followed by beta cell loss over time. Severe diabetic nephropathy has been observed in some NONcNZO10/LtJ diabetic males aged to 49-52 weeks of age (unpublished findings). The TALLYHO/JngJ model has not yet been characterized for diabetic complications. Although the T2D syndrome in NONcNZO10/LtJ is phenotypically very similar to that in TALLYHO, the genetics are distinct.

These polygenic models are, however, not without their disadvantages. Unlike the monogenic models, no wildtype control differing only in a single gene is available for comparison. Further, the male sex bias in syndrome severity, although demonstrable in the monogenic models, particularly on certain inbred strain backgrounds *(9)*, is extreme in the polygenic models. That is, although females develop IGT and obesity, they resist development of hyperglycemia. In the case of the NONcNZO10/LtJ strain, NON/LtJ males maintained on a chow diet not containing more than 6% w/w fat can be used as controls as they share ~88% genome identity. On diets with higher fat contents, NON/LtJ males will actually outgain NONcNZO10LtJ males (TJL, unpublished studies). Alternatively, age-matched normoglycemic

NONcNZO10/LtJ females can serve as controls for the effects of hyperglycemia in the males. TALLYHO/Jng mice, like NON/Lt and NZO/HlLtJ, appear to be Swiss-derived strains. Although B6 has been used for comparative purposes in publications, Swiss-derived strains (such as SWR, SJL, or FVB) would presumably be more closely related (TALLYHO/Jng and SJL/J share the same $H2^s$ MHC haplotype). Given that both strains represent threshold models for diabetes penetrance, both are strongly influenced by environmental parameters (discussed later). One of the TALLYHO/Jng obesity QTL on Chr. 6 made congenic on B6 did not outgain B6 male controls fed chow diet; however, the congenic males were more responsive to high-fat diet-induced obesity *(33)*. Despite these shortcomings, utilization of either polygenic model, or an F1 hybrid model, would provide additional support for the efficacy of a given treatment modality under investigation in a way that comparison of two mutations in a common pathway or gene interaction pairing (e.g., ligand/receptor) would not.

10. Models Generated by Gene Targeting ("Knockouts") or Transgenesis

Because advances in molecular manipulation of the mouse genome have been so rapid and extensive, investigators can find genetically engineered mice designed to produce perturbations in glucose homeostasis via disruption or other manipulation in multiple metabolic pathways and tissues. These types of models not only are important to evaluate specific gene function, but also are useful to evaluate the importance of a specific gene function as a drug target for obesity or T2D. Recent reviews are available, particularly for manipulations of the insulin and IGF receptor signaling pathways *(34, 35)*, but the field progresses so rapidly that investigators should query online (see later) for information regarding specific genes of interest for their research applications.

Such molecular manipulations either decrease or increase efficiency of energy metabolism, adiposity, insulin secretion or action, thereby impairing or improving glucose homeostasis. Similarly, numerous targeted mutations or transgenes, when brought onto the DIO-sensitive B6 background, either increase or decrease male sensitivity to development of adiposity, insulin resistance, and IGT. In many cases what is reported as a "new" T2D model should, in fact, be considered as a model of IGT by this author's definition of diabetes stated previously. Certain gene disruptions in homozygous state elicit diabetes shortly after birth (such as the insulin receptor gene), while others, such as the gene encoding Insulin Receptor Substrate-1 (IRS-1), produce only mild phenotypic change. However, new oligogenic models of insulin-resistant T2D without obesity are generated by combining both knockouts in heterozygous state *(36)*.

Targeted mutations are generally transferred from chimeric founders onto either the 129/Sv or B6 genetic background; the severity of the syndrome developing in these engineered models is strongly background dependent *(36)*. Caveats concerning interpretations of results using genetically engineered mice on mixed, undefined backgrounds have been published *(37)*. The necessity to run extensive controls in mice expressing cell-or-tissue-specific transgenes is particularly important when tissue-specific promoters are used to drive expression of the bacteriophage Cre recombinase in pancreatic beta cells *(38)*. Multiple endogenous Cre excision (loxP-like) sites are present in the mouse genome *(39)*, possibly accounting for the unanticipated side effects in certain Cre transgenic insertions reported in the NOD model of Type 1 diabetes *(40)* and alterations in glucose tolerance in B6 mice congenic for a Cre transgene expressing in beta cells *(38)*.

11. Environmental Effects on Model Characteristics

Although often overlooked by users of T2D mouse models, the physical environment exerts a strong effect on model performance. Obviously, dietary macronutrient composition and concentration such as refined sugars *(41, 42)* or saturated fat *(43)* will have a major effect on severity of hyperglycemia or development of obesity in a given model. Thus, the user should adhere to the supplier's recommendations for diet, water treatment, and bedding when receiving a model for testing. The importance of the enteric flora in relation to energy utilization and on obesity development has recently been demonstrated *(44)*. When the NONc-NZO10/LtJ model was rederived from conventional SPF to full barrier production facilities at TJL, a 6% (w/w) fat-containing chow diet no longer sufficed for the model to achieve the requisite weight gain thresholds necessary for diabesity development. This problem was remedied by increasing the dietary fat content to 11%. For many of the studies wherein gene function is assessed by knockout or knockdown methodologies, it is not uncommon that no significant phenotypic differences are reported when comparisons to wildtype are done using a standard chow diet. Often, feeding a diet with a markedly increased fat content is required to identify an alteration (either exacerbation or attenuation) in glucose tolerance and insulin sensitivity. The reader is reminded that when a targeted mutation made in strain 129/Sv embryonic stem cells is used, and the targeted allele backcrossed into a strain other than 129/Sv (in most cases for T2D research, the backcross is to B6), the targeted allele is introgressed along with linked 129/Sv genes such that any phenotypic alteration may not reflect the loss of the gene under study, but rather, a linked QTL or mutation from the donor 129/Sv genome.

In addition to the dietary environment, other physical parameters need to be considered. The mortality associated with chronic hyperglycemia in the BKS-*Lepr*^{db} model (and the severity of the hyperglycemia) can be attenuated by frequent box changes to maintain as dry a substratum as possible. In addition to its sensitivity to the diabetogenic action of moderate increases in dietary fat, the NONcNZO10LtJ model has been found to be extremely sensitive to handling stress such that a strong placebo effect has been observed in response to multiple treatments by gavage. Thus, care should be taken to minimize stress in the vivarium; e.g., numbers of people accessing the room, noise level, etc. Following receipt from a vendor, mice should be acclimatized to a room and to handling prior to initiation of critical experiments. When male mice are grouped for experiments, they should ideally be randomized. However, in practice, it is advisable to keep males together from weaning to avoid the fighting that often occurs when new cohorts are forced by randomization.

12. How to Identify the Right Mouse Strain "Presensitized" for Your Specific Application?

Many of the subphenotypes associated with the Metabolic Syndrome, IGT, and T2D in humans are individually represented in various inbred mouse strains, or in certain genetically manipulated stocks. Knowledge of which strains or genetically manipulated stocks manifest a desired subphenotype can be of central importance if the goal is to identify the mouse most likely to achieve the experimental goal. As an example, certain inbred strains (DBA/2, FVB/N, KK/Hl) are "presensitized" to development of albuminuria in response to chronic hyperglycemia, whereas others are much more resistant (e.g., B6). Both the DBA/2 and certain KK substrains are prone to aging-associated vascular mineralization in heart and kidney, a feature that may contribute to their "presensitized" state. Finally, as noted earlier, the KK/HlJ strain has been identified to express multiple traits associated with the Metabolic Syndrome and thus males are "presensitized" to development of T2D. A search of MEDLINE will reveal to the interested investigator references for similar strain surveys that identify which inbred strains are particularly susceptible to development of diet-induced atherosclerosis or obesity *(7)*. With regard to

DIO, B6, NON, and AKR males are known to be particularly susceptible, whereas A/J, SWR, BKS, and 129/Sv have been reported as resistant.

In addition to MEDLINE, a variety of online resources are available to help guide the investigator through available models and particular strain characteristics of inbred mice that may be helpful in guiding user decision making. The websites maintained by the major distributors provide extensive information regarding available mouse resources. The Mouse Phenome Project Database maintained at TJL has been discussed earlier. The Mouse Genome Informatics website at TJL provides entry into a host of useful websites for additional information regarding inbred strains and genetically manipulated stocks. The Induced Mutant Resource at TJL provides information on a considerable number of the transgenic and "knockout" stocks on the TJL campus.

The International Mouse Strain Resource site (http://www.informatics.jax.org/imsr/index.jsp) is a searchable online database of extant mouse strains and genetically engineered stocks available worldwide. There is an online forum for topics in mouse genetics that is viewed by investigators with broad experience in mouse biology (mgi-list@lists.informatics.jax.org). Technical specialists associated with the major distributors can be queried directly as to performance characteristics of the various models at each institution. At TJL, the customer support staff interacts with the research staff to provide technical information based upon on-site experience. Finally, informative courses offered at TJL and elsewhere are an excellent means for interacting with experts in a specific area, as well as acquiring specialized techniques necessary for in-depth phenotyping (http://www.jax.org/courses/events/current.do).

Obviously, what may be the ultimate determinant of which mice or mouse models are chosen is the availability of the mice. Regretfully there are many more mouse models of metabolic syndrome and T2D in the literature than have been made available for distribution. Publishing on a new model carries the obligation of research resource sharing - a model can only be exploited productively when it is passed into multiple investigators' vivaria.

References

1. Breyer MD, Bottinger E, Brosius FC, et al. (2005). Diabetic nephropathy: of mice and men. *Adv Chronic Kidney Dis* **12(2)**: 128–145
2. Odom DT, Dowell RD, Jacobsen ES, et al. (2007). Tissue-specific transcriptional regulation has diverged significantly between human and mouse. *Nat Genet* **39(6)**: 730–732
3. Pelleymounter MA, Cullen MJ, Healy D, et al. (1998). Efficacy of exogenous recombinant murine leptin in lean and obese 10- to 12-mo-old female CD-1 mice. *Am J Physiol* **275**(4 Pt 2): R950–R959
4. Mathews CE, Leiter EH. (2004). Rodent models of spontaneous diabetes. In: Kahn CR, Weir GC, King GL, Jacobson AM, Moses

AC, Smith RJ, editors. Joslin's Diabetes Mellitus. 14th ed. Philadelphia, PA: Lippincott Williams & Wilkins; pp. 291–327

5. Ueda H, Ikegami H, Kawaguchi Y, et al. (2000). Age-dependent changes in phenotypes and candidate gene analysis in a polygenic animal model of Type II diabetes mellitus; NSY mouse. *Diabetologia* **43**: 932–938
6. Makino S, Yamashita H, Kunimoto K, et al. (1992). Breeding of the NON mouse and its genetic characteristics. In: Sakamoto N, Hotta N, Uchida K, editors. Current Concepts of a New Animal Model: The NON Mouse. Tokyo: Elsevier Science Publishers B. V.; pp. 4–10
7. Svenson KL, Von Smith R, Magnani PA, et al. (2007). Multiple trait measurements in 43 inbred mouse strains captures the phenotypic diversity characteristic of human populations. *J Appl Physiol* **102(6)**: 2369–2378
8. Herberg L, Leiter EH. (2001). Obesity/diabetes in mice with mutations in the leptin or leptin receptor genes. In: Sima AAF, Shafrir E, editors. Animal Models of Diabetes: A Primer. Amsterdam: Harwood Academic Publishers; pp. 63–107
9. Leiter EH, Herberg L. (1997). The polygenetics of diabesity in mice. *Diabetes Rev* **5(2)**: 131–148
10. Freeman H, Shimomura K, Horner E, et al. (2006). Nicotinamide nucleotide transhydrogenase: a key role in insulin secretion. *Cell Metab* **3(1)**: 35–45
11. Freeman HC, Hugill A, Dear NT, et al. (2006). Deletion of nicotinamide nucleotide transhydrogenase: a new quantitative trait locus accounting for glucose intolerance in C57BL/6J mice. *Diabetes* **55(7)**: 2153–2156
12. Chua Jr. S, Herberg L, Leiter EH. (2007). Obesity/diabetes in mice with mutations in the leptin or leptin receptor genes. In: Shafrir E, editor. Animal Models of *Diabetes: Frontiers in Research.* Boca Raton: CRC-Taylor and Francis Press; pp. 61–102
13. Togawa K, Moritani M, Yaguchi H, et al. (2006). Multidimensional genome scans identify the combinations of genetic loci linked to diabetes-related phenotypes in mice. *Hum Mol Genet* **15(1)**: 113–128
14. Clee SM, Attie AD. (2007). The genetic landscape of type 2 diabetes in mice. *Endocr Rev* **28(1)**: 48–83
15. Collin GB, Maddatu TP, Sen S, et al. (2005). Genetic modifiers interact with Cpefat to affect body weight, adiposity, and hyperglycemia. *Physiol Genomics* **22**: 182–190
16. Coleman DL. (1978). Obese and diabetes: two mutant genes causing diabetes-obesity syndromes in mice. *Diabetologia* **14**: 141–148
17. Naggert JK, Mu M-L, Frankel WF, et al. (1995). Genomic analysis of the C57BL/Ks mouse strain. *Mammal. Genome* **6**: 131–133
18. Clee SM, Yandell BS, Schueler KM, et al. (2006). Positional cloning of Sorcs1, a type 2 diabetes quantitative trait locus. *Nat Genet* **38(6)**: 688–693
19. Luo N, Liu SM, Liu H, et al. (2006). Allelic variation on chromosome 5 controls beta cell mass expansion during hyperglycemia in leptin receptor deficient diabetes mice. *Endocrinology* **147**: 2287–2295
20. Reifsnyder PC, Churchill G, Leiter EH. (2000). Maternal environment and genotype interact to establish diabesity in mice. *Genome Res* **10(10)**: 1568–1578
21. Fam BC, Andrikopoulos S. (2007). The New Zealand obese mouse: polygenic model of obesity, glucose intolerance, and the metabolic syndrome. In: Shafrir E, editor. *Animal Models of Diabetes: Frontiers in Research,* 2nd edn. Boca Raton: CRC Press, Taylor & Francis Group; pp. 139–158
22. Ortlepp JR, Kluge R, Giesen K, et al. (2000). A metabolic syndrome of hypertension, hyperinsulinaemia and hypercholesterolaemia in the New Zealand obese mouse. *Eur J Clin Invest* **30(3)**: 195–202
23. Jurgens HS, Neschen S, Ortmann S, et al. (2007). Development of diabetes in obese, insulin-resistant mice: essential role of dietary carbohydrate in beta cell destruction. *Diabetologia* **50(7)**: 1481–1489
24. Qiao JH, Xie PZ, Fishbein MC, et al. (1994). Pathology of atheromatous lesions in inbred and genetically engineered mice. Genetic determination of arterial calcification. *Arterioscler Thromb* **14(9)**: 1480–1497
25. Leiter EH, Lee CH. (2005). Mouse models and the genetics of diabetes: is there evidence for genetic overlap between type 1 and type 2 diabetes? *Diabetes* **54**(Suppl 2): S151–S158
26. Reifsnyder PC, Leiter EH. (2002). Deconstructing and reconstructing obesity-induced diabetes (diabesity) in mice. *Diabetes* **51(3)**: 825–832
27. Pan H-J, Reifsnyder PC, Vance DE, et al. (2005). Pharmacogenetic analysis of rosiglitazone-induced hepatosteatosis in new mouse models of type 2 diabetes. *Diabetes* **54(6)**: 1854–1862
28. Kim JH, Stewart TP, Soltani-Bejnood M, et al. (2006). Phenotypic characterization of

polygenic type 2 diabetes in TALLYHO/JngJ mice. *J Endocrinol* **191(2)**: 437–446

29. Kim JH, Sen S, Avery CS, et al. (2001). Genetic analysis of a new mouse model for non-insulin-dependent diabetes. *Genomics* **74(3)**: 273–286
30. Leiter EH, Reifsnyder PC. (2004). Differential levels of diabetogenic stress in two new mouse models of obesity and type 2 diabetes. *Diabetes* **53**(Suppl 1): S4–S11
31. Leiter EH, Reifsnyder PC, Zhang W, et al. (2006). Differential endocrine responses to rosiglitazone therapy in new mouse models of type 2 diabetes. *Endocrinology* **147**(2): 919–926
32. Cho YR, Kim HJ, Park SY, et al. (2007). Hyperglycemia, maturity-onset obesity, and insulin resistance in NONcNZO10/LtJ males, a new mouse model of type 2 diabetes. *Am J Physiol Endocrinol Metab* **293(1)**: E327–E336
33. Kim JH, Stewart TP, Zhang W, et al. (2005). The Type 2 diabetes mouse model TallyHo carries an obesity gene on chromosome 6 that exaggerates dietary obesity. *Physiol Genomics* **22(2)**: 171–181
34. LeRoith D, Gavrilova O. (2006). Mouse models created to study the pathophysiology of Type 2 diabetes. *Int J Biochem Cell Biol* **38(5-6)**: 904–912
35. Kadowaki T. (2000). Insights into insulin resistance and type 2 diabetes from knockout mouse models. *J Clin Invest* **106(4)**: 459–465
36. Kulkarni RN, Almind K, Goren HJ, et al. (2003). Impact of genetic background on development of hyperinsulinemia and diabetes in insulin receptor/insulin receptor substrate-1 double heterozygous mice. *Diabetes* **52(6)**: 1528–1534
37. Leiter EH. (2002). Mice with targeted gene disruptions or gene insertions for diabetes research: problems, pitfalls, and potential solutions. *Diabetologia* **45(3)**: 296–308
38. Lee JY, Ristow M, Lin X, et al. (2006). RIP-Cre revisited, evidence for impairments of pancreatic beta-cell function. *J Biol Chem* **281(5)**: 2649–2653
39. Semprini S, Troup TJ, Kotelevtseva N, et al. (2007). Cryptic loxP sites in mammalian genomes: genome-wide distribution and relevance for the efficiency of BAC/PAC recombineering techniques. *Nucleic Acids Res* **35(5)**: 1402–1410
40. Leiter EH, Reifsnyder PC, Driver J, et al. (2007). Unexpected functional consequences of xenogeneic transgene expression in beta cells of NOD mice. *Diabetes Obes Metab* **9**(Suppl 1): 14–22
41. Leiter EH, Coleman DL, Eisenstein AB, et al. (1981). Dietary control of diabetes pathogenesis in C57BL/KsJ-db/db diabetes mice. *Metabolism* **30**: 554–562
42. Leiter EH, Coleman DL, Ingram DK, et al. (1983). Influence of dietary carbohydrate on the induction of diabetes in C57BL. KsJ-db/db diabetes mice. *J Nutr* **113**: 184–195
43. Surwit RS, Feinglos MN, Rodin J, et al. (1995). Differential effects of fat and sucrose on the development of obesity and diabetes in C57BL/6J and A/J mice. *Metabolism* **44(5)**: 645–651
44. Turnbaugh PJ, Ley RE, Mahowald MA, et al. (2006). An obesity-associated gut microbiome with increased capacity for energy harvest. *Nature* **444(7122)**: 1027–1031

Chapter 2

Nutritional Models of Type 2 Diabetes Mellitus

Beverly Sara Mühlhausler

Summary

In order to better understand the events which precede and precipitate the onset of type 2 diabetes (T2DM) several nutritional animal models have been developed. These models are generated by manipulating the diet of either the animal itself or its mother during her pregnancy and, in comparison to traditional genetic and knock out models, have the advantage that they more accurately reflect the aetiology of human T2DM. This chapter will discuss some of the most widely used nutritional models of T2DM: Diet-induced obesity (DIO) in adult rodents, and studies of prenatal and postnatal nutrition in offspring of mothers fed a low-protein diet or overnourished during pregnancy. Several common mechanisms have been identified through which these nutritional manipulations can lead to metabolic disease, including pancreatic beta-cell dysfunction, impaired insulin signalling in skeletal muscle and the excess accumulation of visceral adipose tissue and consequent deposition of non-esterified fatty acids in peripheral tissues resulting in peripheral insulin resistance. The following chapter will discuss each of these nutritional models, their application and relationship to human aetiology, and will highlight the important insights these models have provided into the pathogenesis of T2DM.

Key words: Type 2 diabetes, Obesity, Insulin resistance, Animal models, Nutrition, High-fat diet, Programming

1. Introduction

Whilst the human is undoubtedly the model of choice when studying the pathophysiology of human disease, the study of the underlying mechanisms of disease in living humans has a number of logistical and ethical limitations. Therefore, to better understand the events which precede and precipitate the onset of type 2diabetes (T2DM) there is a need to develop in vivo animal models of this disease. The commonly used genetic models of T2DM, including (*ob/ob* and *db/db* mice and Zucker *fa/fa* rats), have been useful in understanding some of the mechanisms which

C. Stocker (ed.), *Type 2 Diabetes,* Methods in Molecular Biology, vol. 560
DOI 10.1007/978-1-59745-448-3_2, © Humana Press, a part of Springer Science+Business Media, LLC 2009

may contribute to altered glucose and insulin metabolism; however, none of these is an ideal disease model, since these gene mutations are extremely rare in human populations *(1)*. Similarly, experimental animal models of T2DM induced by chemical destruction or removal of a portion of the pancreas *(2)* are not representative of the aetiology of T2DM in humans, which, is typically preceded by obesity *(3, 4)*. This has led to the development of several nutritional animal models, by manipulating the diet of either the animal itself, or its mother during her pregnancy. The following chapter will present an overview of the most widely utilised nutritional models, their application and relationship to human aetiology, including some of the most important insights into the pathogenesis of T2DM which have been provided by each. The limitations of each model will also be discussed in each case.

2. Diet-Induced Obesity

A significant proportion of T2DM in human populations is linked to an excessive accumulation of body fat, particularly in the abdominal region *(4–6)*. This fact makes the diet-induced obesity model (DIO) particularly relevant for studying the underlying mechanisms through which an excessive accumulation of body fat and/or an excessive dietary fat intake can lead to the development of insulin resistance and T2DM. The two most widely used models for the study of obesity-induced T2DM are high-fat feeding in rodents and the sand rat (*Psammomys obesus*).

2.1. Diet-Induced Obesity: Rats and Mice

The DIO rodent model involves a regimen in which healthy, non-obese mice or rats are provided with ad libitum access to a highly palatable high-fat, high-energy diet. C57BL/6J mice were originally selected for this model because in early studies these mice developed clear-cut diabetes more rapidly than other strains fed the same high-fat diet, suggesting that this mouse had a genetic predisposition to T2DM *(7)*. Typically, C57BL/6J (B6) males are maintained on these diets for 8 to 12 weeks and, as a result, become obese, mildly to moderately hyperglycaemic and develop impaired glucose tolerance *(7)*. Similarly, Wistar and Sprague Dawley rats have been the model of choice for studying the metabolic effects of diet-induced obesity in the rat *(1)*.

The use of high-energy diets to induce obesity in laboratory animals for the purpose of studying obesity-related disorders has been widely adopted, and the scope of these diets is now quite extensive, ranging from an oil-based diet to free access to a variety of human junk foods, including pies, cakes and chocolate *(8–10)*.

Despite this variation in the amount and source of dietary fat, all high-fat diets are associated with the emergence of hyperphagia, rapid weight gain and excess body fat accumulation *(8–10)*. Irrespective of the precise nature of the diet, diet-induced obesity results in many of the same changes as seen in human obesity, including the development of central and peripheral leptin and insulin resistance *(8)*, and in the altered expression of adipokines which are known to contribute to the regulation of peripheral insulin sensitivity, in particular adiponectin and resistin *(11)*.

DIO rodent models have been widely utilised in order to investigate the defects within specific tissues which may contribute to the development of insulin resistance in obese individuals. By comparing the profile of gene expression and protein content in specific tissues of DIO mice with those from lean controls using micro-array or 2D gel electrophoresis, it is possible to very quickly identify genes which may be involved in the development of T2DM. Using this approach, DIO was shown to be associated with a reduced pancreatic abundance of enzymes involved in clearance of reactive oxygen species, providing a potential mechanism for the deterioration of pancreatic function seen in the later stages of T2DM *(12)*, with adipocyte hypertrophy *(13)* and the induction of hepatic steatosis and hepatic insulin resistance *(14)*, which again resembles the human obese state (**Fig. 1**).

It is now widely accepted that the susceptibility to developing obesity and T2DM varies between individuals, and there is considerable interest in understanding the genetic and physiological basis of this difference. This question has been addressed using an adaptation of the DIO model in which adult Sprague Dawley rats are fed a purified diet with a moderately high fat content. The rats are subsequently selected as either obesity prone or obesity resistant according to their response (i.e. degree of weight gain and increase in percentage body fat) on the high-energy diet *(15)*. The obesity-prone rats typically eat approximately 16% more calories over the first 30 days compared to the obesity-resistant strain and exhibit a phenotype comparable to human metabolic syndrome, including glucose intolerance, hyperinsulinaemia and T2DM *(15, 16)*. Selective breeding has enabled these researchers to generate obesity-resistant and obesity-prone strains, and to study these two populations in order to determine factors, which may underlie an increased propensity to obesity *(17, 18)*. This is a useful model, in that it provides a means of distinguishing between the effects due to high dietary fat content as distinct from those related to effects of excess body fat.

The major advantage of the DIO model lies in the fact that these rats share many of the same characteristics as humans with obesity-related diabetes ('diabesity'). These therefore provide a model for measuring the cellular events through which excess accumulation of body fat and/or excessive dietary fat intake

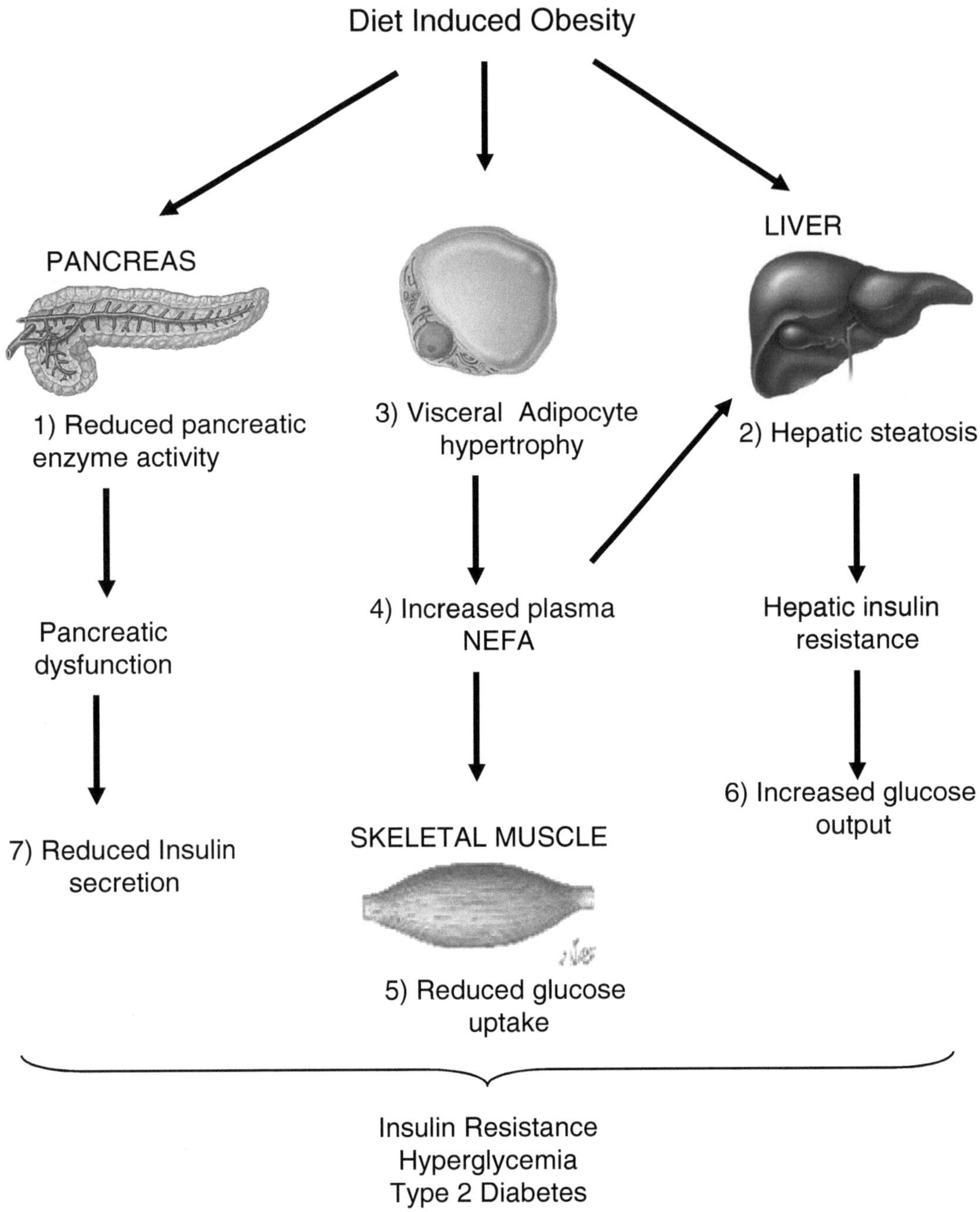

Fig. 1. Summary of proposed mechanisms involved in the development of type 2 diabetes in models of diet-induced obesity in adult rodents. Increased dietary fat intake is associated with (1) reduced activity of pancreatic enzymes, leading to impaired pancreatic function and reduced insulin secretion, and (2) increased accumulation of lipids in the liver (hepatic steatosis) which results in hepatic insulin resistance and increased hepatic glucose output. In addition, increased accumulation of adipose tissue in the visceral compartment (3) results in increased plasma concentrations of non-esterified free fatty acids (NEFAs) (4), and deposition of these NEFAs in liver and skeletal muscle, further contributing to insulin resistance in these tissues. Together, this results in an impaired glucose uptake by skeletal muscle (5), increased hepatic glucose output (6) and impaired insulin secretion (7) and precipitates the development of whole-body insulin resistance and type 2 diabetes.

result in the degradation of insulin action in key insulin-sensitive tissues. Another advantage of this model is that DIO mice and rats can now be ordered directly from commercial suppliers. Whilst this is obviously more expensive than an in-house option, it does have the potential to save the researcher the 8-12 weeks that it would normally take to generate the DIO rodents. In addition, a variety of high-fat diets are now available from commercial animal feed manufacturers.

Whilst the DIO model has many positive attributes, it also has some potential limitations. Perhaps the major limitation is the lack of standardisation of the feeding regimen of different studies, which has meant that the phenotype of fat-fed animals varies between experiments. The high-fat diets which have been used consist of anywhere from 20 to 60% energy content from fat, and the type of fat (i.e. animal versus plant) also varies between studies *(1)*, and there is no clear indication of which type of high-fat feeding represents the best model of the metabolic disturbances seen in human obesity. It is therefore important to consider both the type of dietary intervention (i.e. the proportion of energy derived from fat and type of fat in the diet) and the precise phenotype of the strain under investigation when interpreting results and extrapolating these data to humans.

2.2. Diet-Induced Obesity: *Psammomys obesus*

The sand rat (*Psammomys obesus*) has been another popular model for studying the degradation of metabolic function associated with obesity. This is an attractive model because the sand rat under laboratory conditions rapidly develops obesity when fed a standard laboratory chow, which is considerably less expensive than custom-made high-fat diets. Many of the pathophysiological changes found in the obese sand rat are similar to those seen in human type 2 diabetic patients *(19)*, and this model therefore appears to provide an appropriate nutritional model of human T2DM. When provided with ad libitum access to laboratory chow the adult sand rat progresses through from normoglycaemia and normoinsulinaemia, to hyperinsulinaemia with marked insulin resistance, followed by pronounced hyperinsulinaemia with hyperglycaemia and, after a further 6-10 weeks of chow feeding, gradual beta-cell degradation and disappearance of beta-cell insulin which eventually results in severe insulin deficiency and overt diabetes *(20)*. The obese sand rat exhibits profound insulin resistance in both skeletal muscle and liver, and provides an attractive model for studying the mechanisms, which underlie the development of diabetes in human obesity *(21)*. Studies utilising this model have reported that GLUT4 protein content is reduced in skeletal muscle, resulting in a reduced peripheral glucose uptake and hyperglycaemia *(20)*. In addition, hepatic PEPCK activity is increased, suggesting that the ability of insulin to inhibit hepatic glucose production is impaired *(22)*. Extensive use has been made of the obese sand rats for the purpose of testing potential T2DM drugs, including tyrosine phosphatase inhibitors and glucagon-like peptide-1 (GLP-1) analogues *(20)*.

The major limitations of this model are that the sand rat exhibits insulin resistance even when fed on a low-energy diet, suggesting that the physiology of this desert-adapted animal may not be entirely comparable with humans. The link between weight gain and the development of insulin resistance in this model has yet to be clearly defined; however, the phenotype is normalised by dietary restriction. Nevertheless, this model has been utilised extensively for the study of obesity-induced diabetes and continues to provide important insights into the cellular defects, which contribute to the development of central and peripheral insulin resistance (**Fig. 1**).

3. Prenatal Nutritional Models of T2DM

The foetal or developmental origins of adult disease hypothesis states that insults during critical windows of development results in adaptive changes within foetal tissues and organ systems, which have lifetime consequences for the health of an individual. The hypothesis was first derived from studies of the Hertfordshire birth cohort by Professor David Barker in the early 1990s which showed that there was an inverse relationship between birth weight and the incidence of cardiovascular disease in adult life *(23)*. This was followed by a series of studies in human populations which all demonstrated that being of low birth weight was associated with an increased incidence of adult metabolic and cardiovascular disease *(24, 25)*.

The Dutch Winter Hunger Famine was a 5-month period in World War II during which the food supply to Amsterdam, Holland, was severely restricted, resulting in a substantial decrease in the daily energy intake of the population *(26)*. Subsequent studies of the children of women who were pregnant during the famine showed that those exposed to famine in the last 5 months of gestation had a significantly greater incidence of glucose intolerance, obesity, and T2DM in adult life compared to those children whose mothers were not exposed to the famine *(26, 27)*. Similarly, early studies in infants of diabetic mothers clearly showed that exposure to high glucose levels in the pre- and perinatal period was associated with an increased incidence of hyperglycaemia and T2DM in the offspring in postnatal life *(28)*. These studies provided the first evidence that exposure to an inappropriately low, or inappropriately high, nutrient supply during early development was associated with a permanent alteration of metabolic function in the offspring. An increasing number of epidemiological and experimental animal studies have since continued to highlight the importance of both the prenatal and early postnatal nutritional environment for the determination of later metabolic health *(25, 29, 30)*.

Together, these studies have clearly demonstrated that a low birth weight followed by a period of accelerated postnatal growth or a high birth weight, as a consequence of prenatal overnutrition, are each associated with an increased propensity towards the development of insulin resistance, glucose intolerance and T2DM in adult life *(31–33)*. As a result, both spontaneous and experimentally induced foetal growth restriction (in utero growth restriction (IUGR)) and prenatal overnutrition in animal models have been widely employed in order to understand the physiological basis of reduced insulin sensitivity. It has been demonstrated that global undernutrition in the pregnant rodent is also associated with later onset of T2DM in the offspring *(34)*. This is, however, considered to be largely a consequence of impaired insulin secretion rather than defects in insulin signalling *(35)*, and is therefore not the most appropriate model for the pathophysiological process which contribute to T2DM in the majority of human patients.

3.1. The Maternal Low-Protein Model

The maternal low-protein model is one of the most extensively studied models of foetal growth restriction. In this model, pregnant dams are fed a diet containing approximately 8% of energy as protein, compared to approximately 20% in controls, and this is associated with low birth weight in the offspring, followed by accelerated postnatal growth *(29, 36)*. The period of rapid postnatal growth is due to enhanced insulin sensitivity in the period immediately after birth; however, this is not maintained beyond the early postnatal period, and the offspring develop insulin resistance by the age of 15 months and frank T2DM by 17 months *(33, 37)*, and the deterioration of metabolic function is accelerated by a postnatal high-fat diet *(38)*. The phenotype of the low-protein offspring has many similarities with that of human type 2 diabetics, including insulin resistance, altered regulation of hepatic glucose output and pancreatic dysfunction *(29)*. As a result, this model has been used extensively to explore and characterise the cellular defects within the insulin signalling pathway which may contribute to reduced insulin sensitivity. These studies have demonstrated that prenatal exposure to a low-protein diet results in defects in several peripheral insulin-sensitive tissues, which are central to the maintenance of glucose homeostasis. In the pancreas, the islets of Langerhans are smaller and exhibit a reduced insulin secretion in response to amino acid stimulation *(39)*. Whilst there is no obvious defect in glucose-stimulated insulin release in offspring fed a control chow diet post-weaning, a reduction in the capacity of glucose to stimulate insulin release emerges if these offspring are fed on a high-fat diet post-weaning. The liver of the low-protein offspring is unresponsive to the actions of glucagon, and insulin stimulates, rather than suppresses, hepatic glucose output *(40)*. Moreover, adipose cells exhibit increased basal and insulin-stimulated glucose uptake, leading to an increased accumulation of fat in the visceral compartment and ectopic fat storage in liver and skeletal muscle, which further contributes to the peripheral insulin resistance *(41)* (**Fig. 2**).

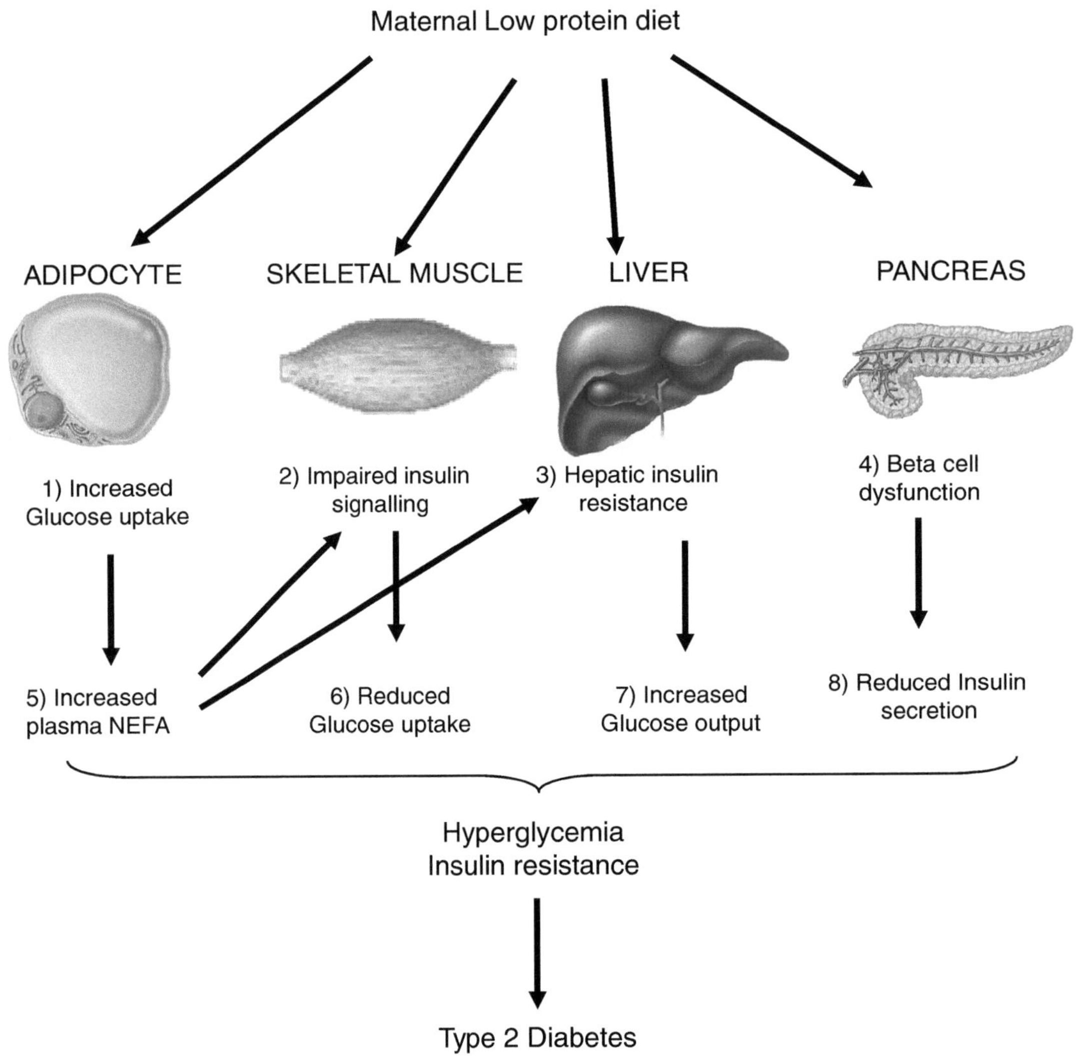

Fig. 2. Summary of mechanisms proposed to contribute to the programming of type 2 diabetes of offspring in the maternal low-protein model. Prenatal exposure to a low-protein diet results in (1) an increased capacity for glucose uptake by visceral adipocytes (2) impaired insulin signalling in skeletal muscle, (3) hepatic insulin resistance and (4) impaired pancreatic function. The increased glucose uptake by visceral adipocytes results in an increased accumulation of visceral adipose tissue, resulting in elevated plasma concentrations of non-esterified free fatty acids (NEFAs) (5) which are deposited in peripheral tissues (liver and skeletal muscle), further reducing insulin sensitivity. This reduced insulin sensitivity is associated with impaired glucose uptake by skeletal muscle (6), increased glucose output by the liver (7) and reduced insulin secretion by the pancreas (8), resulting in peripheral hyperglycaemia, insulin resistance and type 2 diabetes.

Given that muscle represents the major site of postprandial glucose disposal, it is not surprising that changes in the functional characteristics of muscle fibres during the perinatal period are important in the programming of insulin resistance and diabetes (**Fig. 2**). Isolated muscle strips from these low-protein animals exhibit enhanced basal and insulin-stimulated glucose uptake, and this increase in insulin sensitivity is associated with a twofold increase in the abundance of insulin receptors in muscle membranes *(42)*. By 15 months of age, however, there is a decrease in the insulin sensitivity of glucose uptake in skeletal muscle from the group exposed to the low-protein diet in utero *(43)*. This impaired insulin action is not associated with changes in the expression of either the insulin receptor or GLUT4, but is associated with a decrease in the abundance of signalling molecules downstream of the insulin receptor, including the zeta-isoform of protein kinase C, an isoform that is involved in GLUT4-mediated glucose transport *(43)* and p85 PI3K *(44)* (**Fig.** 2). In addition to defects in insulin signalling, it has also been reported that prenatal undernutrition is associated with impaired mitochondrial biogenesis and impaired mitochondrial oxidative capacity in skeletal muscle, which has previously been associated with reductions in insulin sensitivity in this tissue *(45, 46)*.

Whilst these studies have provided important insights into the cellular defects which contribute to deteriorations in insulin sensitivity in peripheral tissues, it is still unclear whether these defects are the same as those seen in human T2DM, which typically develops secondary to increased body fat accumulation. There is recent evidence that the mechanisms involved in the prenatal programming of insulin resistance may be quite distinct from those in insulin resistance which develops in response to diet-induced obesity *(35)*. Nevertheless, the obvious importance of the early environment in determining metabolic health in later life may well explain why it is that some individuals are more susceptible to insulin resistance than others at the same degree of body fatness.

3.2. Prenatal Overnutrition, Postnatal Obesity and T2DM

There is increasing evidence that prenatal exposure to a high plane of nutrition is also associated with an increased risk of obesity and T2DM in postnatal life. The rat and the sheep represent the two main animal models which have been utilised thus far for investigating the effects of prenatal overnutrition on the offspring. Unlike the low-maternal low-protein model, however, the role of defects within the insulin signalling pathway in models of maternal overnutrition or high-fat feeding remains largely unexplored. Studies to date have suggested that the deterioration of metabolic function in these individuals is associated with altered development of pancreatic beta-cells, mitochondrial dysfunction and programming of the central appetite-regulating network *(10, 47, 48)*. Several studies have also suggested that the deterioration of metabolic function may be secondary to the increased accumulation of adipose tissue in these offspring (**Fig. 3**) *(48, 49)*; however, it is not clear whether this is the case in all models of prenatal overnutrition.

In the rat, maternal high-fat feeding results in disturbed glucose homeostasis in the offspring at weaning and in adult life, including an impaired glucose tolerance and reduced whole-body insulin sensitivity. Patel and colleagues found that feeding rats on a high-fat chow during pregnancy and lactation resulted in offspring that were significantly heavier than controls, had elevated plasma concentrations of insulin, glucose, free fatty acids and triglycerides and exhibited glucose intolerance *(47)*. When they investigated the pancreatic islets in these animals, they found that those from male offspring exhibited an increased insulin secretary response at low glucose concentrations compared to controls, suggesting that high-fat feeding resulted in altered pancreatic development *(50)*. This was also the case in a separate study, in which feeding pregnant rats a high-fat diet during pregnancy and lactation was associated with hyperglycaemia and evidence of compromised beta-cell function in the weanling offspring *(51)*. Similarly, the offspring of Sprague-Dawley rats fed a lard-rich diet during pregnancy and lactation exhibited whole-body insulin resistance and a reduced glucose-stimulated insulin secretion in isolated islets at 9 months *(10)*, again supporting the thesis that maternal high-fat feeding is associated with impaired pancreatic function in the offspring (**Fig. 3**).

In the sheep, feeding ewes approximately 55% above their maintenance energy requirements in late pregnancy results in an increase in foetal glucose and insulin concentrations in the last third of gestation *(52)*, and is associated with an increased accumulation of subcutaneous adipose tissue at the end of the first month of postnatal life *(52)*. The offspring of overfed ewes exhibit elevated glucose concentrations during the first month of postnatal life *(52)*, although whether this is associated with reduced insulin sensitivity during this period has yet to be determined.

Fig. 3. (continued) The increased accumulation of body fat contributes to metabolic dysfunction by elevating plasma non-esterified free fatty acid (NEFA) concentrations (4) which are deposited in skeletal muscle and liver, resulting in insulin resistance in these tissues (5) and (6). Recent evidence suggests that epigenetic changes which occur before birth (7) may also play a role in metabolic programming after prenatal overnutrition. Together, these changes result in peripheral insulin resistance and, ultimately, type 2 diabetes.

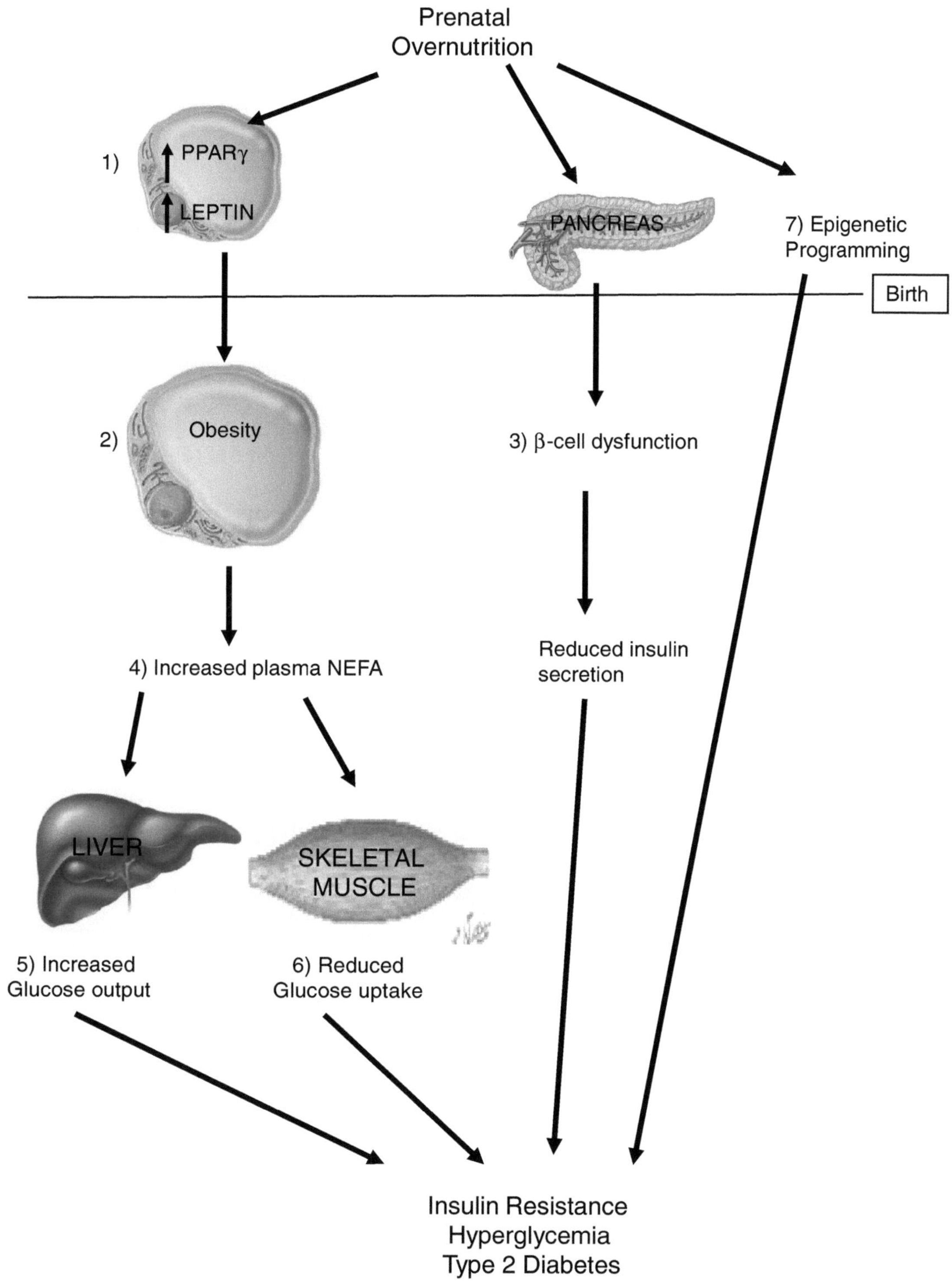

Fig. 3. Potential mechanisms contributing to the programming of type 2 diabetes following prenatal overnutrition. It has been demonstrated that prenatal overnutrition is associated with an increased lipogenic capacity of adipose cells (1), which results in increased fat accumulation after birth (2) and predisposes these offspring to obesity in later life. In addition, prenatal high-fat diets result in impaired pancreatic development and beta-cell dysfunction in postnatal life (3).

4. Possible Mechanisms for Metabolic Programming

4.1. The Adipocyte

In large animal models there is evidence that exposure to prenatal overnutrition or undernutrition can act to permanently alter the function of adipocytes and result in an increased lipogenic capacity in adipose depots in postnatal life. In sheep, which have a similar profile of adipose cell development to humans, exposure to increased glucose concentrations in late foetal life increases the expression of genes within adipose cells that are responsible for promoting lipid storage and forming new adipocytes *(53)*. This is associated with increased adipose tissue mass by the end of the first month of life, due primarily to an increase in adipocyte cell size *(48)*. In pigs, adipocytes exposed to high glucose levels before birth also exhibit a dramatic increase in their capacity for lipogenesis *(54)* and this precedes their development of obesity *(55)*. These findings have since been supported by work in rodents, in which maternal junk food feeding during pregnancy and lactation in rats and an obesogenic diet during this same period in mice were each associated with increased adiposity and increased expression of lipogenic genes and insulin-independent glucose transporters in the perirenal adipose depot *(49, 56)*. It would therefore appear that fat cells exposed to an excess substrate supply during critical windows in their development have an increased capacity for storing lipid in postnatal life. This enhanced lipogeneic capacity would render these individuals more likely to store excess energy in the form of fat, and increase their susceptibility to weight gain, obesity and, consequently, to the excess deposition of fatty acids in liver and skeletal muscle, resulting in peripheral insulin resistance, hyperglycaemia and, ultimately, type 2 diabetes (**Fig. 3**).

In individuals exposed to low nutrient levels before birth, adipocyte development is initially sacrificed in favour of essential organs *(25, 57)*. If an in utero ‘restricted’ individual is born into a postnatal environment where nutrient supply is no longer constrained, a period of ‘catch-up’ fat deposition ensues, mainly in the visceral adipose depot *(58)*. These individuals are therefore at increased risk of visceral obesity *(59)* and, consequently, to the development of insulin resistance and T2DM *(60)*. It is the increased accumulation of visceral adipose tissue that has also been demonstrated in animal models of IUGR, including the sheep, guinea pig and rodent *(61–63)*. Therefore, exposure of the developing adipocyte to sub-optimal nutrition, particularly of the visceral adipose tissue which is the first adipose depot to develop in sheep and humans *(64, 65)*, also appears to play a critical role in defining an individual’s propensity for accumulating visceral body fat later in life, i.e. the fat pattern linked to increased risk of metabolic dysfunction *(6)*.

4.2. Mitochondrial Biogenesis

Mitochondria play a central role in the regulation of cellular energy metabolism, and impaired mitochondrial function and reduction in mitochondrial oxidative capacity in skeletal muscle have been associated with the onset of insulin resistance and T2DM both in experimental animal models and in human subjects *(66)*. In experimental animal studies, both diet-induced obesity and prenatal undernutrition have been associated with impaired mitochondrial biogenesis and reduced abundance of oxidative enzymes in skeletal muscle. Importantly, there is evidence that the reduction of mitochondrial biogenesis in adult rats exposed to prenatal undernutrition precedes the development of insulin resistance and glucose intolerance in this model *(45, 46)*, therefore implicating impaired mitochondrial function in the causal pathway linking prenatal undernutrition to later metabolic disease. The role of mitochondrial dysfunction in metabolic programming has yet to be explored in large animal models, and the potential role of mitochondrial dysfunction in the development of T2DM remains an important area for investigation.

4.3. Epigenetics

The concept that changes in phenotype could be elicited by modification of the DNA in the absence of changes in DNA sequence, i.e. epigenetic changes, provides a new basis for understanding of phenotypic programming. The two most well-characterised epigenetic modifications include both DNA methylation and histone acetylation, which act to suppress gene expression *(67, 68)*. Recent evidence has demonstrated that exposure to an either an excession or deficient nutrient supply during early development may result in epigenetic modifications in the foetus which have the potential to permanently alter the function of important metabolic systems. Waterland and colleagues demonstrated that when mice with a genetic tendency towards obesity were fed a standard diet during pregnancy, the degree of obesity in the offspring increased progressively with each generation. This effect was, however, completely abolished if mice were fed a diet high in methyl groups (which increases DNA methylation) during pregnancy, and the offspring remained lean. These findings suggested that reduced DNA methylation in genes which play a role in the regulation of energy balance and fat storage, as a result of early nutritional programming, may contribute to the later development of obesity and metabolic disease *(69)*. There is also increasing evidence that exposure to a sub-optimal nutrient supply before birth can also alter methylation of a series genes involved in growth and energy homeostasis, and that this may explain the link between foetal growth restriction and later metabolic dysfunction *(67, 68)*.

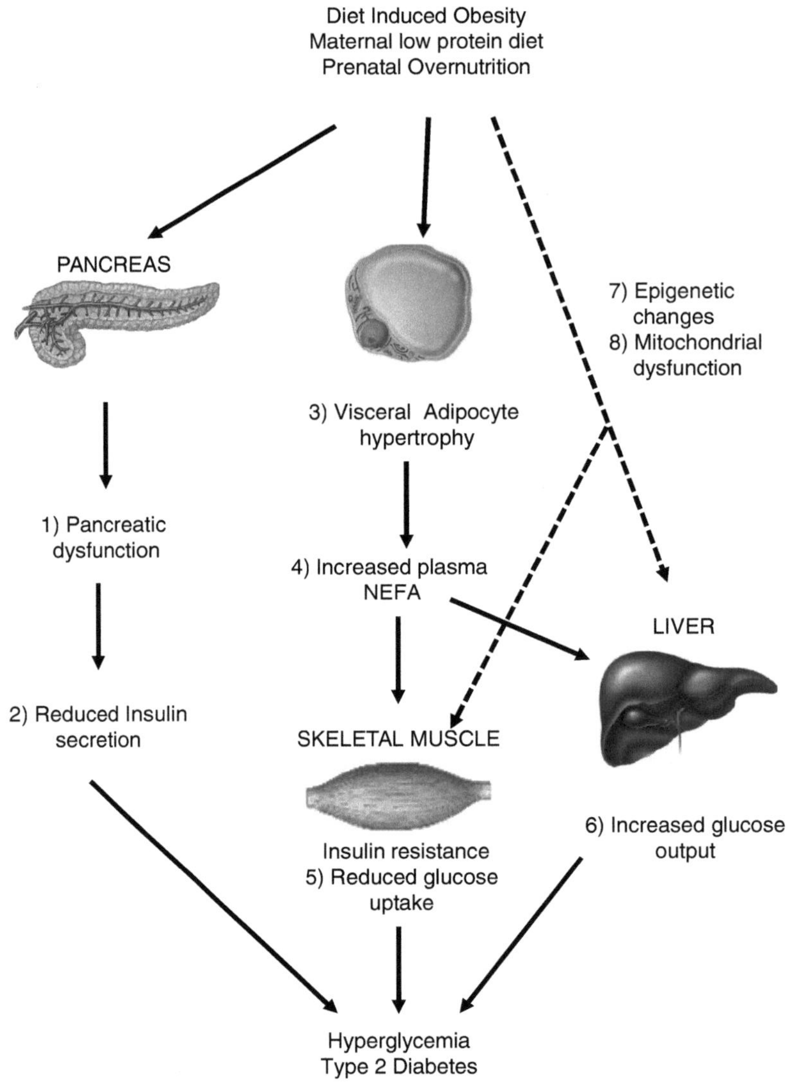

Fig. 4. Summary of common mechanisms identified in all nutritional models of type 2 diabetes. Both diet-induced obesity and prenatal nutritional interventions are associated with pancreatic dysfunction (1) and impaired insulin secretion (2), which contributes to peripheral hyperglycaemia. In addition, adipocyte hypertrophy, in particular within the visceral compartment (3), is associated with increased circulating concentrations of non-esterified free fatty acids (NEFA) (4) which, when deposited in liver and skeletal muscle, are associated with the development of insulin resistance in these tissues and, consequently, reduced glucose uptake by skeletal muscle (5) and increased hepatic glucose output (6). In addition, recent evidence suggests that epigenetic changes and mitochondrial dysfunction in liver and skeletal muscle may also contribute to development of metabolic disorders.

5. Summary

The dramatic increase in the incidence of T2DM over the past decade has highlighted the need to better understand the pathophysiology of this disease. The use of animal models which mimic the disease progression in humans is essential in order to investigate the cellular mechanisms which contribute to the deterioration of insulin metabolism in key insulin-sensitive tissues. This criterion is not fulfilled by genetic models, or models in which the pancreas is surgically ablated, since these causes account for only a relatively minor proportion of the humans who will develop T2DM. A number of nutritional models of T2DM have now been developed, and have made a significant contribution to our current understanding of the cellular defects which emerge in insulin-sensitive tissues in response to an excess accumulation of body fat or excessive intake of dietary fat, and which result in the development of peripheral insulin resistance. It has also become clear that exposure to either inappropriately high or inappropriately low levels of nutrition *in utero* is associated with an increased susceptibility to T2DM in adult life, and that the detailed study of the cellular and molecular defects in these offspring has the potential to provide novel insights into why some individuals are more prone to the development of insulin resistance and T2DM than others. The study of diet-induced obesity and models of prenatal undernutrition and overnutrition has revealed several common mechanisms which contribute to the onset of insulin resistance and T2DM in these different models (**Fig. 4**), and this has provided important insights into the aetiology of type 2 diabetes in humans and has identified possible targets for intervention. As with all animal models, it is important to recognise that animal data may not always be directly extrapolated to the human situation, where other factors, in particular socioeconomic status and demographic variations, also contribute to risk of metabolic disease *(70)*. It is therefore important to exercise caution when extrapolating results to human clinical practice. Nevertheless, it is clear that nutritional studies in the animal models discussed in this chapter have been critical in shaping our current understanding of the pathophysiology of T2DM and offer significant opportunities for identifying and testing potential clinical interventions.

References

1. Buettner, R., Scholmerich, J., and Bollheimer, L. C. (2007). High-fat diets: modeling the metabolic disorders of human obesity in rodents. *Obesity* **15**, 798–808
2. Portha, B., Blondel, O., Serradas, P., McEvoy, R., Giroix, M. H., Kergoat, M., and Bailbe, D. (1989),. The rat models of non-insulin dependent diabetes induced by neonatal streptozotocin. *Diabetes Metab* **15**, 61–75
3. Bray, G. A. (2004). Medical consequences of obesity. *J Clin Endocrinol Metab* **89**, 2583–2589
4. Goralski, K. B. and Sinal, C. J. (2007). Type 2 diabetes and cardiovascular disease: getting to the fat of the matter. *Can J Physiol Pharmacol* **85**, 113–132
5. Smith, S. R., Lovejoy, J. C., Greenway, F., Ryan, D., deJonge, L., de la Bretonne, J., Volafova, J., and Bray, G. A. (2001). Contributions of total body fat, abdominal subcutaneous adipose tissue compartments, and visceral adipose tissue to the metabolic complications of obesity. *Metabolism* **50**, 425–435
6. Ravussin, E. and Smith, S. R. (2002). Increased fat uptake, impaired fat oxidation, and failure of fat cell proliferation result in

ectopic fat storage, insulin resistance, and type 2 diabetes. *Ann N Y Acad Sci* **967**, 363–378

7. Surwit, R. S., Kuhn, C. M., Cochrane, C., McCubbin, J. A., and Feinglos, M. N. (1988). Diet-induced type II diabetes in C57BL/6J mice. *Diabetes* **37**, 1163–1167
8. Roberts, C. K., Berger, J. J., and Barnard, R. J. (2002). Long-term effects of diet on leptin, energy intake, and activity in a model of diet-induced obesity. *J Appl Physiol* **93**, 887–893
9. Bayol, S. A., Farrington, S. J., and Stickland, N. C. (2007). A maternal 'junk food' diet in pregnancy and lactation promotes an exacerbated taste for 'junk food' and a greater propensity for obesity in rat offspring. *Br J Nutr* **98**, 843–851
10. Taylor, P. D., McConnell, J., Khan, I. Y., Holemans, K., Lawrence, K. M., Asare-Anane, H., Persaud, S. J., Jones, P. M., Petrie, L., Hanson, M. A., and Poston, L. (2005). Impaired glucose homeostasis and mitochondrial abnormalities in offspring of rats fed a fat-rich diet in pregnancy. *Am J Physiol Regul Integr Comp Physiol* **288**, R134–R139
11. Woods, S. C., Seeley, R. J., Rushing, P. A., D'Alessio, D., and Tso, P. (2003). A controlled high-fat diet induces an obese syndrome in rats. *J Nutr* **133**, 1081–1087
12. Qiu, L., List, E. O., and Kopchick, J. J. (2005). Differentially expressed proteins in the pancreas of diet-induced diabetic mice. *Mol Cell Proteomics* **4**, 1311–1318
13. Corbett, S. W., Stern, J. S., and Keesey, R. E. (1986), Energy expenditure in rats with diet-induced obesity. *Am J Clin Nutr* 44, 173–180
14. Yaqoob, P., Sherrington, E. J., Jeffery, N. M., Sanderson, P., Harvey, D. J., Newsholme, E. A., and Calder, P. C. (1995), Comparison of the effects of a range of dietary lipids upon serum and tissue lipid composition in the rat. *Int J Biochem Cell Biol* 27, 297–310
15. Levin, B. E., Hogan, S., and Sullivan, A. C. (1989), Initiation and perpetuation of obesity and obesity resistance in rats. *Am J Physiol Regul Integr Comp Physiol* **256**, R766–R771
16. Clegg, D. J., Benoit, S. C., Reed, J. A., Woods, S. C., Dunn-Meynell, A., and Levin, B. E. (2005). Reduced anorexic effects of insulin in obesity-prone rats fed a moderate-fat diet. *Am J Physiol Regul Integr Comp Physiol* **288**, R981–R986
17. Levin, B. E., Dunn-Meynell, A. A., Balkan, B., and Keesey, R. E. (1997). Selective breeding for diet-induced obesity and resistance in Sprague-Dawley rats. *Am J Physiol Regul Integr Comp Physiol* **273**, R725–R730
18. Tkacs, N. C. and Levin, B. E. (2004). Obesity-prone rats have preexisting defects in their counterregulatory response to insulin-induced hypoglycemia. *Am J Physiol Regul Integr Comp Physiol* **287**, R1110–R1115
19. Wassink, A. M., Olijhoek, J. K., and Visseren, F. L. (2007), The metabolic syndrome: metabolic changes with vascular consequences. *Eur J Clin Invest* 37, 8–17
20. Shafrir, E., Ziv, E., and Kalman, R. (2006). Nutritionally induced diabetes in desert rodents as models of type 2 diabetes: Acomys cahirinus (spiny mice) and P*sammomys obesus* (desert gerbil). *ILAR J* **47**, 212–224
21. Kaiser, N., Nesher, R., Donath, M. Y., Fraenkel, M., Behar, V., Magnan, C., Ktorza, A., Cerasi, E., and Leibowitz, G. (2005). Psammomys obesus, a model for environment-gene interactions in type 2 diabetes. *Diabetes* **54**, S137–S144
22. Maislos, M., Medvedovskv, V., Sztarkier, I., Yaari, A., and Sikuler, E. (2006). Psammomys obesus (sand rat), a new animal model of non-alcoholic fatty liver disease. *Diabetes Res Clin Pract* **72**, 1–5
23. Barker, D. J. P., Bull, A. R., Osmond, C., and Simmonds, S. J. (1990). Fetal and placental size and risk of hypertension in adult life. *Br Med J* **301**, 259–262
24. Hales, C. N. and Barker, D. J. P. (2001). The thrifty phenotype hypothesis. *Br Med Bull* **60**, 5–20
25. McMillen, I. C. and Robinson, J. S. (2005), Developmental origins of the metabolic syndrome: prediction, plasticity, and programming. *Physiol Rev* **85**, 571–633
26. Ravelli, A. C., van der Meulen, J. H., Osmond, C., Barker, D. J., and Bleker, O. P. (1999). Obesity at the age of 50 y in men and women exposed to famine prenatally. *Am J Clin Nutr* **70**, 811–816
27. Ravelli, A. C. J., van der Meulen, J. H. P., Michels, R. P. J., Osmond, C., Barker, D. J. P., Hales, C. N., and Bleker, O. P. (1998). Glucose tolerance in adults after prenatal exposure to famine. *Lancet* **351,** 173–177
28. Pettit, D. J. and Knowler, W. C. (1998). Long-term effects of the intrauterine environment, birth weight, and breast-feeding in Pima Indians. *Diabetes Care* **21**, B138–B141
29. Ozanne, S. E. (2001). Metabolic programming in animals: Type 2 diabetes. *Br Med Bull* 60, 143–152
30. Armitage, J. A., Khan, I. Y., Taylor, P. D., Nathanielsz, P. W., and Poston, L. (2004), Developmental programming of the metabolic syndrome by maternal nutritional imbalance: how strong is the evidence from experimental

models in mammals?. *J Physiol (Lond)* **561**, 355–377

31. Bavdekar, A., Yajnik, C., Fall, C., Bapat, S., Pandit, A., Deshpande, V., Bhave, S., Kellingray, S., and Joglekar, C. (1999). Insulin resistance syndrome in 8-year-old Indian children: small at birth, big at 8 years, or both?. *Diabetes* **48**, 2422–2429
32. McMillen, I. C., Adam, C. L., and Muhlhausler, B. S. (2005). Early origins of obesity: programming the appetite regulatory system. *J Physiol* **565**, 9–17
33. Hales, C. N. and Barker, D. J. P. (2001). The thrifty phenotype hypothesis: type 2 diabetes. *Br Med Bull* **60**, 5–20
34. Holemans, K., Verhaeghe, J., Dequeker, J., and Van Assche, F. A. (1996). Insulin sensitivity in adult female rats subjected to malnutrition during the perinatal period. *J Soc Gynecol Investig* **3**, 71–77
35. Thompson, N. M., Norman, A. M., Donkin, S. S., Shankar, R. R., Vickers, M. H., Miles, J. L., and Breier, B. H. (2007). Prenatal and postnatal pathways to obesity: different underlying mechanisms, different metabolic outcomes. *Endocrinol Metab Clin North Am* **148**, 2345–2354
36. Ozanne, S. E., Jensen, C. B., Tingey, K. J., Storgaard, H., Madsbad, S., and Vaag, A. A. (2005). Low birthweight is associated with specific changes in muscle insulin-signalling protein expression. *Diabetologia* **48**, 547–552
37. Hales, C. N., Desai, M., Ozanne, S. E., and Crowther, N. J. (1996). Fishing in the stream of diabetes: from measuring insulin to the control of fetal organogenesis. *Biochem Soc Trans* **24**, 341–350
38. Petry, C. J., Ozanne, S. E., Wang, C. L., and Hales, C. N. (1997). Early protein restriction and obesity independently induce hypertension in 1-year-old rats. *Clin Sci (Lond)* **93**, 147–152
39. Snoeck, A., Remacle, C., Reusens, B., and Hoet, J. J. (1990). Effect of a low protein diet during pregnancy on the fetal rat endocrine pancreas. *Biol Neonate* **57**, 107–118
40. Ozanne, S. E., Smith, G. D., Tikerpae, J., and Hales, C. N. (1996). Altered regulation of hepatic glucose output in the male offspring of protein-malnourished rat dams. *Am J Physiol Endocrinol Metab* **270**, E559–E564
41. Ozanne, S. E., Nave, B. T., Wang, C. L., Shepherd, P. R., Prins, J., and Smith, G. D. (1997). Poor fetal nutrition causes long-term changes in expression of insulin signaling components in adipocytes. *Am J Physiol Endocrinol Metab* **273**, E46–E51
42. Ozanne, S. E., Wang, C. L., Coleman, N., and Smith, G. D. (1996). Altered muscle insulin sensitivity in the male offspring of protein-malnourished rats. *Am J Physiol Endocrinol Metab* 271, E1128–E1134
43. Ozanne, S. E., Olsen, G. S., Hansen, L. L., Tingey, K. J., Nave, B. T., Wang, C. L., Hartil, K., Petry, C. J., Buckley, A. J., and Mosthaf-Seedorf, L. (2003). Early growth restriction leads to down regulation of protein kinase C zeta and insulin resistance in skeletal muscle. *J Endocrinol* **177**, 235–241
44. Ozanne, S. E., Jensen, C. B., Tingey, K. J., Storgaard, H., Madsbad, S., and Vaag, A. A. (2005). Low birthweight is associated with specific changes in muscle insulin-signalling protein expression. *Diabetologia* **48**, 547–552
45. Wadley, G. D., Siebel, A. L., Cooney, G. J., McConell, G. K., Wlodek, M. E., and Owens, J. A. (2008). Uteroplacental insufficiency and reducing litter size alters skeletal muscle mitochondrial biogenesis in a sex-specific manner in the adult rat. *Am J Physiol Endocrinol Metab* **294**, E861–E869
46. Siebel, A. L., Mibus, A., De Blasio, M. J., Westcott, K. T., Morris, M. J., Prior, L., Owens, J. A., and Wlodek, M. E. (2008). Improved lactational nutrition and postnatal growth ameliorates impairment of glucose tolerance by uteroplacental insufficiency in male rat offspring. *Endocrinology* **149**, 3067–3076
47. Srinivasan, M., Katewa, S. D., Palaniyappan, A., Pandya, J. D., and Patel, M. S. (2006). Maternal high-fat diet consumption results in fetal malprogramming predisposing to the onset of metabolic syndrome-like phenotype in adulthood. *Am J Physiol Endocrinol Metab* **291**, E792–E799
48. Muhlhausler, B. S., Adam, C. L., Findlay, P. A., Duffield, J. A., and McMillen, I. C. (2006). Increased maternal nutrition alters development of the appetite-regulating network in the brain. *FASEB J* **20**, 1257–1259
49. Samuelsson, A.-M., Matthews, P. A., Argenton, M., Christie, M. R., McConnell, J. M., Jansen, E. H. J. M., Piersma, A. H., Ozanne, S. E., Twinn, D. F., Remacle, C., Rowlerson, A., Poston, L., and Taylor, P. D. (2008). Diet-induced obesity in female mice leads to offspring hyperphagia, adiposity, hypertension, and insulin resistance: a novel murine model of developmental programming. *Hypertension* **51**, 383–392
50. Srinivasan, M., Aalinkeel, R., Song, F., Mitrani, P., Pandya, J. D., Strutt, B., Hill, D. J., and Patel, M. S. (2006). Maternal hyperinsulinemia predisposes rat fetuses for hyperinsuline-

mia, and adult-onset obesity and maternal mild food restriction reverses this phenotype. *Am J Physiol Endocrinol Metab* **290**, E129–E134

51. Cerf, M. E., Williams, K., Chapman, C. S., and Louw, J. (2007). Compromised beta-cell development and beta-cell dysfunction in weanling offspring from dams maintained on a high-fat diet during gestation. *Pancreas* **34**, 347–353
52. Muhlhausler, B. S., Roberts, C. T., McFarlane, J. R., Kauter, K. G., and McMillen, I. C. (2002). Fetal leptin is a signal of fat mass independent of maternal nutrition in ewes fed at or above maintenance energy requirements. *Biol Reprod* **67**, 493–499
53. Muhlhausler, B. S., Duffield, J. A., and McMillen, I. C. (2007). Increased maternal nutrition stimulates peroxisome proliferator activated receptor-{gamma} (PPAR{gamma}), adiponectin and leptin mRNA expression in adipose tissue before birth. *Endocrinology* **148**, 878–885
54. Kasser, T. R., Martin, R. J., and Allen, C. E. (1981). Effect of gestational alloxan diabetes and fasting on fetal lipogenesis and lipid deposition in pigs. *Biol Neonate* **40**, 105–112
55. Ezekwe, M. O. and Martin, R. J. (1980). The effects of maternal alloxan diabetes on body composition, liver enzymes and metabolism and serum metabolites and hormones of fetal pigs. *Horm Metab Res* **12**, 136–139
56. Bayol, S. A., Simbi, B. H., Bertrand, J. A., and Stickland, N. C. (2008). Offspring from mothers fed a 'junk food' diet in pregnancy and lactation exhibit exacerbated adiposity that is more pronounced in females. *J Physiol* **586**, 3219–3230
57. Padoan, A., Rigano, S., Ferrazzi, E., Beaty, B. L., Battaglia, F. C., and Galan, H. L. (2004). Differences in fat and lean mass proportions in normal and growth-restricted fetuses. *Am J Obstet Gynecol* **191**, 1459–1464
58. Crescenzo, R., Samec, S., Antic, V., Rohner-Jeanrenaud, F., Seydoux, J., Montani, J.-P., and Dulloo, A. G. (2003). A role for suppressed thermogenesis favoring catch-up fat in the pathophysiology of catch-up growth. *Acta Paediatr* **52**, 1090–1097
59. Ibanez, L., Ong, K., Dunger, D. B., and de Zegher, F. (2006). Early development of adiposity and insulin resistance after catch-up weight gain in small-for-gestational-age children. *J Clin Endocrinol Metab* **91**, 2153–2158
60. Jaquet, D., Gaboriau, A., Czernichow, P., and Levy-Marchal, C. (2000). Insulin resistance early in adulthood in subjects born with intra-uterine growth retardation. *J Clin Endocrinol Metab* **85**, 1401–1406
61. Ozanne, S. E. (2001). Metabolic programming in animals. *Br Med Bull* **60**, 143–152
62. Kind, K. L., Clifton, P. M., Grant, P. A., Owens, P. C., Sohlstrom, A., Roberts, C. T., Robinson, J. S., and Owens, J. A. (2003). Effect of maternal feed restriction during pregnancy on glucose tolerance in the adult guinea pig. *Am J Physiol Regul Integr Comp Physiol* **284**, R140–R152
63. De Blasio, M. J., Gatford, K. L., McMillen, I. C., Robinson, J. S., and Owens, J. A. (2006). Placental restriction of fetal growth increases insulin action, growth and adiposity in the young lamb. *Endocrinology* **148**, 1350–1358
64. Alexander, G. (1978). Quantitative development of adipose tissue in foetal sheep. *Aust J Biol Sci* **31**, 489–503
65. Merklin, R. J. (1973). Growth and distribution of human fetal brown fat. *Anat Res* **178**, 637–646
66. Højlund, K., Mogensen, M., Sahlin, K., and Beck-Nielsen, H. (2008), Mitochondrial dysfunction in type 2 diabetes and obesity. *Endocrinol Metabol Clin North Am* **37**, 713–731
67. Junien, C., Gallou-Kabani, C., Vigé, A., and Gross, M. S. (2005). Nutritional epigenomics: consequences of unbalanced diets on epigenetics processes of programming during lifespan and between generations. *Ann Endocrinol (Paris)* **66**, S19–S28
68. Gallou-Kabani, C. and Junien, C. (2005). Nutritional epigenomics of metabolic syndrome: new perspective against the epidemic. *Diabetes* **54**, 1899–1906
69. Waterland, R. A., Travisano, M., Tahiliani, K. G., Rached, M. T., and Mirza, S. (2008).Methyl donor supplementation prevents transgenerational amplification of obesity. *Int J Obes* **32**, 1373–1379
70. Haslam, D. W. and James, W. P. (2005). Obesity. *Lancet* **366**, 1197–1209

Chapter 3

The Isolation and Purification of Rodent Pancreatic Islets of Langerhans

Jacqueline F. O'Dowd

Summary

This chapter describes the detailed protocol for the isolation and purification of islets of Langerhans from rodent pancreas using collagenase digestion. The first step of the process is to separate and isolate the insulin-producing islets of Langerhans from the rest of the pancreas. The pancreas is excised from the animal, trimmed of non-pancreatic tissues before being inflated and chopped into small pieces. The connective tissue is then broken down with a collagenase enzyme solution to selectively digest the bulk of the exocrine tissue while leaving the endocrine islets intact and separated from their surrounding non-islet tissue. Once this process is completed, the islets of Langerhans are separated from the remaining mixture by centrifugation and purified by the means of hand picking. Once isolated, the subsequent islets can be used for a number of experimental processes.

Key words: Islets of Langerhans, Insulin, Isolation, Endocrine pancreas, β-Cell, Collagenase

1. Introduction

The pancreas gland is located in the abdomen behind the stomach and on the posterior abdominal wall surrounded by the liver and intestine. It is composed of both exocrine and endocrine tissue. Embedded throughout the exocrine glandular tissue, clusters of secretory endocrine cells called the islets of Langerhans secrete hormones directly into the bloodstream. Discovered in 1869 by the German pathological anatomist Paul Langerhans, the islets of Langerhans constitute only 1-3% of the total pancreatic volume *(1)* but fulfil a vital role in glucose homeostasis. The number of islets within a human pancreas can range from 200,000 to almost 2 million. Each islet itself can range in size from a cluster of

C. Stocker (ed.), *Type 2 Diabetes,* Methods in Molecular Biology, vol. 560
DOI 10.1007/978-1-59745-448-3_3, © Humana Press, a part of Springer Science+Business Media, LLC 2009

a few cells less than 40 μm in diameter to ovoids of 400 μm in diameter *(2)*. Within the pancreas, islets are not randomly distributed: small islets (160 nm or less, in diameter) tend to be scattered throughout the exocrine tissue, while larger islets, 250 nm or more in diameter, appear to be located near larger ducts and blood vessels *(3)*.

The ability to isolate islets from the pancreas enables investigators to use them in a number of downstream applications. Once isolated, islets of Langerhans can be maintained as viable units for extended periods of time in tissue culture or they can be used in more acute experiments investigating aspects of mechanistic functionality. Isolated islets have long been used for the static and perfusion incubations to assess hormone release in response to compounds, but recent advances such as RNA interference (RNAi), a powerful and convenient tool for studying gene function, mean that the ability to isolate islets is a useful tool that allows investigators to gather functional information without using cell lines.

Islets are isolated by a modification of the method originally described by Lacy in 1967 using enzymatic digestion with a relatively crude preparation of collagenase *(4)*. The less fibrous nature of the rodent pancreas, as compared to man, makes the release of islets easier and allows for the preferential use of less purified collagenase preparations in many laboratories. The first step of the process is to remove the pancreas from the animal and trim it of non-pancreatic tissues. The pancreas is then inflated to increase the surface area and the connective tissue digested with collagenase. After digestion is complete the mixture is centrifuged to separate the islets from non-islet tissue. The pellet is then resuspended in physiological saline. A small sample of the resuspended pellet is then placed on a black petri dish containing more buffer. The black background of the petri dish allows the white islets to be visible under a dissection microscope with an external light source. Islets are then purified by hand picking using a very fine glass pipette. The picking procedure is repeated twice to ensure no carryover of unwanted exocrine tissue debris. It is very important that the islets being isolated are intact and relatively pure. Contamination of islets with acinar cells when used for functional studies may lead to a high level of proteases that will later influence islet integrity and functionality during incubation. The highest level of purity is required if protein or RNA is to be extracted from the isolated islets as any contamination of the preparation with acinar cells will cause spurious data to be obtained.

In this chapter, a method for the isolation of islets of Langerhans from the pancreas by enzymatic digestion and then harvesting by hand-picking individual islets will be described. Although the process of hand-picking islets is both time consuming and labour intensive this method gives islet preparations with the highest purity.

2. Materials

2.1. Reagents

1. Collagenase (Type XI, Sigma) (*see* **Note 1**).
2. Buffered saline solution: either Gey and Gey or Krebs Ringer buffer supplemented with 1 mM $CaCl_2$, 4 mM glucose and gassed with CO_2:O_2 (95:5).
   (a) Gey and Gey Buffer-111 mM NaCl, 27 mM $NaHCO_3$, 5 mM KCl, 1 mM $CaCl_2$, $MgCl_2$, 0.3 mM $MgSO_4$, 1.18 mM Na_2HPO_4, 0.29 mM KH_2PO_4 and 4 mM d-glucose gassed to pH 7.4 by CO_2:O_2 (95:5).

A ten times stock solution without KCl, $CaCl_2$, $MgCl_2$, $MgSO_4$, KH_2PO_4 and D-glucose can be made and kept for 1 month at room temperature.

3. RPMI-1640 culture medium.

2.2. Equipment

1. Sterilised forceps.
2. Sterilised scissors: One for skin incision and another for removal of pancreas from adjacent tissue and another for chopping the pancreas into pieces.
3. 10 mL syringe.
4. 25 G needle.
5. 15 mL polypropylene tubes.
6. 25 mL glass measuring beaker.
7. 50 mL conical flask with lid.
8. Water bath with shaker.
9. Plastic Pasteur pipette.
10. 90 mm petri dish painted 'in house' with two layers of black enamel paint to ensure a darkened background to visualise and pick islets against.
11. Dissection microscope.
12. External light source.

3. Methods

3.1. Islet Isolation

1. For islets isolated from normal rats (150-180 g) use two animals per isolation or three normal mice (*see* **Note 2**).
2. Just prior to dissection, euthanise the donor rodent by an appropriate technique.
3. Make a V-incision starting at the genital area, move the bowel to the left side of the open rodent. This will expose the pancreas, which is tan in colour and can be easily differentiated from the surrounding fat as can the spleen.
4. Using forceps to grasp the spleen, gently push up and back the stomach.
5. Cut the pancreas away from the surrounding fat and where attached at the small intestine.
6. Remove the pancreas from the body and place the pancreas, still attached to the spleen, into 100 mL of Gey and Gey in a Petri dish and cut away from the spleen, any retained fat, lymph nodes and other non-pancreatic tissues.
7. Inflate the pancreas by inserting a 25 gauge needle attached to a 10-mL syringe into the pancreas and injecting Gey and Gey solution into all the folds of the tissues so that the pancreas increases in size, thus creating a larger surface area.
8. Place the pancreata into a glass 50 mL beaker and chop using scissors until all the pieces are approximately the same size (1 mm × 1 mm).
9. Transfer the contents to a 15 mL tube and centrifuge for 5 min at 100 × *g*. After centrifugation, remove the supernatant, which contains fat, and transfer the pellet to a 15 mL conical tube.
10. Digest the pancreas with collagenase type XI (1-2 mg/pancreas) in a 1:1 mixture of Gey and Gey solution in order to release islets from exocrine tissue.
11. Place the conical tube in a shaking water bath at 37°C and shake at 800 oscillations per minute until the solution appears 'milky' and most of the pieces of pancreas are digested (approximately 5-10 min - time varies with strain and age of the animal). During this time take up a small amount (approximately 400 μL) in a plastic pipette and examine under a dissecting microscope to confirm whether islets are free from the exocrine tissue. If there are no islets visible continue the shaking by hand and repeat the process (*see* **Note 3**). Normally, a total shaking time of 6-8 min is sufficient to release the bulk of free islets.

12. Place the contents of the conical flask and stop the digestion by adding 15 mL of cold buffer.
13. Centrifuge at 500 × *g* for 5 min to remove the collagenase in the solution.
14. Aspirate the supernatant and resuspend the pellet in 15 mL of the isolation buffer.
15. Add a sample of the resuspended pellet (1 mL) to a blackened 90 mm Petri dish, add buffer to the top of the Petri dish and mix with a plastic Pasteur pipette.
16. Using a dissection microscope and an external light source, handpick and count individual islets using a drawn-out glass pipette (*see* **Note 4**).
17. Only pick clean and intact islets free of exocrine tissues (*see* **Note 5**).
18. Repeat the picking procedure at least twice.
19. Incubate the islets with isolation buffer in a 37°C water bath until use. Always use the islets within 30 min to 1 h after isolation.
20. While the yield of islets is variable, approximately 600-1200 islets are obtainable from two Wistar rats and 400 from three mice with this method (*see* **Note 6**).

3.2. Islet Culturing

For certain experimental protocols it may be necessary to culture the isolated islets. When culturing it is important to handle the islets under aseptic conditions and use sterile tubes and flasks.

1. Wash the islets with sterile Gey and Gey solution.
2. Resuspend groups of 200 islets in RPMI-1640 containing 11.1 mM glucose (*see* **Note 7**) and transfer to a 6-well cell culture plate.
3. Incubate the islets in a humidified culture incubator with 5% CO2; 95% air.

4. Notes

1. A wide variety of collagenase preparations are available for islet isolation, but in our experience Collagenase Type XI from Sigma-Aldrich is best suited for isolations. This crude collagenase isolated from *Clostridium histolyticum* is actually a mixture of several different enzymes (collagenase, neutral proteases, clostripain, and caseinase) that act together to break down tissue. While collagenase Type XI has one of the

highest collagenase activities not every batch is equivalent, and it is usually appropriate to test small quantities from several different batches before choosing to make a bulk purchase.

2. The age and weight of the animals can influence the numbers of islets of Langerhans obtained. Rats heavier than 180 g often yield fewer islets per pancreas. Although younger animals can give high yields the islets obtained from these animals should be considered from a 'juvenile' stage of development.
3. If no islets are isolated or isolated islets are not intact, the islets are over-digested. This can be prevented by decreasing the collagenase digestion time or collagenase concentration (*see* **step 10**).
4. Normal bore pipettes draw up too much liquid as islets are picked, so drawn pipettes are preferential. Draw glass pipettes by heating in a Bunsen flame. Once the glass begins to give, pull sharply to yield pipettes with a bore of approximately 1 mm.
5. If most of the islets are not discrete and difficult to isolate (*see* **step 15**) the exocrine tissues are under-digested. In order to overcome this problem increase the collagenase digestion time (*see* **step 10**) and/or increase the collagenase concentration (*see* **step 10**) and ensure vigorous shaking of the vial to disrupt the pancreas (*see* **step 11**).
6. The yield of islets will vary depending on the age and strain. Diabetic and older animals will have reduced numbers. Digestion continues as the hand-picking selection proceeds; therefore, speed is important. Islets should be collected within 15-20 min and the entire isolation completed within 45 min to 1 h of removal of the organ.
7. The culture medium can be altered depending on the experimental conditions required.

References

1. Hellerstrom, C. (1984). The life story of the pancreatic β-cell. *Diabetologia* **26**(6): 393–400
2. Lifson, N., K. Kramlinger, R. Mayrand and E. Lender (1980). Blood flow to the rabbit pancreas with special reference to the islets of Langerhans. *Gastroenterology* **79**(3): 466–473
3. Bonner-Weir, S. and L. Orci. (1982). New perspectives on the microvasculature of the islet of Langerhans in the rat. *Diabetes* **31**(10): 883–889
4. Lacy, P. and M. Kostianovsky (1967). Method for the isolation of intact islets of Langerhans from the rat pancreas. *Diabetes* **16**(1): 35–39

Chapter 4

The Measurement of Insulin Secretion from Isolated Rodent Islets of Langerhans

Anna L. Nolan and Jacqueline F. O'Dowd

Summary

Insulin secretion plays an essential part in the modulation of glucose homeostasis. Pancreatic β cells are extremely sensitive to small changes in the concentration of glucose, peptides, hormones and fatty acids and insulin secretion is stimulated in response to these factors. The measurement of insulin secretion from isolated islets with either initiators or potentiators is a useful tool for investigating their efficacy in vitro without using cell lines, which can be subject to modification. Static islet incubation is a fast and powerful tool for the investigation of dose-response curves in response to insulin secretagogues, while islet perifusion experiments are useful for the investigation of the kinetics of insulin secretion. These two methods for measuring insulin secretion from isolated rodent islets of Langerhans are described in detail in this chapter.

Key words: Islets of Langerhans, Insulin secretion, Static, Perifusion, β-cell, Two phase

1. Introduction

Hormone secretion is a frequently measured end-point following islet isolation and can provide an accurate and reproducible index of islet cell function. The secretion of insulin from the pancreatic islets of Langerhans modulates the control of glucose homeostasis. Substances that provoke insulin release (secretagogues) are frequently divided into two main groups, initiators and potentiators. The initiators, such as glucose and fatty acids, directly induce insulin secretion, whereas potentiators such as glucagon-like peptide 1 (GPL-1) do so only in the presence of an elevated concentration of glucose. The most important initiator of insulin

C. Stocker (ed.), *Type 2 Diabetes,* Methods in Molecular Biology, vol. 560
DOI 10.1007/978-1-59745-448-3_4, © Humana Press, a part of Springer Science+Business Media, LLC 2009

secretion is D-glucose. Other fuel initiators include D-glyceraldehyde and D-mannose, the amino acids arginine and leucine, fatty acids and ketone bodies.

The insulin secretory response to glucose has been documented widely in several mammalian species, both in vitro and in vivo. In vitro studies demonstrate that pancreatic β-cells are acutely sensitive to small changes in extracellular glucose concentrations. Isolated islets incubated with a range of glucose concentrations show a dose-dependent pattern of insulin release. Both the perfused pancreas and the perifused islet studies have demonstrated that the time course of response to glucose is biphasic with a rapid initial spike, followed by an abrupt fall *(1)*. A more prolonged second phase continues with the duration of the stimulus. Insulin is released during the first phase from granules closest to the plasma membrane *(2)*, which is soon significantly depleted. The secondary rise in insulin reflects the considerable amount of newly synthesised insulin that is released immediately. In β-cells, glucose not only functions as a physiological stimulus but also as a metabolisable fuel. Nutrient-induced insulin release by glucose is due to the activation of specific receptors located on the β-cell plasma membrane *(3)*. The metabolic hypothesis of glucose-stimulated insulin release from β cells is shown in **Fig. 1**.

The use of isolated islets is a physiological way of investigating the effects of initiators and potentiators on insulin secretion. Isolated, rodent and human, islets can be maintained as viable units in culture or used in more acute experiments to monitor functionality. Using freshly isolated islets is potentially more physiological than using a cell line such as RINm5F, which possess an intracellular insulin content of only 1% of that of freshly isolated rat β-cells. Moreover, many cell lines are unresponsive to glucose *(4)*, although what is becoming clear is that the phenotype of these primary endocrine cells can change during islet culture.

In this chapter we aim to describe two methods for the successful measurement of insulin secretion from isolated islets in vitro. Using a static measurement of insulin secretion, it is possible to identify compounds that can initiate or potentiate insulin secretion in a dose-dependent manner. This method gives the researcher an opportunity to examine numerous concentrations and conditions from the same batch of isolated islets. In contrast perifusion experiments can be used to identify the timed kinetics of insulin secretion, for example, if the stimulation of insulin secretion is acute (in which it activates sharply before tailing off) or if insulin secretion is continuous for the duration of the islet treatment. Both methods are useful in determining the action of various compounds on insulin secretion in isolated islets of Langerhans, improving our understanding of the mechanisms of insulin secretion and aiding in the development of novel insulin secretagogues.

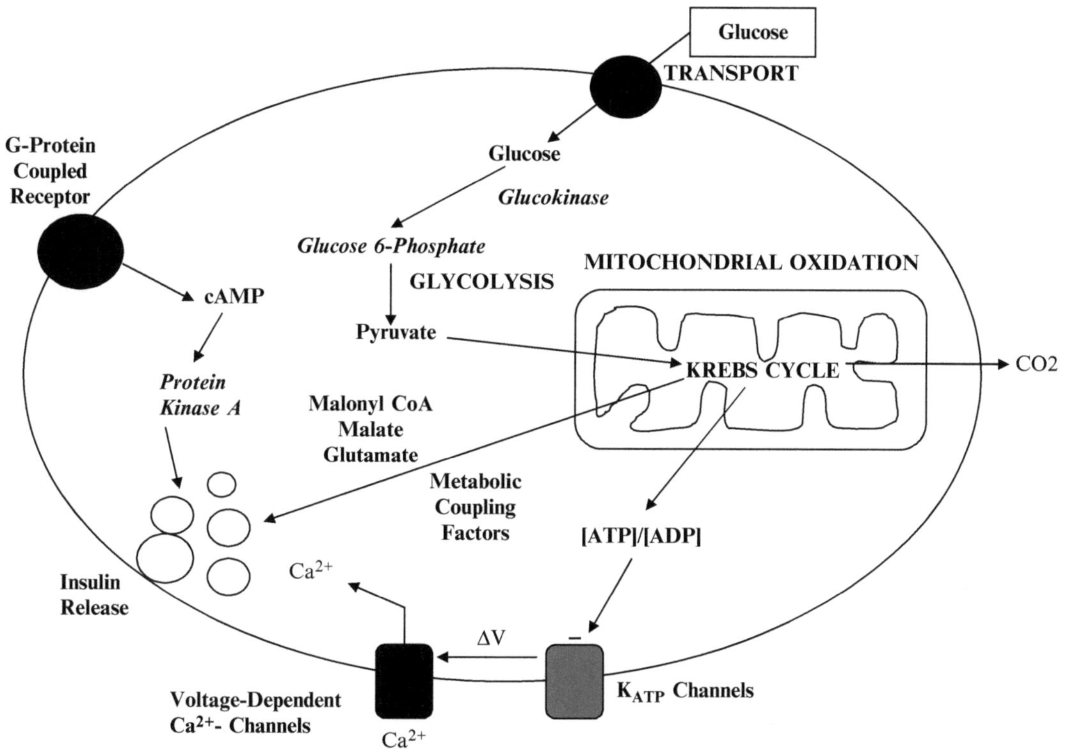

Fig. 1. Glucose control of insulin secretion. Glucose stimulates insulin secretion via two mechanisms (**a**) Type 2 glucose transporters (GLUT2) mediate the entry of glucose into β-cells. Glucose is then phosphorylated by the rate-limiting enzyme glucokinase. The modified glucose is further metabolised providing energy for synthesis of ATP. An increased ATP: ADP ratio causes the ATP-gated potassium channels in the cellular membrane to close up, preventing potassium ions from crossing the cell membrane. The ensuing decrease in negative charge inside the cell leads to the depolarisation of the cell and the activation of voltage-gated calcium channels, which transport calcium ions into the cell. The increase in intracellular calcium concentration triggers exocytosis of insulin granules. (**b**) Insulin granules in a reserve pool undergo acidification to augment the secretion process.

2. Materials

2.1. Static Measurements of Insulin Secretion

1. Buffered saline solution: Gey and Gey *(5)* or Krebs Ringer buffer supplemented with 1 mM $CaCl_2$, 4 mM glucose and gassed with CO_2:O_2 (5:95).
2. Tissue culture media: RPMI 1640 or DMEM containing the desired glucose concentration, 2 mM L-glutamine, 100 U/ml penicillin, 100 μg/ml streptomycin and 1% BSA. Store the media at 4°C and warm to 37°C before use.
3. Bovine Serum Albumin (Fraction V).
4. Penicillin-streptomycin solution (100 U/ml penicillin, 100 μg/ml streptomycin).

2.2. Measurement of Insulin Secretion Using a Perifusion System

For insulin secretion measurements by perifusion, a perifusion system must be established, maintaining the temperature of the islets and the buffer at 37°C and collecting fractions at 1-min intervals. A diagram illustrating the schematics of how this system is setup is shown in **Fig. 2**. The infusion system is designed to allow the addition of compounds midperifusion and to remove compounds at specific time points.

1. Two pumps, one set at 1 ml/min, the second at 10 µl/min. A consistent pattern of flow with minimal pressure change across each cycle of the pump is required for this apparatus.
2. An incubator set to 37°C (Stewart Scientific) (*see* **Note 1**).
3. PVC tubing, approximately 1.85 mm in diameter.
4. Plastic male and female hose barbs (2 mm in width at the bottom and 11 mm at the top (Cole-Palmer, U.K)). A glass wool plug is placed at the bottom to prevent the islets from coming out of the hose barbs but allowing the continuous unimpeded flow of buffer.
5. 25-G needle.
6. Fraction collector.
7. Buffered saline solution: Gey and Gey or Krebs Ringer buffer supplemented with 1 mM $CaCl_2$, 4 mM glucose and gassed with CO_2:O_2 (5:95).

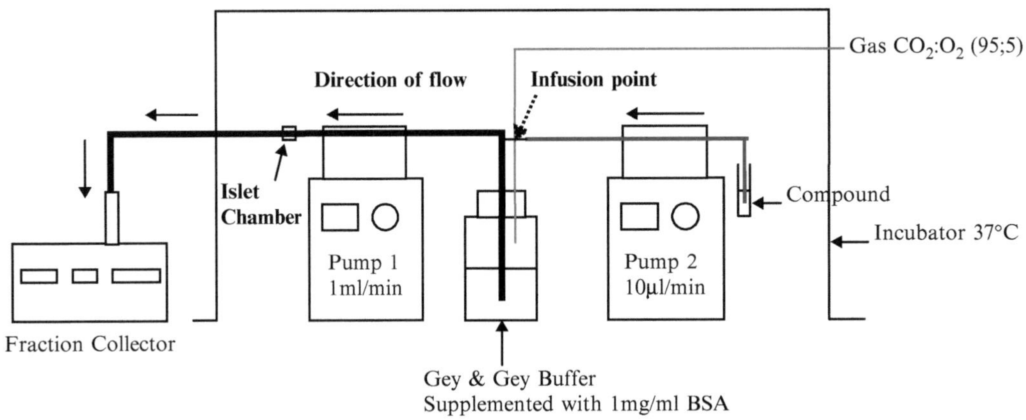

Fig. 2. Schematic of the perifusion system setup. Both pumps, tubing containing islets and perifusion buffer should be placed in a clear incubator set to 37°C. The perifusion buffer is continuously gassed during the islet perifusion using a gas line that needs to be put in place before entering the incubator. The perifusion system should be equilibrated for at least 30 min prior to placing islets into the system.

3. Methods

For the majority of functional studies of glucose-induced insulin secretion in vitro, purity may not be as critical a criterion as the purity required for RNA or protein extraction because insulin is released only from the β-cells and their activity can, therefore, be studied independent of any other cell types that may be present. Nevertheless it is important to note that any contamination of the preparation with exocrine tissue can interact with the insulin secretary responsiveness of the islets and should be avoided if possible.

Despite the collagenase digestion procedure not directly altering the responsiveness of islet cells to glucose or other nutrients, it may proteolyse cell surface receptors thereby affecting the response to agents acting on the cell surface *(6)*. It is therefore advantageous, for some pharmacological studies, to culture the islets for a period of 12-18 h prior to functional experiments to allow the replacement of receptors that have undergone proteolysis during collagenase treatment *(7)*.

3.1. Static Measurements

3.1.1. Static Incubations

Static incubation conditions are preferable when studying dose-response curves or for a wide range of different experimental treatments in a single experiment.

1. Place each pool of isolated islets into a black-bottomed petri dish for the final hand picking selection round of purified endocrine cells. Dilute these with ice-cold Gey and Gey solution during this final islet selection process.
2. At the end of the selection place ten of islets (*see* **Note 2**) into a 2.5 ml borosilicate glass tube (*see* **Note 3**).
3. Allow the islets to settle and add the experimental compound at 100× concentration if calculating a dose-response curve for a compound.
4. Add Gey and Gey buffer supplemented with 1 mg/ml BSA and differing glucose concentrations supplemented with media to give a final volume of 0.5 ml (*see* **Note 4**).
5. Gas the tubes with CO_2:O_2 (5:95) and cap (*see* **Note 5**).
6. Place the tubes in a water bath set to 37°C for 1 h.
7. After the 1 h incubation, remove the lids from the tubes and cool the tubes on ice prior to sampling for the measurement of hormone secretion (*see* **Note 6**).
8. Store the supernatant at 4°C before the analysis.
9. Isolated islets incubated with a range of glucose concentrations show a typical dose-dependent pattern of insulin release as shown in **Fig. 3**.

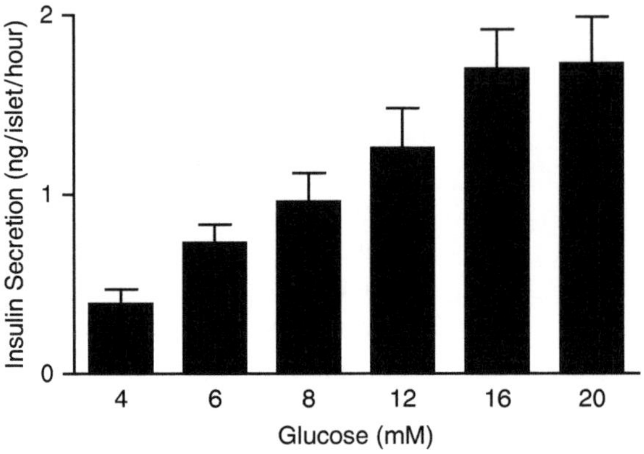

Fig. 3. Isolated islets show a dose-dependent increase in insulin secretion in response to changing glucose levels. Rat islets were isolated and groups of ten were placed in 0.5 ml of incubation buffer containing varying concentrations of glucose for 1 h. Samples of the incubation media were then assayed for insulin using a radioimmunoassay.

3.1.2. Short-Term Islet Incubation

Where a period of culture may be appropriate, it is necessary to work under aseptic conditions and use sterile tubes and flasks during the islet isolation procedure. Here we describe the method for the short-term culture of islets after isolation.

1. Wash the islets with sterile RPMI-1640 by repeated centrifugation at 200 × *g* for 45 s and resuspend the islets in fresh sterile medium containing antibiotics (penicillin (100 U/ml) plus streptomycin (100 μg/ml)) for a minimum of five occasions.
2. At the end of the washing period place 200 isolated islets into a 12-well plate in the relevant sterile culture medium (*see* **Note 7**).
3. Incubate the islets for the desired length of time at 37°C and 5% CO_2; 95% air (*see* **Note 8**).
4. Following incubation to the experimental medium, harvest the buffer samples from the incubated islets.
5. Centrifuge the media at 800 × *g* for 5 min and remove the supernatant, store at 4°C prior to the analysis of insulin secretion.
6. Measure the insulin levels in triplicate samples by radioimmunoassay (RIA) or ELISA. Dilute samples with assay buffer if necessary. For static islet incubations dilute sample medium 1:4 with insulin assay buffer in order to fit within a standard curve ranging from 5 to 0.02 nmol/l for RIA.

3.2. Perifusion Measurements

Perifusion allows for the dynamics of secretion to be measured. Set up the islet perifusion system as shown in **Fig. 2**. The system should be set to 37°C at least 1 h prior to the experiment. Place the isolated islets in a 15-ml falcon tube in a water bath at 37°C. The buffered saline solution should also be prewarmed to 37°C.

1. Connect the buffered saline solution to the first pump (*see* **Note 9**) using the tubing and set the pump to 1 ml/min; gas the main stock of buffer with CO_2:O_2 (5:95) to retain a constant pH of 7.4.
2. Connect the tubing from pump 1 to the fraction collector and the islet chamber as shown in **Fig. 2**. The glass wool should be placed in the bottom of the islet chamber to prevent the escape of islets but allow the flow of buffer.
3. Pre-set pump 2-10 μl/min and infuse the test compounds that will be removed or those that are in short supply.
4. Ensure that the tubing between pump 1 and the buffered saline contains an area of re-sealable rubber tubing which will be the incision point for the compounds injected from pump 2.
5. Switch on the pumps and allow the buffer to circulate until the tubing is full of buffer and then stop the flow.
6. Place the previously isolated islets in the chambers on top of the glass wool (100 islets/chamber) and connect to the pump 1 tubing.
7. Pre-run the perifusion system for 30 min before starting collection in order to stabilise the islets in the system. Compounds that need to be removed from the system during the experiment can be added using pump 2 and an infusion needle (*see* **Note 10**). An example of a perfusion experiment is shown in **Fig. 4**.
8. Set up the fraction collector to collect samples every 1 or 2 min depending on the experimental protocol.
9. Store the samples at 4°C prior to analysis of insulin secretion.
10. Rates of insulin secretion are usually measured by radioimmunoassay directly from the collected samples without dilution and expressed as nmol/l/100 islets/minute from the standard curve.
11. The response to glucose is biphasic with an initial rapid spike followed by a more prolonged second phase that continues with the duration of the stimulus as seen in **Fig. 5**.
12. At the end of each experiment, wash the tubing with sterile water for 2 h and dismantle from the pumps.

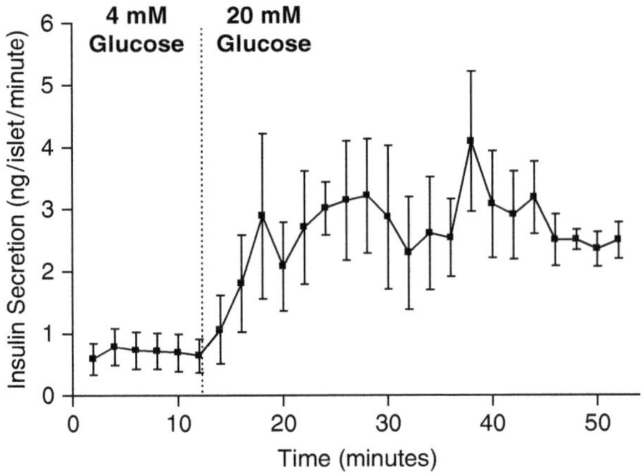

Fig. 4. Insulin secretion from isolated islets following perfusion. Isolated rat islets showed an increase in insulin secretion in response to 20 mM glucose using the perifusion system.

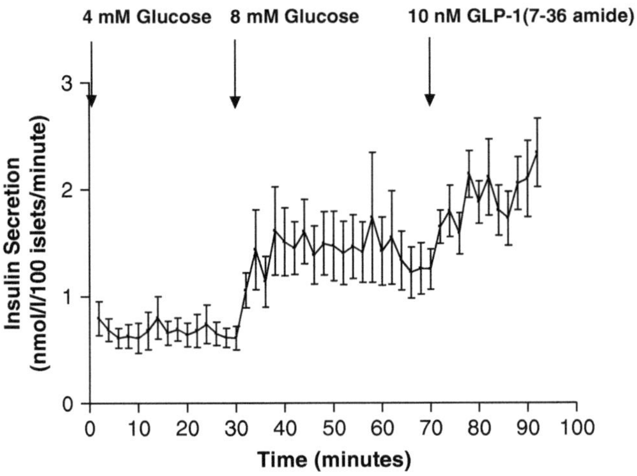

Fig. 5. Biphasic insulin secretion following perfusion. The response to glucose is biphasic with an initial rapid spike followed by a more prolonged second phase that continues with the duration of the stimulus using the perifusion system.

4. Notes

1. The incubator should be constructed from clear acrylic polymer to give total visibility of samples at all times. The chamber used has the advantage of not having a base, so it can be placed directly over the samples.
2. Groups of ten islets are routinely used for static experiments but a minimum of three islets may be used.

3. Standard microfuge tubes (1.5 ml volume) also work well.
4. Select the purified islets in a consistent minimal volume of buffer when transferring to the tube. It is important that the volume of the tubes does not differ significantly.
5. The incubation tubes are flushed with a stream of gas by placing a pipette tip onto a flexible tube attached to the gas outlet and displacing the air for a period of at least 5 s.
6. It is critical not to remove any of the islets during this procedure and a sampling volume of 50 μl allows this to be achieved readily.
7. The culture medium of choice depends upon the precise experimental conditions required. For measurements of insulin secretion, nutrient responsiveness can be maintained effectively when RPMI-1640 medium is used containing 11.1 mM glucose.
8. Culturing islets overnight may cause a loss of approximately 10% in islet number viability.
9. The limiting factor to islet perifusion is the number of channels available on the peristaltic pump. Four or eight channel pumps are most frequently used although higher channel numbers are possible.
10. Prepare the test reagents as a stock solution made up at a concentration 100 times that required and then infuse this at a rate 100 times lower than the pump 1 (i.e., if the main perifusion system is operating at 1 ml/min, the infusion rate of test reagents will be 10 μl/min). Use of the infusion system allows the introduction and removal of test reagents at defined times within the protocol.

References

1. Grodsky, G.M., Curry, D.L., Bennett, L.L. and Rodrigo, J.J. (1968). Factors influencing different rates of insulin release in vitro. *Acta Diabetol Lat* **5**(1):140–161.
2. Lacey, P.E. (1970) Beta cell secretion - from the standpoint of a pathobiologist. *Diabetes* **19**:895–905.
3. Matschinsky, F.M., Landgraf, R., Ellerman, J. and J. Kotler-Brajtburg. (1972). Glucoreceptor mechanisms in islets of Langerhans. *Diabetes* **21**(2 Suppl):555–69.
4. Ulrich, A.B., Schmid, B. M., Standop, J., Schneider, M. B. and Pour, P. M. (2002). Pancreatic Cell Lines: A Review. *Pancreas* **24**(2):111–120.
5. Gey, G.O. and Gey, M.K. (1936). Maintenance of human normal cells in continuous culture: preliminary report; cultivation of mesoblastic tumors and normal cells and notes on methods of cultivation. *Am. J. Cancer* **27**:45–76.
6. Bottino, R., Balamurugan, A.N. and Tse, H. (2004). Response of human islets to isolation stress and the effect of antioxidant treatment. *Diabetes* **53**:2559–2568.
7. Abdelli, S., Ansite, J., Roduit, R., Borsello, T., Matsumoto, I., Sawada, T., Allaman-Pillet, N., Henry, H., Beckmann, J.S., Hering, B.J. and Bonny, C. (2004). Intracellular stress signaling pathways activated during human islet preparation and following acute cytokine exposure. *Diabetes* **53**:2815–2823.

Chapter 5

The Incubation and Monitoring of Cell Viability in Primary Rat Islets of Langerhans and Pancreatic β-Cell Lines

Noel G. Morgan, Eleftheria Diakogiannaki, and Mark A. Russell

Summary

This chapter describes a method to measure the viability of isolated intact islets of Langerhans from rat pancreas and considers the use of isolated islets and of pancreatic beta-cell lines to study cell viability following culture. The islet isolation method is based on the use of preparations of collagenase to selectively digest the bulk of the exocrine tissue while leaving the endocrine islets intact and separated from their surrounding acini. The islets can be obtained in relatively pure form and are suitable for use in hormone secretion assays as well as for measurement of cell viability. They can be cultured if required and viability maintained for periods of days to weeks. Beta-cell lines are useful for study of the control of cell viability although their secretory capacity is usually altered compared to primary islet cells. Islet cell death can be estimated in a number of ways using either direct or more indirect means. Some methods will distinguish between apoptotic and necrotic death while others offer a more generic index of changes in viability.

Key words: Islets of Langerhans, Insulinoma cells, Insulin, Glucagon, Endocrine pancreas, Apoptosis, Necrosis

1. Introduction

The islets of Langerhans represent distinct clusters of cells distributed throughout the body of the pancreas each of which operates as a functionally autonomous unit. Individual islets have a defined cellular anatomy and, in rodents, this comprises a central core of insulin-secreting β-cells, surrounded by a mantle of other endocrine (secreting, for example, glucagon, somatostain or pancreatic polypeptide) and non-endocrine (e.g. endothelial cells, macrophages and dendritic cells) cells *(1, 2)*. In man, this organisation is retained but the core of β-cells may be subdivided

C. Stocker (ed.), *Type 2 Diabetes,* Methods in Molecular Biology, vol. 560
DOI 10.1007/978-1-59745-448-3_5, © Humana Press, a part of Springer Science+Business Media, LLC 2009

such that the mantle of non-β-cells penetrates into the interior of the islet to a greater extent than in rodents *(3)*.

Islet isolation requires that approximately 98% of the total mass of pancreatic tissue is discarded, since the endocrine cells comprise only about 2% of the mass. Thus, one critical aspect to be considered when isolating islets is the final level of purity required. Indeed, even when islets are obtained in a highly pure form, it remains true that the cell population is heterogeneous (as indicated earlier) and that biochemical data should be interpreted cautiously to reflect this heterogeneity. This is a particular issue when monitoring the effects of exogenous agents on islet cell viability since measurements of cell death will not usually allow the differentiation of beta from non-beta cells in the preparations. For this reason, many studies of beta-cell viability are performed with clonal insulinoma cell lines since these represent a homogeneous population of insulin-secreting cells. The cells often have altered secretory functions compared to primary islets, but they are a more useful model for studies of cell death. A range of cell lines are available which are derived from a variety of species (e.g. hamster (HIT-T15 *(4)*) mouse (MIN6 *(5)*; βTC-3 *(6)*) and rat (RINm5F *(7)*, BRIN-BD11 *(8)*, INS-1 *(9)*). Unfortunately, no successful human β-cell lines have been developed so far that are suitable for long-term use in tissue culture.

The goal of islet isolation techniques is to release the individual islets from their surrounding exocrine tissue and to harvest them with their original architecture intact in a relatively pure form. The process of harvesting can be achieved in a number of ways and density gradient methods are used in many laboratories. However, we still prefer to hand-pick individual islets since, ultimately, this method yields preparations with the highest purity. Once isolated, rodent and human islets can be maintained as viable units for extended periods of time in tissue culture or they can be used in more acute experiments to monitor short-term functionality. It is clear that the phenotype of the endocrine cells can change during islet culture (depending on factors such as the glucose concentration), and this should be considered when deciding on the most appropriate experimental system for in vitro studies.

The majority of methods designed to achieve islet isolation from mammalian pancreas rely on enzymatic digestion to release the islets from the bulk of the tissue. Preparations of collagenase are frequently used for this purpose *(10, 11)* and the most successful isolations are often achieved with relatively impure enzyme fractions which probably reflects the multiplicity of proteins involved in stabilising the structure of the pancreas. For human islet isolation, enzyme preparations containing well-defined protease activities have been developed *(12)* and these offer certain advantages over less well-characterised fractions (notably consistency of performance) but, for rodent pancreas, the less well-fractionated collagenase preparations remain valuable (not least because that are usually much less expensive).

Hormone secretion is a frequently measured end-point following islet isolation and can provide an accurate and reproducible index of islet function. As far as can be determined, the collagenase digestion procedure does not directly alter the responsiveness of islet cells to glucose or other nutrients although it can affect the response to agents acting on cell surface receptors which may become proteolysed during the isolation procedure. Thus, for some pharmacological studies, it may be advantageous to allow the islets to "recover" during a brief period of tissue culture (12-18 h) prior to study of their functional activity. As an example, we have observed that the potency of somatostatin to inhibit glucose-induced insulin secretion is increased following a brief period of culture *(13)*, and this probably reflects the replenishment of receptors for this hormone that have suffered proteolysis during collagenase treatment.

Increasingly, islet cell viability also represents an important end-point measurement, even in relatively acute studies, and it is important to consider this aspect of islet function in addition to secretory activity. There are a variety of methods to monitor islet cell viability, ranging from global indices such as the reduction of dyes in response to changes in mitochondrial dehydrogenase activity (as exemplified by MTT and its variants *(14)*) to more specific markers of apoptotic pathway activation (e.g. annexin-V disposition *(15)*). The precise choice of marker can place a very different requirement on the final islet preparation since large-scale changes in metabolic activity might still be measurable across a cell population, even when individual cellular responses vary, whereas markers of apoptosis may require analysis at the level of individual cells in order to yield appropriately accurate data. Thus, deliberate islet dispersion could prove to be the final step of an experiment in which great pains have been taken to maintain the islet structure at earlier stages.

2. Materials

1. Hanks' balanced salt solution.
2. Collagenase (Type XI - Sigma).
3. Islet incubation buffer: NaCl (111 mM) $NaHCO_3$ (27 mM) KCl (5 mM) $MgCl_2$ (1 mM) Na_2HPO_4 (1 mM) $MgSO_4$ (0.3 mM) KH_2PO_4 (0.2 mM) $CaCl_2$ (1 mM) glucose (2.5 mM) of pH 7.4.

4. Phosphate-buffered saline (PBS): NaCl (137 mM) Na_2HPO_4 (10 mM) KCl (27 mM) of pH 7.4.
5. RPMI-1640 culture medium.
6. Annexin-V-Cy3 apoptosis detection kit (Sigma).
7. CaspACE™ FITC-VAD-FMK In Situ Marker (Promega).
8. Penicillin-streptomycin solution.
9. Trypsin-EDTA solution.
10. Trypan blue.
11. Hoechst 33342.
12. Propidium iodide.
13. CellTiter96 Aqueous One Solution Reagent (Promega).
14. Bovine serum albumin; crude fraction V - not treated to remove fatty acids. (MP Biomedical).
15. Bovine serum albumin; fraction V - fatty acid free (MP Biomedical).
16. Annexin V-FITC Apoptosis Detection Kit 1 (BD Pharmingen).
17. RNase; DNase-free (Roche).

3. Methods

3.1. Isolation of Rat Islets of Langerhans

A wide variety of collagenase preparations are available for islet isolation but, in our laboratory, Collagenase Type XI from Sigma-Aldrich is employed routinely. The method described as follows represents a typical procedure for islet isolation from male Wistar rats of body weight 150-180 g. Following euthanasia two choices present themselves. Either the pancreas can be cannulated via the bile duct and retro-perfused in situ with a collagenase solution or, alternatively, the organ can be dissected from the animal (together with the spleen) and processed entirely on the bench. In situ cannulation can provide higher islet yields (probably because more of the organ is accessible) but, for ease and speed of preparation, direct removal of the organ prior to processing still offers advantages and remains our method of choice.

1. Once isolated from the animal, trim the pancreas to remove the spleen together with any retained fat and lymph nodes and place into a black-bottomed Petri dish under illumination from a cold light source.
2. Lift the organ gently from the dish surface with forceps and inject with approximately 20 mL of ice-cold Hanks' balanced salt solution until fully distended.

3. Transfer to a 25-50 mL glass beaker and chop finely with scissors to yield pieces of tissue approximately 1 mm^3 in size (*see* **Note 1**).
4. Discard any excess liquid and transfer to a 10 mL conical centrifuge tube to which ice-cold Hanks' solution is added to bring the final volume to 10 mL. Centrifuge the tube gently (100 × *g*) for 30 s and transfer the tissue directly to a Nalgene 25 mL conical flask.
5. Add solid collagenase powder (5-8 mg according to the batch) directly to the flask and adjust the final volume of ice-cold Hanks' solution to yield a collagenase concentration of approximately 1 mg/mL, as judged by eye.
6. Cap the flask and transfer to a side-arm flask shaker (*see* **Note 2**) and hold in a water batch at 37°C. Shake the flask vigorously for 5 min and monitor digestion.
7. Once optimal digestion is achieved, transfer the mixture to a 10 mL conical test tube and dilute by the addition of ice-cold Hanks' solution.
8. Centrifuge the tube at 500 × *g* for 30 s and discard the supernatant. Add 10 mL ice-cold Hanks' solution and resuspend the pellet with the aid of a polystyrene Pasteur pipette.
9. Transfer small portions of the digest (approximately 2 mL at a time) to a black-bottomed Petri dish and dilute with 20 mL ice-cold Hanks' solution. View the mixture under a dissecting microscope using cold light illumination and select the islets by hand-picking with a finely drawn glass Pasteur pipette (*see* **Note 3**).
10. Groups of 5-10 islets are collected in a minimal volume of buffer solution and transferred into a second tube containing fresh ice-cold Hanks' solution (*see* **Note 4**). Successive groups of islets are selected and added until all islets are recovered (*see* **Note 5**).

3.2. Islet Cell Viability

Determination of islet cell viability is an increasingly popular goal and a variety of methods are available. These can either provide information about the overall extent of viability or yield more specific information about the induction of necrosis and apoptosis (generally based on fluorescence microscopy techniques). A major hurdle with all the available methods is to identify individual endocrine cell types and to study the process in intact islets. The use of confocal microscopy provides one means to analyse viability within intact islets, but many workers still prefer to disperse the islets after incubation and to analyse the resultant cell suspension. The latter can yield more directly quantitative data, but it also runs the risk of altering the measure(s) of viability during the dispersion process, which inevitably requires both mechanical and enzymatic disruption. Nevertheless, this represents the method of choice in many laboratories.

1. Following incubation of groups of islets (usually between 50 and 100 islets per group) under appropriate experimental conditions, recover the islets by centrifugation (500 × *g* for 30 s).
2. Wash the pellet in PBS and re-suspend in trypsin-EDTA (250-500 μL depending on islet number) prior to incubation at 37°C for approximately 10 min. During the incubation, pipette the islets gently for 10-15 s at 2 min intervals to aid dispersion.
3. Following dispersion, centrifuge the cells at 500 × *g* for 30 s and re-suspend.
4. For the measurement of apoptosis, fluorescent CaspACE™ substrates can provide reliable data with minimal background staining. The substrate is provided to the cell as a membrane permeant ester. Resuspend islet cells in 25 μL of PBS and an equal volume of diluted CaspACE™ solution to yield a final concentration of 10 μM of the substrate.
5. Incubate the cells in the dark for 20 min at 37°C and then centrifuge at 3,000 × *g* for 5 min.
6. Wash the cell pellet in 200 μL of phosphate-buffered saline (PBS).
7. Resuspend the final pellet in 50 μL of PBS, and apply to a microscope slide coated with poly-L-lysine and incubate at room temperature for 5 min.
8. Cover the cells with a coverslip and view under a fluorescence microscope to detect stained cells. A total of at least 1,000 cells should be counted for each experimental condition and the percentage of apoptotic cells (fluorescently labelled) determined.

An alternative method makes use of a combination of annexin-V-Cy3 and 6-carboxyfluorescein diacetate (6-CFDA) to detect live, apoptotic and necrotic cells *(15)*. The approach is similar up to the point of islet cell dispersion (**Subheading 3.2**, **step 3**) but then proceeds as follows:

1. Wash the cell suspension in 200 μL of PBS and then resuspend to achieve a final cell concentration of about 10^6 cells/mL. 100 islets should yield approximately 50,000 cells after dispersion; thus, a volume of 50 μL would be used.
2. Transfer this to a poly-L-lysine-coated microscope slide and wash the cells three times with 100 μL binding buffer (provided in the assay kit).
3. Add 50 μL of double staining solution (containing both dyes) and incubate for 10 min at room temperature in the dark.

4. Wash the cells a further five times with 100 μL of binding buffer.
5. View the cells under fluorescence illumination and determine the number of viable (green) apoptotic (green with a red halo around the plasma membrane) and necrotic (red throughout) cells.

3.3. Measurement of the Viability of Clonal Insulinoma Cell Lines

As outlined earlier, it is frequently more convenient to make use of one or more of the various types of insulinoma cell that are available in order to determine the effects of defined agents or incubation conditions on the viability of β-cells. A number of methods are available and most are applicable to any of the cell types in common usage (HIT-T15; MIN6; β-TC3; RINm5F; BRIN-BD11; INS-1).

3.3.1. Vital Dye Staining

Vital dyes provide a convenient and rapid method for estimation of cell viability which can be quantified readily. Most commonly, trypan blue is used as a routine screening dye since this is excluded from viable cells (it is actively pumped out across the plasma membrane) and it can be visualised easily using a standard laboratory microscope.

1. Following incubation, collect the culture medium from the cell culture plates as this will contain any detached cells (detachment is often an early response to loss of viability).
2. Wash the plates with PBS and add Trypsin-EDTA to each plate or well and incubate for 2-3 min at 37°C to free all adherent cells.
3. Harvest the adherent and floating cells by centrifugation at 200 × *g* for 5 min.
4. Resuspend the cell pellet in 250 μL of RPMI-1640 plus 250 μL Trypan blue (0.4% in PBS) (*see* **Note 6**).
5. Count the number of viable (unstained) and dead cells (blue) using a haemocytometer and express the number of dead cells as a percentage of the total cell population for each condition.

3.3.2. Fluorescence Microscopic Assays of Cell Viability

Fluorescence-based assay methods are useful as a means to distinguish between apoptotic, necrotic and viable cells within a culture.

1. Prior to treatment with the relevant test reagents grow the cells on sterile glass cover slips (22 mm × 22 mm) which have been inserted into the wells of one or more 6-well plates (*see* **Note 7**).
2. Following incubation, aspirate the medium and replace with a mixture of 50 μg/mL Hoechst 33342 dye and 5 μg/mL propidium iodide dissolved in PBS.
3. Incubate the cells in the dark for 5 min at 37°C.

4. Recover the coverslips from the plates using forceps and examine the staining patterns under a fluorescent microscope equipped with blue and green filters.
5. Calculate the percentages of viable cells (pale blue), apoptotic (dark or fluorescent blue) and necrotic (pink) cells after counting at least 100 cells of randomly chosen fields for each experimental condition (*see* **Note 8**).

3.3.3. Methanethiosulphonate-Based Proliferation Assay

Methanethiosulphonate (MTS) (or a variant, MTT) assays are frequently reported as measures of either cell proliferation or cell viability. However, this is something of an overstatement since these assays actually measure mitochondrial dehydrogenase activity and, while this usually correlates with cell number, it is only an indirect measure of viability. Nevertheless, the method is easy to apply and can serve as a useful means to gain information about possible changes in viability since it can be applied easily in 96-well plates thereby allowing a variety of incubation conditions to be studied in as single experiment.

1. Culture the cells in 96-well plates and after incubation for the desired time with the appropriate reagents discard the culture medium.
2. Mix the CellTiter96® AQueous One Solution Reagent (Promega) at a ratio of 1:5 with culture medium and add directly in the culture wells at volume of 100 μL/well.
3. Incubate the cells with the mixture at 37°C for 1 h and read the absorbance at 490 nm with an ELISA plate reader (*see* **Note 9**). The absorbance value is taken to be proportional to the number of viable cells in the culture.

3.3.4. Flow Cytometric Assays of Cell Viability

DNA Fragmentation

During the process of cell death, cellular DNA frequently becomes cleaved from a high molecular weight to lower molecular weight forms, and this can be monitored by flow cytometry as a measure of ongoing changes in viability. The appearance of low molecular weight DNA is frequently equated with evidence of apoptosis, but it should be noted that DNA fragmentation is not specifically diagnostic since this can also occur during necrosis.

1. Following incubation harvest both adherent and non-adherent cells (*see* **Subheading 3.3.1**) into appropriate tubes (*see* **Note 10**). Centrifuge these at 200 × *g* for 5 min and carefully decant the supernatant and discard (*see* **Note 11**).
2. Resuspend the pellet immediately in 200 μL PBS.
3. Fix the cells by slowly adding 1 mL of ice-cold 70% Ethanol in PBS to each tube, and incubating on ice for 30 min.
4. After incubation centrifuge the tubes for 5 min at 200 × *g*. Decant the supernatant and resuspend the stained cells in 1 mL 20 μg/mL propidium iodide (PI) which is supplemented

with 5 μL RNase, DNase-free (*see* **Note 12**) and incubated at 37°C for 30 min.

5. Following incubation, analyse the samples by flow cytometry according to the manufacturer's instructions (which will depend on the instrument being used). A histogram plotting PI intensity against cell number will provide a profile of the sample population's cell-cycle status. Cells exhibiting fragmented DNA are found in a sub-G_0/G_1 population. Information can be also obtained on the percentage of cells within the G_0/G_1, S and G_2/M phases.

Fluorescence Methods for Estimation of Cell Viability

As an alternative to DNA integrity, the induction of apoptosis can be measured more directly using various fluorescent dyes. Typically, PI is used in parallel with Annexin-V conjugated to fluorophores such as FITC. This method then allows the proportion of healthy, early apoptotic and late apoptotic or necrotic cells to be calculated.

1. Incubate, harvest and centrifuge the cells as described in **Subheading 3.3.4, step 1**.
2. Resuspend the pellet in 100 μL 1× binding buffer (*see* **Note 13**).
3. Add 5 μL of 50 μg/mL propidium iodide and 5 μL of 400 ng/mL Annexin V-FITC to each tube and briefly mix. Incubate at room temperature, in the dark, for 15 min.
4. Add an additional 400 μL (*see* **Note 14**) of 1× binding buffer per tube and analyse by flow cytometry according to the instrument being used. Populations of cells that are negative for Annexin V and PI are defined as healthy, while those positive for Annexin V but negative for PI are early apoptotic and those positive for both Annexin V and PI are either late apoptotic or necrotic (*see* **Note 15**).

3.4. Incubation with Fatty Acids as a Means to Simulate Lipotoxicity

One area of particular interest at present is the effect of fatty acids on beta-cell viability since this may recapitulate some of the changes that occur during the process of "lipotoxicity" in vivo. Thus, a method that is commonly employed to alter β-cell viability is to incubate cells in the presence of various fatty acids. Combinations of the methods described can be employed to monitor viability, but it is important that fatty acids are prepared appropriately. In particular, it is important that complexes of fatty acids are formed with albumin prior to incubation since this reproduces most closely the likely free concentrations achieved in vivo. One important issue to note here is that some batches of bovine serum albumin exert significant toxicity without the addition of exogenous fatty acids. The reasons for this are unclear but it is important to test each batch in viability experiments before embarking on fatty acid studies. Bovine serum albumin controls should also be run alongside all test conditions as a matter of routine.

1. Prepare stock solutions of 50 mM of the appropriate long chain *saturated* fatty acids by dissolving the fatty acids in 50% ethanol during heating to 70°C for 5 min.
2. Prepare *mono-unsaturated* fatty acids by mixing with 90% ethanol at room temperature to produce stock solutions of 90 mM.
3. Make up a solution of 10% (10 g per 100 mL) fatty acid-free bovine serum albumin by dissolution of BSA in PBS.
4. Bind the appropriate volumes of the fatty acid preparations to 10% fatty acid-free BSA by incubation for 1 h at 37°C.
5. Add the mixture to RPMI-1640 medium (containing 11 mM glucose) deprived of foetal calf serum. The final concentrations present in the cell environment should be 1% for BSA and 0.5% for ethanol. Control cells receive vehicle alone.
6. Seed cells into 6-well plates and incubate for 24 h in complete RPMI-1640 medium prior to the beginning of the experiment. Following this period, replace the culture medium with the fatty acid/BSA complex (in RPMI-1640 devoid of foetal calf serum) and incubate as appropriate. Determine cell viability using any of the methods described.

4. Notes

1. This part of the procedure can seem laborious but chopping to achieve a uniform texture and size is critical to the ultimate success of the digest.
2. High-intensity shaking is important to islet yield.
3. Glass pipettes are drawn by heating in a Bunsen flame and pulled by hand to yield pipettes with a bore of approximately 1 mm. Larger bore pipettes are undesirable as too much liquid is likely to be drawn up as each islet is picked.
4. Pipettes can be coated with silane to prevent islets sticking to the internal glass but it is preferable to develop a picking technique in which the groups of islets are kept within the region of minimum bore and are not allowed to reach the collar of the pipette.
5. The method usually yields approximately 500 islets per pancreas and, at this stage, the islets should be free of exocrine contamination.

6. Trypan blue selectively colours dead cells blue, whereas it is excluded from living cells which therefore remain unstained.
7. Sterile chambered coverslips are also available but their cost is relatively high and they offer few obvious advantages.
8. Hoechst 33342 penetrates the plasma membrane of all cells, staining the DNA blue. Propidium iodide can penetrate the cells only when their plasma membrane is damaged, leading to fluorescent pink staining of the nucleus.
9. The assay measures the conversion of a tetrazolium salt into a soluble formazan product by viable cells in proliferation (MTT assays are equivalent but produce an insoluble formazan product which must be solubilised prior to measurement). The amount of formazan formed is proportional to the population of viable cells in the culture and is determined spectrophotometrically at 490 nm.
10. We use 12 × 75 mm polypropylene tubes from Sarstedt; however, these can be varied according to the flow cytometer being used.
11. Whenever discarding the supernatant it is important to be careful to prevent the pellet from dislodging or fracturing.
12. Propidium iodide can bind to RNA making it essential to use an RNase in order to measure only its binding to DNA.
13. This is diluted from 10× Binding Buffer provided in the BD Pharmingen apoptosis detection kit cited in the material section.
14. This volume may need to be altered to allow steady flow of cells through the cytometer to achieve optimal detection.
15. To confirm apoptosis, it is useful to use several time-points to determine whether the late apoptotic/necrotic population is progressing through apoptosis.

References

1. Orci, L. (1985). The insulin factory: a tour of the plant surroundings and a visit to the assembly line. *Diabetologia* **28**, 528–546
2. Baetens, D., Malaisse-Lagae, F., Perrelet, A., and Orci, L. (1979). Endocrine pancreas: three-dimensional reconstruction shows two types of islets of Langerhans. *Science* **206**, 1323–1325
3. Cabrera, O., Berman, D.M., Kenyon, N.S., Ricordi, C., Berggren, P.-O., and Caicedo, A. (2006). The unique cytoarchitecture of human pancreatic islets has implications for islet cell function. *Proc. Natl. Acad. Sci. U.S.A.* **103**, 2334–2339
4. Ashcroft, S.J., Hammonds, P., and Harrison, D.E. (1986). Insulin secretory responses of a clonal cell line of simian virus 40-transformed B cells. *Diabetologia* **29**, 727–733
5. Miyazaki, J., Araki, K., Yamato, E., Ikegami, H., Asano, T., Shibasaki, Y., Oka, Y., and Yamamura, K. (1990). Establishment of a pancreatic beta cell line that retains glucose-inducible insulin secretion: special reference to expression of glucose transporter isoforms. *Endocrinology* **127**, 126–132
6. D'Ambra, R., Surana, M., Efrat, S., Starr, R.G., and Fleischer, N. (1990). Regulation of insulin secretion from beta-cell lines derived

from transgenic mice insulinomas resembles that of normal beta-cells. *Endocrinology* **126**, 2815–2822

7. Praz, G.A., Halban, P.A., Wollheim, C.B., Blondel, B., Strauss, A.J., and Renold, A.E. (1983). Regulation of immunoreactive insulin release from a rat cell line (RINm5F). *Biochem. J.* **210**, 345–352
8. McClenaghan, N.H., Barnett, C.R., Ah-Sing, E., Abdel-Wahab, Y.H., O'Harte, F.P., Yoon, T.W., Swanston-Flatt, S.K., and Flatt, PR. (1996). *Diabetes* **45**, 1132–1140
9. Asfari, M., Janjic, D., Meda, P., Li, G., Halban, P.A., and Wollheim, C.B. (1992). Establishment of 2-mercaptoethanol-dependent differentiated insulin-secreting cell lines. *Endocrinology* **130**, 167–178
10. Lacy, P.E. and Kostianovsky, M. (1967). Method for the isolation of intact islets of Langerhans from the rat pancreas. *Diabetes* **16**, 35–39
11. Montague, W. and Taylor, K.W. (1968). Pentitols and insulin release by isolated rat islets of Langerhans. *Biochem J.* **109**, 333–370
12. Antonioli, B., Fermo, I., Cainarca, S., Marzorati, S., Nano, R., Baldissera, M., Bachi, A., Paroni, R., Ricordi, C., and Bertuzzi, F. (2007). Characterization of collagenase blend enzymes for human islet transplantation. *Transplantation* **84**, 1568–1575
13. Hurst, R.D. and Morgan, N.G. (1990). Evidence for differential effects of noradrenaline and somatostatin on intracellular messenger systems in rat islets of Langerhans. *J. Mol. Endocrinol.* **4**, 231–237
14. Janjic, D. and Wollheim, C.B. (1992). Islet cell metabolism is reflected by the MTT (tetrazolium) colorimetric assay. *Diabetolgia* **35**, 482–485
15. Elliott, J., Scarpello, J.H.B., and Morgan, N.G. (2002). Differential effects of genistein on apoptosis induced by fluoride and pertussis toxin in human and rat pancreatic islets and RINm5F cells. *J. Endocrinol.* **172**, 137–143

Chapter 6

In Vitro Culture of Isolated Islets of Langerhans: Analysis of Function

Anna L. Nolan

Summary

In vitro culture has been well defined as a useful tool to improve survival and functionality of isolated islets of Langerhans. Evaluation of islet morphology and function is essential prior to use for experimental investigations. Novel techniques such as co-culture and the use of matrices have been shown to improve islet survival and functional viability, and can enhance the purity of the islet preparations, which is particularly important prior to experimental use or patient transplantation.

Key words: Islets of Langerhans, Culture, Foetal bovine serum, Islet survival, Matrices, Matrigel, Fibronectin, Laminin

1. Introduction

Optimizing culture conditions of isolated islets of Langerhans, from either human or rodent donors, can vastly improve their functionality and survival. However, stringent conditions are required to maintain their viability. Islets isolated from the surrounding exocrine tissue have been exposed to digestive enzymes, a reduction in temperature, inadequate oxygen supply, extensive dilution, and mechanical stress. Prolonged pancreatic digestion can lead to extensive islet damage and hence a period of culture is often employed after isolation to restore viability and improve functionality *(1, 2)*. A period of culture can be used to purify islet preparations, which is particularly important when islets are to be used for transplantation into patients with type I diabetes where cell number is important *(3)*. In vitro culture has also been shown to improve the insulin secretory capacity of isolated

C. Stocker (ed.), *Type 2 Diabetes,* Methods in Molecular Biology, vol. 560
DOI 10.1007/978-1-59745-448-3_6, © Humana Press, a part of Springer Science+Business Media, LLC 2009

islets from diabetic subjects *(4)*. However, there is a potential risk of infection when culturing islets which should be considered. Recently, novel techniques such as co-culture and the use of three-dimensional matrices have been employed in an attempt to improve islet survival and functional viability *(3)*. It has been shown that the number of islets that survive culture procedures is greater when matrices are utilized. However, tissue loss can occur when retrieving islets from matrices due to reduced diffusion of nutrients and waste products across the matrix *(3)*. Culturing islets is a vital requirement for the study of the in vitro function of beta cells in diabetes research. Investigations into the effects of both nutrients and therapeutic compounds on insulin secretion, islet function, and viability are essential components of basic islet biology research.

2. Materials

2.1. Transportation of Adult Human Islets

1. Transportation medium: HAM F10 containing 6.1 mM glucose and supplemented with 0.5% BSA, 0.08 mg/mL benzylpenicillin, and 0.1 mg/mL streptomycin.
2. Vessel: 50 mL sterile tubes.

2.2. Evaluation of Islet Structure and Function

1. 1× PBS.
2. Human fibrinogen (80 mg/mL stock made in PBS).
3. Human thrombin (50 U/mL stock made in 40 mM $CaCl_2$).
4. Parafilm® M Barrier Film.
5. Microscope slides (Superfrost).
6. Solutions and buffers for hematoxylin (Gill's Formula) and eosin (1% w/v).

2.3. Culture of Adult Islets

The materials required for islet culture are determined according to the donor species. The media requirements for rat islets are different compared with those used for human islets. Commonly RPMI-1640 is used for rat islets and CMRL-1066 for human islets.

1. Tissue incubator with automatically controlled temperature at 37°C, humidified air of 5% CO_2.
2. Either RPMI-1640 or CMRL-1066.
3. 2 mM L-glutamine.
4. 10% foetal bovine serum.
5. 100 U/mL penicillin.
6. 100 μg/mL streptomycin.

2.4. Culture of Islets Using Matrices

A number of different matrices have been investigated for co-culture with islets. Many studies have shown that the culture of islets within a matrix can lead to the differentiation of islet cells. This chapter will outline the use of matrigel matrices to improve the functionality of the isolated islets, and to enhance insulin secretion and islet cell morphology. This section will also cover two of the most common matrices used for culture, namely fibronectin and laminin. The consistency of these matrices will depend heavily on the desired purpose of the islet culture. Recovery techniques for the appropriate use in either transplantation or functional experiments are also suggested.

2.4.1. Matrigel

1. Matrigel is the most widely used matrix for islet culture. Matrigel™ Matrix is a solubulized basement membrane preparation extracted from an Engelbreth-Holm-Swarm mouse sarcoma, a tumor rich in extracellular matrix proteins. Its major component is laminin, but it also contains collagen IV, heparan sulfate proteoglycans, and entactin 1. At room temperature, BD Matrigel™ Matrix polymerizes to produce a biologically active matrix material resembling the mammalian cellular basement membrane *(5)*. BD Matrigel™ (BD Biosciences) is used either undiluted or diluted (1:2) in serum-free culture medium. Matrigel should be aliquoted and multiple freeze/thaw cycles prevented. Aliquots can be stored at either –20 or –80°C freezers until use.
2. BD™ Cell Recovery Solution BD Biosciences, for use when recovering cultured islets from BD Matrigel™ (stored at 4°C).

2.4.2. Fibronectin and Laminin

Fibronectin, a product of most mesenchymal and epithelial cells, is a widely distributed glycoprotein consisting of two subunits, each approximately 250 kDa linked by a disulfide bond *(6)*. Laminin is a large major glycoprotein in the basement membrane (900 kDa) and is composed of three polypeptide chains with a multidomain structure.

1. Fibronectin and laminin diluted in sterile water to a concentration of 1 mg/mL and stored in a –20°C freezer.
2. 20 mM sodium carbonate pH 9.7.
3. BD™ Cell Recovery Solution (BD Biosciences) or 2% trypsin solution.

3. Methods

3.1. Transport of Adult Human Islets

Before handling adult human islets, ethical approval is required and patient medical background information must be examined for potential exposure to pathogen and infectious agents. Donor gender, date of birth, and the date and time of isolation must be included so one can fully assess the islets and ascertain any potential adverse outcomes.

3.2. Evaluation of Islet Structure and Function

To evaluate whether islets remain physiologically functional following isolation and culture, a detailed examination of morphology and function needs to be performed, as this will enable the researcher to determine islet quality.

3.2.1. Fixation, Embedding, and Staining for Microscopy

1. Select 300 islets either by approximation or by hand picking using a stereomicroscope.
2. Place the islets in a 1.5 mL sterile eppendorf tube and wash by adding 500 μL of 1× PBS and centrifugation at 800 × *g* for 5 min.
3. Carefully remove the PBS and resuspend the islets in a further 500 μL 1× PBS, repeat this wash step.
4. Add 50 μL of human fibrinogen onto a 4 cm × 4 cm piece of parafilm, transfer the islets and mix.
5. Add an equal volume of thrombin and allow to congeal. Avoid introducing air bubbles at this stage.
6. Place the congealed islets into an embedding cassette and then into 10% formalin in PBS to fix for 24 h at room temperature.
7. The islets should be embedded in paraffin using standardized equipment and techniques.
8. Paraffin-embedded tissue is generally cut at a thickness of 3 μm. Sections are cut and floated on a warm water bath (45°C) before being placed on microscope slides and then allowed to drain.
9. Hematoxylin and eosin staining can be used to obtain a general impression of islet morphology. Examination of islet structure will identify areas within the islet which are necrotic, indicative of problems within the islet preparation.

3.3. Culture of Adult Islets

1. There are many different protocols for culturing islets from both rodent and human; this section will focus on standard methodology. The methodologies to be used will be dependent upon the experimental question being addressed. Adult islets are usually transported at room temperature and can usually remain at room temperature for 12-18 h. However, islets must be placed in culture for at least 24 h after transportation to allow them to recover. Gloves should always be worn when handling human tissue; all procedures should be performed using sterile techniques and containers containing islets should be opened in a tissue culture hood to prevent contamination (*see* **Note 1**).

2. Upon arrival centrifuge the islets at 800 × *g* for 10 min to remove transportation media (*see* **Note 2**).
3. Add 10 mL of the relevant culture media to the islets and resuspend them using a sterile pipette.
4. Place the resuspended islets in 6-10 cm sterile culture dishes depending on the desired number of islets to be cultured (*see* **Note 3**).
5. Keep the dishes in a humidified incubator at 37°C, and 5% CO_2.
6. Replace the culture media every 2-3 days using a syringe and needle or by removing islets and old media with a pipette followed by centrifugation and resuspension in an appropriate volume of fresh media in new culture dishes.
7. When culturing islets for more than 24 h, a monolayer of fibroblasts usually attaches to the bottom of the culture dish. Islets can be removed from this monolayer by mechanical means using a pipette.

3.4. Islet Culture Using Matrices

3.4.1. Matrigela

1. Thaw the matrigel bottle at 4°C overnight (or until it liquefies).
2. Dilute the matrigel (5-1 mg/mL) in serum-free cold cell culture media. Ensure all sterile pipettes and tubes are cooled to 4°C.
3. Add the matrigel to either 6- or 12-well tissue culture plates. A volume of 150-200 μL/cm^2 is desirable. Allow the plate to sit at room temperature for 1 h or overnight at 4°C.
4. When the matrigel has solidified, wash the plate with 2 mL of culture medium.
5. Plate the islets at 100-500 per well in a six-well plate. Avoid high density cultures. Replace the media every 2-3 days and routinely check islet morphology.
6. To remove islets from the matrigel, use the BD™ Cell Recovery Solution.

3.4.2. Fibronectin and Laminin

Both fibronectin and laminin can be treated in a similar way. However, the reader must optimise the concentrations for their specific experimental design.

1. Gently thaw a frozen aliquot at 4°C and dilute to 0.1-100 mg/mL in 20 mM sodium carbonate pH 9.6.
2. Add between 150 and 200 μL fibronectin or laminin solution to a six-well plate and incubate for 90 min at 37°C.
3. Wash with 2 mL culture media and add approximately 500-1000 islets per well in a six-well plate.
4. Replace the media every 2-3 days.
5. To remove islets from fibronectin or laminin, use either a 2% trypsin solution or the BD™ Cell Recovery Solution.

4. Notes

1. There is a significant potential for contamination when culturing islets. Always ensure that islets or media are not exposed to the air and that containers, bottles of media, and tissue culture dishes are always opened in a class II hood.
2. Disposal of transportation media should be performed under your institute's guidelines for handling potentially contaminated tissue.
3. Pure islet cultures have increased viability in vitro. Islets of low purity, or those which are highly contaminated with undigested exocrine tissue, have poor viability in culture. The simplest way to purify an islet preparation prior to culture is to hand pick islets with a dissecting microscope and a drawn out glass pipette. To identify islet from exocrine tissue, staining with dithizone is usually performed (*see* **Note 4**).
4. To prepare a stock of dithizone solution: dissolve 20 mg of dithizone (diphenylthiocarbazone) in 0.6 mL of 95% ethanol and mix. Add 1-2 drops of ammonium hydroxide and mix (dithizone in solution is bright orange). Add PBS to 0.3 mL of the stock dithizone solution and bring to a final volume of 100 mL. Mix slowly and add 1 M HCl to adjust the pH to 7.4. Add the islets to 2-3 mL of the final dithizone solution in a petri dish and incubate for 1-2 min. Islets will appear red and acinar tissue will remain gray. Prolonged staining will start to colour the acinar tissue.

Acknowledgements

The author would like to thank Dr. Peter diStefano and Dr. Claire J. Stocker for helpful comments and suggestions.

References

1. Bottino R, Balamurugan AN, and Tse H. (2004). Response of human islets to isolation stress and the effect of antioxidant treatment. *Diabetes* **53**: 2559–2568.
2. Abdelli S, Ansite J, Roduit R Borsello T, Matsumoto I, Sawada T, Allaman-Pillet N, Henry H, Beckmann JS, Hering BJ, and Bonny C. (2004). Intracellular stress signaling pathways activated during human islet preparation and following acute cytokine exposure. *Diabetes* **53**: 2815–2823.
3. Murdoch TB, McGhee-Wilson D, Shapiro AM, and Lakey JR. (2004). Methods of human islet culture for transplantation. *Cell Transplantation* **13**: 605–617.
4. Lupi R, Marselli L, Dionisi S, Del Guerra S, Boggi U, Chiaro M, Lencioni C, Bugliani M, Mosca F, Di Mario U, Del Prato S, Dotta F, and Marchetti P. (2004). Improved insulin secretory function and reduced chemotactic properties after tissue culture of islets

from type 1 diabetic patients. *Diabetes Metabolism Research and Reviews* **20930**: 246–251.

5. Kleinman HK and Martin GR. (2005). Matrigel: basement membrane matrix with biological activity. *Seminars in Cancer Biology* **15**: 378–386.
6. Hynes RO and Yamada KM. (1982). Fibronectins: multifunctional modular glycoproteins. *Journal of Cell Biology* **95**: 369–377.

Chapter 7

Single-Cell RT-PCR Identification of Genes Expressed by Human Islet Endocrine Cells

Dany Muller, Peter M. Jones, and Shanta J. Persaud

Summary

Studies of gene expression by different islet endocrine cell populations can provide useful information about signal transduction cascades regulating α-, β- and δ-cell function. Experiments on expression of β-cell gene products are relatively easy to perform in rodent islets as these islets are readily isolated at high purities from the exocrine pancreas; β-cells are the majority cell type and their autofluorescent properties allow them to be purified from non-β-cells by fluorescence-activated cell sorting (FACS). However, the situation is rather more complicated when investigating human islet gene expression profiles as purities of collagenase-isolated human islets are generally less than those of mouse and rat islets; β-cells are less abundant in human islets than they are in rodent islets and conventional FACS purification of human islet β-cells is not possible because of their high background fluorescence. In addition, FACS does not provide pure α- or δ-cell populations from either rodent or human islets. We have developed single-cell RT-PCR protocols to allow identification of genes expressed by human islet α-, β- and δ-cells. This chapter describes these protocols and appropriate steps that should be followed to minimise generation of false-positive amplicons.

Key words: Human islets, α-Cell, β-Cell, δ-Cell, mRNAs, Single-cell RT-PCR, Gene expression, Insulin, Glucagon, Somatostatin

1. Introduction

Islets of Langerhans are small clusters of endocrine cells that are found scattered throughout the pancreas. Islets of most species range in size from 50 to 500 μm and are composed of approximately 2-3,000 cells. Insulin-secreting β-cells are the majority cell type in islets and in rodents they constitute up to 80% of the total islet mass, with most of the remainder being glucagon-secreting α-cells or somatostatin-secreting δ-cells *(1)*. Given that

C. Stocker (ed.), *Type 2 Diabetes,* Methods in Molecular Biology, vol. 560
DOI 10.1007/978-1-59745-448-3_7, © Humana Press, a part of Springer Science+Business Media, LLC 2009

β-cell numbers are considerably higher than those of other cell types in rodent islets it is often assumed that identification of genes expressed by islets represents expression of those genes by β-cells. While this assumption may often be correct, the conclusions from such observations are suggestive rather than definitive and such studies provide no information about gene expression by the minority α- and δ-cells. The endocrine cell composition of human islets is distinct from rodent islets in that β-cells make up approximately 55% of the islet mass, with α- and δ-cells contributing approximately 35–40% and 5–10%, respectively *(1)*. The lower abundance of β-cells in human islets than in rodent islets makes it difficult to draw conclusions from expression studies performed using whole islets.

Mouse and rat islets are commonly used for investigations of gene expression and functional regulation, and although the small size of these rodents precludes retrieval of large numbers of islets (approximately 250 from a mouse and up to 1,000 from a rat) fairly pure β-cell populations can be isolated by FACS purification of dispersed islets *(2)*. Ideally the FACS method could be adapted to obtain purified human islet β-cell populations for gene expression analyses. However, human islets have a high background fluorescence, which means that the autofluorescence methods used to sort rodent islets cannot be readily applied to them. A method using Newport Green, a fluorescent zinc-binding dye, has recently been reported to generate relatively pure (approximately 90%) human β-cell populations *(3)*, but this protocol has not yet been widely adopted by other laboratories. In any case, approximately one in ten cells obtained from such a protocol is a non-β-cell and methods are still not available for retrieval of pure populations of α- and δ-cells.

The protocols described in this chapter use nested RT-PCR amplification of α- β- and δ- cell hormone mRNAs from isolated single human islet cells to identify islet endocrine cell type and the remaining mRNA can then be used to determine whether individual cells also express mRNAs of interest. We have used this method to examine expression of mRNAs for angiotensin receptors *(4)*, cyclooxygenase-2 (COX-2; *(5)*), the calcium-sensing receptor *(6)*, melatonin receptors *(7)* and the insulin receptor signalling cascade *(8, 9)* by human islet cells. Our data indicate that some mRNAs, such as that encoding the angiotensin AT1 receptor, are expressed by α-, β- and δ-cells, while others show cell-specific expression (e.g. COX-2 is expressed by human islet β-cells but is not detectable in α-cells, while melatonin MT1 receptor mRNA can be amplified from α-cells but not β-cells). Given the very high sensitivity of PCR amplifications and the necessity of performing two rounds of PCR with single-cell cDNAs care must be taken to avoid false-positive amplifications: full details and examples are provided here.

2. Materials (see Note 1)

2.1. Cell Dissociation and RNase A Treatment

1. Connaught Memorial Research Laboratories (CMRL)-1066 medium (Invitrogen) supplemented with 10% foetal bovine serum (FBS; Invitrogen) and stored at 4°C.
2. Trypsin (0.25%)/ethylenediamine tetraacetic acid (EDTA; 1 mM) solution (Sigma Aldrich) stored in 1 ml aliquots at −20°C.
3. RNase A (Sigma Aldrich) stored as a 6 mg/mL stock in 100-μL aliquots at −20°C.

2.2. Single-Cell Isolation and Storage

1. Glass microcapillaries are prepared by heating standard glass pipettes and pulling to a diameter of approximately 20 μm.
2. tRNA (Sigma Aldrich) dissolved in water to 100 mg/mL and stored in 50 μL aliquots at −20°C.
3. RNasin (Promega) stored at 40 units/ml in 50 μL aliquots at −20°C.
4. 1,4-dithiothreitol (DTT; Promega) dissolved in dimethyl sulphoxide (DMSO) to 400 mM and stored in 500 μL aliquots at −20°C.
5. Single-cell Lysis Buffer (S-CLB) composition: 0.8% NP-40, 60 μg/mL tRNA, 40 units RNasin, 10 mM DTT, RNase/DNase-free water. Prepare fresh as required.

2.3. Reverse Transcription

1. Oligo d(T)18 (Promega) reconstituted in RNase/DNase-free water to a concentration of 2 μg/μL and stored in 20 μL aliquots at −20°C.
2. Random primers (Promega) reconstituted in RNase/DNase-free water to a concentration of 2 μg/μL and stored in 20 μL aliquots at −20°C.
3. Deoxyribonucleotide tri-phosphates (dNTPs: dATP, dCTP, dGTP and dTTP; Promega) stored in 200 μL aliquots at −20°C.
4. Moloney Murine Leukaemia Virus Reverse Transcriptase (M-MLV RT; Promega) stored in 50 μL aliquots at −20°C.
5. Reverse Transcription Buffer 1 (RTB1) composition: 285 μg/μL oligo d(T)18, 285 μg/μL random primers, 15 μM of each outer reverse primer pre(pro)insulin (PPI), pre(pro)glucagon (PPG), pre(pro)somatostatin (PPS) and insulin receptor (IR), RNase/DNase-free water. Prepare fresh as required.
6. Reverse Transcription Buffer 2 (RTB2) composition: 90.9 mM Tris-HCl (pH 8.3), 136.4 mM KCl, 5.5 mM $MgCl_2$, 18.2 mM DTT, 20 units RNasin, 910 μM dNTPs, 100 units

M-MLV RT, RNase/DNase-free water. Prepare fresh as required.

2.4. First Round of Amplification by PCR

1. GoTaq DNA polymerase (Promega) stored in 20 μL aliquots at –20°C.
2. Polymerase Chain Reaction Mixture 1 (PCR M1) composition: ×1 PCR reaction mixture (Promega), 2.5 units GoTaq DNA polymerase, 150 μM dNTPs, 1.4 mM $MgCl_2$, 0.5 μM of the outer forward primer of interest and 0.25 μM of the corresponding outer reverse primer. Prepare fresh as required.
3. The following outer human primer sequences can be used for amplification of
   PPI: forward 5′-ccctctggggacctgacc-3′, reverse 5′-acaatgccacgcttctgc-3′
   PPG: forward 5′-ccaggcagacccactcag-3′, reverse 5′-ttcaacaatggcgacctc-3′
   PPS: forward 5′-cccagactccgtcagtttc-3′, reverse 5′-gcctcatttcatcctgctc-3′
   IR: forward 5′-tctccaccattcgagtctga-3′, reverse 5′-atgtcatcagccttggcttc-3′
   Store all primers as 10 μM stocks at –20°C (*see* **Note 2**).

2.5. Second Round of Amplification by PCR and PCR Product Visualisation

1. Polymerase Chain Reaction Mixture-2 (PCR M2) composition: ×1 PCR reaction mixture (Promega), 1.5 units GoTaq DNA polymerase, 200 μM dNTPs, 1.5 mM $MgCl_2$, 0.75 μM of the inner forward and reverse primers of interest. Prepare fresh as required.
2. The following inner human primer sequences can be used for re-amplification of
   PPI: forward 5′-aacgaggcttcttctacacac-3′, reverse 5′-ggtacagcattgttccaca-3′
   PPG: forward 5′-cattcacagggcacattcac-3′, reverse 5′-gcttggccttccaaataag-3′
   PPS: forward 5′-gactccgtcagtttctgca-3′, reverse 5′-gcatcattctccgtctggtt-3′
   IR forward 5′-acagttggacggtggtagacat-3′, reverse 5′-cttcatacagcacgatcagacc-3′
   Store all primers as 10-μM stocks at –20°C (*see* **Note 2**).
3. Make a 1% stock of ethidium bromide by adding 100 mg to 10 mL water and wrap the container in foil to protect the contents from light. This solution is stable at room temperature for at least 1 year (*see* **Note 3**).
4. DNA gel-loading buffer (Promega, ×6 stock) stored in 1 mL aliquots at –20°C.
5. Molecular weight standards (Promega) stored in 200 μL aliquots at –20°C.

6. Tris–Borate–EDTA buffer (TBE) stored at room temperature as a ×10 stock and diluted 1:10 with double-distilled water when required.

2.6. Extraction and Sequencing of Amplicons

1. Qiaquick gel extraction kit (Qiagen) contains buffers QG, PE and EB (elution buffer) and Qiaquick spin columns for extraction and elution of PCR-amplified nucleotides from agarose gels.
2. BigDye™ Terminator (Applied Biosystems) contains dNTPs, ddNTPs, DNA polymerase, Mg^{2+} and buffer.
3. Hi-Di™ Formamide sample resuspension solution is from Applied Biosystems.

3. Methods

The methods described assume the availability of approximately 20 collagenase-isolated human islets (*(10)*; *see* **Note 4**) of high purity (>80%). The islet preparation should be as pure as possible to minimise carryover of pancreatic exocrine cells. Dissociation of 20 islets will provide in excess of 20,000 cells. Cell number is not rate limiting for this protocol, but the time that it takes to retrieve and wash the cells means that an individual operator is likely to obtain no more than 100 individual cells from one group of 20 islets. If the islets are of a purity considerably lower than 80% the proportion of non-endocrine cells that are retrieved will increase and this will necessitate screening of larger numbers of cells to obtain the appropriate numbers of α- β- and δ-cells that are required for mRNA analyses of interest. Each cell that is retrieved will provide sufficient material for analysis of islet hormone gene expression (PPG, PPI, PPS) and two other mRNAs of interest (*see* **Fig. 1**).

3.1. Cell Dissociation and RNase A Treatment

1. Select 20 isolated human islets using a 200 μL Gilson pipette or a fine glass capillary under a standard binocular microscope (*see* **Note 5**).
2. Transfer the islets into a 1.5 mL RNase/DNase-free Eppendorf tube.
3. Dissociate the islets into a cell suspension using 200 μL trypsin/EDTA for 3–5 min at 37°C, and pipette up and down several times each minute to aid the dissociation process.
4. Add 1 mL of CMRL-1066 medium supplemented with 10% FBS and 60 μg/mL RNase A and gently disperse the cells at room temperature by pipetting up and down twice.

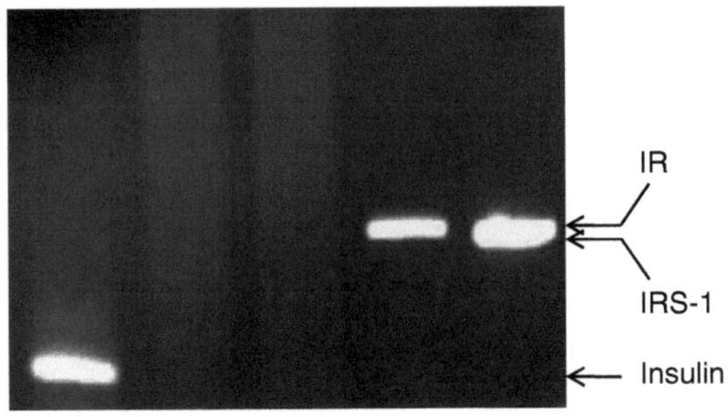

Insulin	+	--	--	--	--
Glucagon	--	+	--	--	--
Somatostatin	--	--	+	--	--
IR	--	--	--	+	--
IRS-1	--	--	--	--	+

Fig. 1. Endocrine cell identification and analysis of mRNAs of interest. Human islet single-cell cDNA underwent PCR amplifications using primers for mRNAs encoding insulin, glucagon, somatostatin, IR and IRS-1, as shown by the "+" symbols. Amplification of a product with the insulin primers, but not with glucagon and somatostatin primers indicated that the cDNA had been obtained from a β-cell. This human β-cell expressed mRNAs encoding both IR and IRS-1, as indicated by the generation of amplicons of the appropriate sizes. Product identities were confirmed by nucleotide sequencing.

5. Incubate the cell suspension in the presence of RNase A for 15 min at 37°C in a water bath to degrade RNA released from lysed cells.
6. Transfer 500 μL of the cell suspension to a 90 mm diameter bacterial dish pre-filled with 12 mL of CMRL-1066 medium supplemented with 10% FBS (*see* **Note 6**).
7. The remaining cell suspension can be kept in a tissue culture incubator (37°C, 5% CO_2) for 2-4 h and used later if required.

3.2. Single-Cell Isolation and Storage

1. One by one, select individual single cells under a zoom stereo microscope (×20 or ×40 objective; *see* **Fig. 2**) using a fine glass microcapillary (*see* **Notes 5** and 7).
2. Transfer each cell in a drop of PBS (15 μL) containing 5.5 mM glucose and supplemented with 5% FBS.
3. Wash each cell by flushing it in and out of the microcapillary three times using the same drop of PBS.
4. Repeat this washing step another three times using three additional drops of 15 μL PBS supplemented with 5.5 mM glucose and 5% FBS.
5. Using a new microcapillary, transfer the cell into another 15 μL drop of PBS (containing 5.5 mM glucose, no FBS) and wash it three more times (*see* **Note 8**).

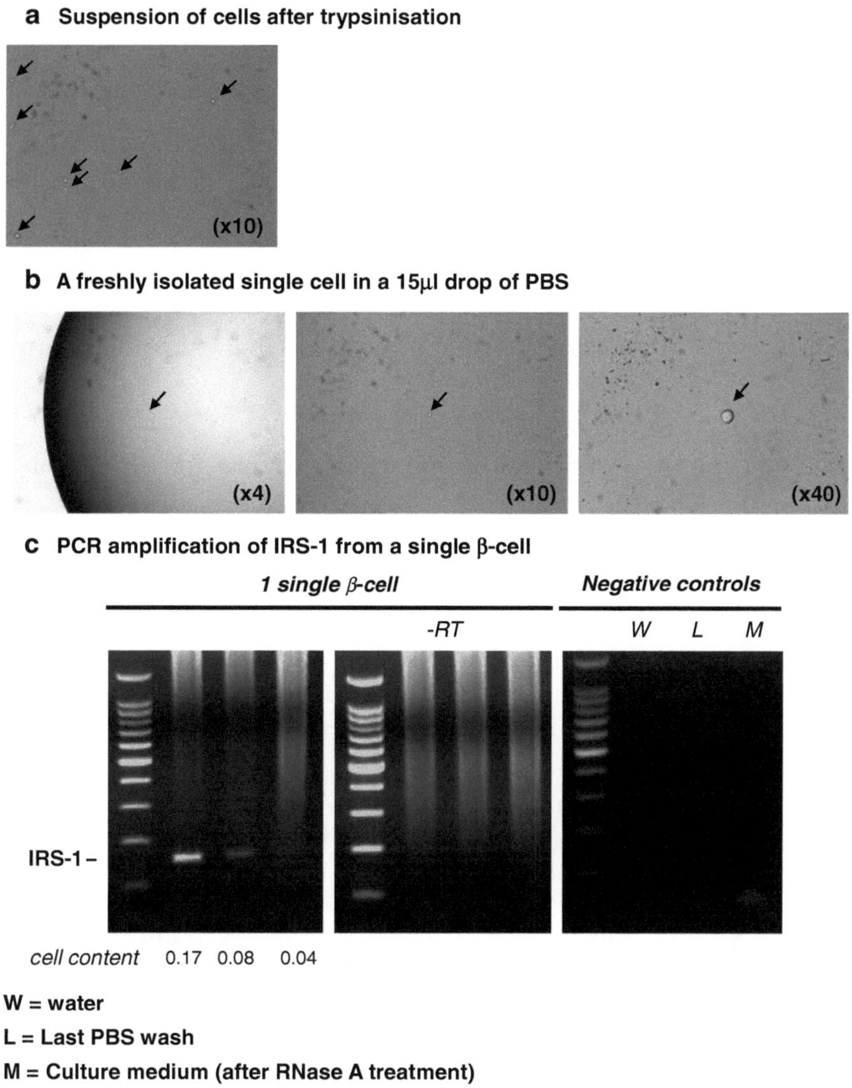

Fig. 2. Validation of single-cell isolation procedure and RT-PCR amplification. Images obtained under a phase-contrast microscope showing (**a**): a suspension of cells that was obtained after trypsinisation, and (**b**): one isolated single cell that was transferred in a 15 μL drop of PBS. (**c**) Typical ethidium-bromide-stained agarose gels showing the sensitivity of the single-cell RT-PCR technique using serial dilutions of the content of one single β-cell. The *left panel* shows that IRS-1 could be easily amplified in a two-round PCR reaction using as little as 1/6 (~17%) of the content of a cell, and a product was also obtained when cDNA from 1/12 (~8%) of a cell was used. Control reactions, in which mRNA was used instead of a cDNA template (-RT), were used to check that genomic contamination could not contribute to product synthesis (*middle panel*). To verify that extracellular contamination with mRNA released from damaged cells during the isolation procedure could not account for product synthesis, additional control reactions containing culture medium (after RNase A treatment) or 0.5 μL of the last PBS wash were used instead of mRNA for reverse transcription (*right panel*).

6. Transfer the cell into another 15 μL drop of PBS (containing 5.5 mM glucose, no FBS).
7. Wash the cell twice in the drop of PBS and, using the same microcapillary, transfer the cell in a minimum volume of PBS

(approximately 0.5 μL) to a RNase/DNase-free 200 μL PCR tube containing 5 μL S-CLB.

8. Transfer Eppendorf tubes, each containing a single cell in a final volume of approximately 5.5 μL, to liquid nitrogen for storage.

3.3. Reverse Transcription

1. Retrieve the tubes containing single cells from the liquid nitrogen; store and thaw on ice.
2. Add 3.5 μL of RTB1 to each tube, on ice.
3. Incubate for 5 min at 72°C using either a hot plate or a PCR machine.
4. Place the tubes on ice for 1 min.
5. Centrifuge at room temperature for 2-5 s using a bench Eppendorf centrifuge at 1,000 × *g*.
6. Add 11 μL of RTB2 to each tube on ice.
7. Incubate for 50 min at 42°C followed by 15 min incubation at 72°C using a PCR machine.
8. Cool the tubes down to 4°C on ice, centrifuge at room temperature for 2-5 s using a bench Eppendorf centrifuge at 1,000 × *g* and place the tubes on ice. The final volume should be 20 μL.
9. The complementary DNAs (cDNAs) can be used immediately or stored at –20°C for several weeks or at –80°C for months.

3.4. First Round of Amplification by PCR

1. PPI, PPG and PPS cDNA amplifications are performed separately using 3 μL of the reverse transcription mixture. IR cDNAs are amplified in a fourth Eppendorf tube using 5 μL of the same reverse transcription solution (*see* **Note 9**).
2. Add 45 μL of PCR M1 to each PCR tube.
3. Make up the volume to 50 μL with RNase/DNase-free water where necessary.
4. The denaturation stage is performed at 95°C for 3 min.
5. PPI, PPG and PPS amplifications are achieved by performing 38 cycles of the following protocol: 95°C for 30 s, 56°C for 30 s and 72°C for 30 s. IR amplification is performed by 45 cycles at 95°C for 30 s, 58°C for 30 s and 72°C for 45 s.

3.5. Second Round of Amplification by PCR and PCR Product Visualisation

1. Add 3 μL of the first round PCR product to 27 μL PCR M2 using another set of RNase/DNase-free Eppendorf tubes. Keep the remaining first round PCR products at –20°C in case a problem arises during the second round of PCR amplification.
2. Use the inner PCR primers to perform the second round of PCR amplification for PPI, PPG and PPS using 38 cycles and

the following protocol: 95°C for 30 s, 56°C for 30 s and 72°C for 30 s. IR cDNA is re-amplified using inner primers for 45 cycles and the following protocol: 95°C for 30 s, 58°C for 30 s and 72°C for 30 s (*see* **Note 10**).

3. Prepare a 1.8% (w/v) agarose gel by dissolving 0.9 g agarose in 50-mL TBE buffer and heating until complete dissolution in a microwave oven. When the gel has cooled down sufficiently it can be held with gloves, supplemented with 5 μL of 1% ethidium bromide and poured into a horizontal gel tank. Add the well former and leave to polymerise for about 30 min.
4. Add 15 μL of the final PCR products to 3 μL of ×6 DNA gel-loading buffer. Add 8 μL of the molecular weight standard and 7 μL of DNase/RNase-free water to 3 μL of ×6 DNA gel-loading buffer.
5. Load 16 μL of the PCR products and 16 μL of the molecular weight standard onto ethidium bromide-supplemented 1.8% agarose gels. Separate the nucleotides in TBE buffer at constant voltage (70 V) until the dye front has migrated to approximately the final 25% of the gel.
6. Remove the gel from the apparatus and visualise amplicons under UV light (*see* **Note 11**).

3.6. Extraction and Sequencing of Amplicons

1. Excise DNA fragments of interest from the agarose under UV light using clean scalpels and place the amplified products into individual 1.5 mL RNAse/DNase-free Eppendorf tubes.
2. Weigh the gel slices and add three volumes of Buffer QG to one volume of gel slice (*see* **Note 12**).
3. Incubate gel slices at 50°C for 10 min and upon complete dissolution add one gel volume of 100% isopropanol and mix.
4. Add the mixtures to QIAquick spin columns, centrifuge for 1 min, 17,900 × *g*, discard the flow through and repeat this process after adding 500 μL Buffer QG.
5. Add 750 μL of Buffer PE to the columns, centrifuge twice for 1 min, 17,900 × *g* and discard the flow through.
6. Add 30 μL of Buffer EB (elution buffer) to the columns, centrifuge for 1 min, 17,900 × *g* and collect the eluates (approximately 28 μL per column) into 1.5 mL Eppendorf tubes.
7. Quantify the amount of DNA in each eluate spectrophotometrically (*see* **Note 13**)
8. For a 200 bp PCR product add 8 ng of DNA (*see* **Note 14**), 4 μL BigDye Terminator, 2 μL PCR primer (1 μM) and make up the volume to 10 μL with water.

9. Carry out PCR amplification for 25 cycles using the following protocol: 96°C for 15 s, 55°C for 15 s and 60°C for 30 s.
10. Add 10 μL of water to each reaction to make a final volume of 20 μL.
11. Add 60 μL of 100% ethanol and 5 μL of 135 mM EDTA, incubate at room temperature for 10 min then centrifuge for 30 min, 2,100 × *g* at 4°C.
12. Wash with 200 μL of 70% ethanol; then dry the samples in a vacuum centrifuge.
13. Redissolve the samples in 15 μL of Hi-Di Formamide-loading buffer and separate the nucleotides using an autosequencer (*see* **Note 15**).
14. Use an appropriate database (e.g. Entrez PubMed nucleotide BLAST) to determine the degree of sequence homology between the amplicon nucleotide sequences obtained and those predicted for the primers used.

3.7. Positive and Negative Controls

1. At least one positive and two negative controls should be used for each PCR procedure. To ensure that the PCR reaction is successful and that the final PCR products are of the right size, 2 μL of human islet cDNA can be used as a template in **Subheading 3.4** as a positive control. False positives are discriminated by the use of a control in which 5 μL of non-reverse transcribed single-cell extract is used as template in **Subheading 3.4** instead of complementary DNA and 5 μL of the last PBS wash (**Subheading 3.2**) is used to rule out amplification of products obtained from lysed cells (*see* **Notes 8** and **16**).

4. Notes

1. Unless otherwise stated all solutions should be prepared in RNase/DNase-free water in RNase/DNase-free tubes.
2. The protocols may also be applied to mouse or rat islets or islets derived from other species such as pig (using appropriate species-specific primers).
3. Care should be taken when handling ethidium bromide as it is a strong mutagen, and it may also be carcinogenic.
4. Human islets are isolated from cadaver organ donors with the appropriate ethical approvals.
5. Islets are retrieved using an Olympus SZ40 microscope (final magnification ×20 to ×40) and single cells are selected with a Nikon SMZ1000 zoom stereo microscope (final

magnification ×200 to ×400). Other suitable microscopes may be used.

6. Cell suspensions are transferred to uncharged bacterial Petri dishes to minimise cell adhesion.
7. It is critical to ensure that single cells are transferred so that RNA is extracted from individual cells. This can be established by a visual approach (photographs of an isolated single cell in a drop of PBS are shown in **Fig. 2**). It is worth bearing in mind that ~2% of human islet cells co-express insulin and glucagon while ~1% of cells express both glucagon and somatostatin *(9)*, so a minority of single cells will contain mRNAs for more than one islet hormone.
8. Sequential washing stages with PBS are essential to minimise carryover of RNA or genomic DNA from lysed cells, which may lead to false-positive amplification. The use of 5 μL of the last PBS wash and non-reverse transcribed cell extract can be used as negative controls (**Subheading 3.7**), as can cell culture medium. **Figure 2** shows that products are not amplified when water, the last PBS wash or culture medium after RNase A treatment (*right panel*), or single β-cell extracts in the absence of reverse transcriptase (*middle panel*) are used as PCR templates, in this instance with primers for human insulin receptor substrate-1 (IRS-1). When dilutions of β-cell cDNA were used with these primers a product of the appropriate size is amplified (*left panel*). The use of the appropriate negative controls in the same reactions allows confidence in analysis of product generation with cDNA, thus providing evidence that IRS-1 is expressed by β-cells.
9. Identification of islet endocrine cells expressing insulin receptors is described in this chapter. Once the cell type has been determined by reactions using PPI, PPG and PPS primers the remaining cDNA can be used for identification of up to two additional mRNAs (*see* **Fig. 1**).
10. The nested PCR approach described here is necessary for detection of mRNAs of interest in individual cells as the number of copies of mRNA available for amplification from a single cell is limiting. It is therefore advisable to perform serial dilution experiments with groups of pooled cells of a particular phenotype to determine the threshold for detection of amplicons of interest. For example, experiments using three separate groups of ten β-cells indicate that the threshold for detecting β-cell IRS-1 is between 1/10 (10%) and 1/20 (5%) of an individual cell (**Fig. 3**, *left panels*). These observations can be confirmed in parallel experiments using serial dilutions of single β-cells: Fig. 3 (*right panels*) show that the IRS-1 threshold detection was between 1/12

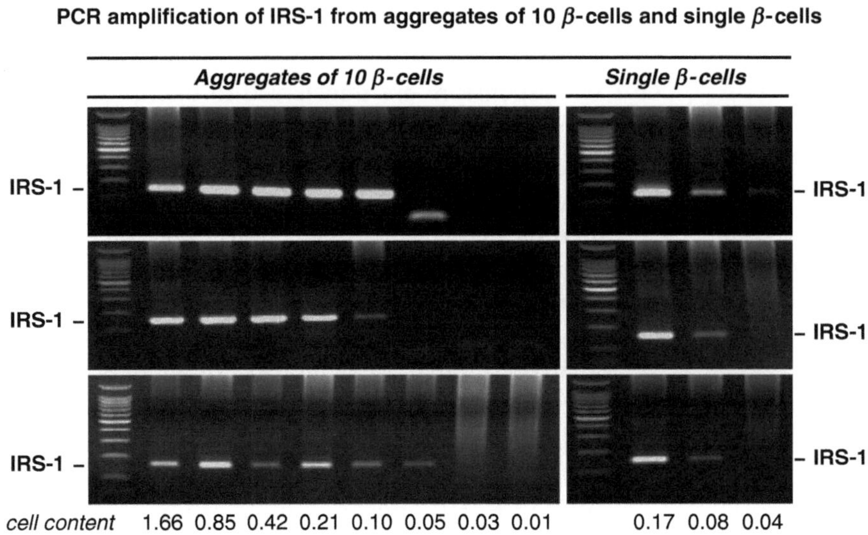

Fig. 3. Threshold determination for single-cell RT-PCR amplification. Serial dilution experiments of RNA extracts isolated from three separate groups of ten pooled β-cells were performed, and IRS-1 cDNA amplified in nested PCR reactions. The left panel shows that the threshold for detection of IRS-1 was between 1/10 (~10% of the content of one cell) and 1/20 (~5% of the content of one cell). Similar results were obtained when serial dilution experiments were carried out with RNA extracts isolated from three separate single cells (*right panel*).

(8%) and 1/24 (4%) of a cell's content. These data indicate slight variations in detection thresholds, but in the protocols described mRNA from between 1/5 and 1/3 of a single cell are used for PCR reactions. This is at least four times more cDNA than the detection threshold, thus providing confidence in the data that are generated.

11. Ethidium-bromide-stained PCR products can be detected using a simple UV plate, or a UV imaging system will allow storage of images. We use the GeneGenius BioImaging System (Syngene).
12. Assume that 100 mg of agarose gel is approximately equivalent to 100 μL.
13. We use the NanoDrop ND-1000 spectrophotometer to quantify DNA using 1 μL of gel eluate. Other spectrophotometers can be used.
14. As a general rule nucleotide sequencing of PCR products requires 4 ng of DNA for every 100 bp of PCR products.
15. We use an Applied Biosystems ABI3130 autosequencer for sequencing PCR products. Other sequencers can be used.
16. Once false positives have been ruled out by the use of appropriate negative controls (**Subheading 3.7**) identification of both PPI mRNA and a mRNA of interest together with confirmation of product identities by sequencing provides direct

evidence that the gene of interest is transcribed in β-cells. Similarly co-amplification of the mRNA with PPG or PPS in distinct cells indicates expression by α- and δ-cells respectively. However, the absence of an appropriate amplicon cannot be used by itself to definitively state that a cell does not express a particular mRNA: it is possible that mRNAs of low copy number may be amplified from some cells of an identified phenotype, but not others. It is therefore essential that multiple cells are used for each mRNA under investigation. Consistent lack of product amplification may indicate that the cell type being used does not express the mRNA or it may be that the levels of expression are below the detection limit. This itself is informative if products are consistently obtained when using the same primers with, for example, α-cells, but not with β-cells.

17. The single-cell PCR protocol detailed in this chapter is time-consuming and other methods have been used to identify localisation of islet mRNAs and proteins. In situ hybridisation *(11–14)* may be used to localise mRNAs to particular cells, but the detection limit is not sufficient to identify mRNAs that show low levels of expression and labelled probes must be synthesised for each mRNA that is to be detected. The single-cell PCR method is therefore advantageous in terms of sensitivity (re-iterative amplification cycles) and the ease of primer preparation. Immunohistochemistry *(15–17)* may be used to identify protein location within cells. However, unlike methods that detect mRNAs, this technique cannot be used to determine if proteins of interest are actually synthesised by the cells in which they are detected. In addition, this technique is dependent on availability and specificity of antibodies, neither of which is limiting for mRNA detection methods. In addition, proteins that are present at low abundance may not be readily detected by immunohistochemistry.

Acknowledgements

The authors are grateful to Dr. S. Pickering for initial advice on appropriate methods for single-cell selection, to Ms. H. Mandefield, the transplantation co-ordinators of South-Thames and King's College Hospital and relatives of the organ donors for human pancreases, and to Professor S. Amiel and Dr. G.C. Huang for provision of isolated human islets. We thank Rongrong Chen for providing details of nucleotide sequencing. Dr. D. Muller was a Diabetes UK RD Lawrence Research Fellow.

References

1. Cabrera, O., Berman, D.M., Kenyon, N.S., Ricordi, C., Berggren, P.O., and Caicedo, A. (2006). The unique cytoarchitecture of human pancreatic islets has implications for islet cell function. *Proc Natl Acad Sci U S A* **103**, 2334–2339
2. Pipeleers, D.G., in't Veld, P.A., Van de Winkel, M., Maes, E., Schuit, F.C., and Gepts, W. (1985). A new in vitro model for the study of pancreatic A and B cells. *Endocrinology* **117**, 806–816
3. Parnaud, G., Bosco, D., Berney, T., Pattou, F., Kerr-Conte, J., Donath, M.Y. et al. (2008). Proliferation of sorted human and rat beta cells. *Diabetologia* **51**, 91–100
4. Ramracheya, R.D., Muller, D.S., Wu, Y., Whitehouse, B.J., Huang, G.C., Amiel, S.A., Karalliedde, J., Viberti, G., et al. (2006). Direct regulation of insulin secretion by angiotensin II in human islets of Langerhans. *Diabetologia* **49**, 221–231
5. Persaud, S.J., Belin, V.D., Muller, D., Asare-Anane, H., Kitsou-Mylona, I., Papadimitriou, A., Burns, C.J., Huang, G.C., et al. (2007). The role of arachidonic acid and its metabolites in insulin secretion from human islets of Langerhans. *Diabetes* **56**, 197–203
6. Gray, E., Squires, P.E., Muller, D., Asare-Anane, H., Huang, G.C., Amiel, S., et al. (2006). Activation of the calcium sensing receptor initiates insulin secretion from human islets of Langerhans: involvement of protein kinases. *J. Endocrinol.* **190**, 703–710
7. Ramracheya, R.D., Muller, D., Squires, P.E., Brereton, H., Sugden, D., Huang, G.C., Amiel, S.A., Jones, P.M., and Persaud, S.J. (2008). Function and expression of melatonin receptors on human pancreatic islets. *J. Pineal Res.* **44**(3), 273–279
8. Muller, D., Huang, G.C., Amiel, S., Jones, P.M., and Persaud, S.J. (2006). Identification of insulin signalling elements in human β-cells: autocrine regulation of insulin gene expression. *Diabetes* **55**, 2835–2842
9. Muller, D., Huang, G.C., Amiel, S., Jones, P.M., and Persaud, S.J. (2007). Gene expression heterogeneity in human islet endocrine cells: the insulin signalling cascade. *Diabetologia* **50**, 1239–1242
10. Huang, G.C., Zhao, M., Jones, P.M., Persaud, S., Ramracheya, R., Lobner, K., et al. (2004). The development of new density gradient media for the purification of human islets and islet quality assessments. *Transplantation* 77, 143–145
11. Brown, C., (1998). In situ hybridization with riboprobes: An overview for veterinary pathologists. *Vet Pathol* **35**, 159–167
12. Le Guellec, D. (1998). Ultrastructural in situ hybridization: A review of technical aspects. *Biology of the Cell* **90**, 297–306
13. Chehadeh, W., Kerr-Conte, J., Pattou, F., Alm, G., Lefebvre, J., Wattre, P., and Hober, D. (2000). Persistent infection of human pancreatic islets by coxsackievirus B is associated with alpha interferon synthesis in β-cells. *J. Virology* **74**, 10153–10164
14. Westermark, G.T., Christmanson, L., Terenghi, G., Permerth, J., Betsholtz, C., Larsson, J., Polak, J.M., and Westermark, P. (1993). Islet amyloid polypeptide: demonstration of mRNA in human pancreatic islets by in situ hybridization in islets with and without amyloid deposits. *Diabetologia* **36**, 323–328
15. Ramos-Vara, J.A. (2005). Technical aspects of immunohistochemistry. *Vet Pathol* 42, 405–426
16. Richardson, C.C., Hussain, K., Jones, P.M., Persaud, S., Lobner, K., Boehm, A., Clark, A., and Christie, M.R. (2007). Low levels of glucose transporters and K_{ATP} channels in human pancreatic beta cells early in development. *Diabetologia* **50**, 1000–1005
17. Squires, P.E., Harris, T.E., Persaud, S.J., Curtis, S.B., Buchan, A.M.J. and Jones, P.M. (2000). The extracellular calcium-sensing receptor on human β-cells negatively modulates insulin secretion. *Diabetes* **49**, 409–417

Chapter 8

Laser Capture Microdissection of Human Pancreatic β-Cells and RNA Preparation for Gene Expression Profiling

Lorella Marselli, Dennis C. Sgroi, Susan Bonner-Weir, and Gordon C. Weir

Summary

Human β-cell gene profiling is a powerful tool for understanding β-cell biology in normal and pathological conditions. The assessment is complicated when isolated islets are studied because of contamination by non-β-cells and the exposure to the trauma of isolation that causes changes in gene expression. These limitations can be overcome by dissecting the β-cells from the pancreatic tissue directly using the laser capture microdissection (LCM) technique. LCM allows the sampling of specific cell types from tissue sections. The technique requires morphological criteria or specific stains for targeted cells, and the protocols must preserve the condition of the sought-after macromolecules. We have developed a protocol of rapid tissue dehydration followed by identification of human β-cells by their intrinsic autofluorescence, which allows laser microdissection for gene-profiling studies.

Key words: Human β-cell, Laser capture microdissection, RNA extraction, RNA integrity, Type 2 diabetes

1. Introduction

Pancreatic β-cells have a specialized phenotype maintained by the expression of a unique set of genes and the suppression of others, but this pattern is altered in diabetes, presumably by hyperglycemia *(1, 2)*. Gene expression studies performed on islets isolated from type 2 diabetic donors allowed identification of alteration in the expression of genes involved in β-cell function *(3, 4)*. However, higher-quality data about β-cell biology in the normal and type 2 diabetic states can be obtained by

C. Stocker (ed.), *Type 2 Diabetes,* Methods in Molecular Biology, vol. 560
DOI 10.1007/978-1-59745-448-3_8, © Humana Press, a part of Springer Science+Business Media, LLC 2009

gene-profiling studies of a pure β-cell population not exposed to the trauma of the isolation procedure and the ischemia of isolated islets that cause changes in gene expression *(5–7)*. The objective can be achieved by dissecting β-cells from the pancreatic tissue directly using the laser capture microdissection (LCM) technique.

LCM allows the sampling of single cells or groups of cells located in histologically complex tissues that can be analyzed for gene or protein expression *(8)*. The technique requires methods for the identification of the target cells, the methods must preserve the macromolecules to be analyzed, and the tissue must be completely dehydrated *(9)*. We have developed a protocol of rapid tissue dehydration and the use of the intrinsic autofluorescence of human β-cells which allows their identification and laser microdissection for gene-profiling studies *(7)*. This is especially useful for human tissue because the islet non-β cells are often found in the center of islets, which means that careful dissection of the green autofluorescence allows avoidance the nonfluorescent non-β-cells. Dissection of β-cells from rodent islets is easier because non-β-cells are restricted to the islet mantle and rarely found in the islet cores *(1, 2)*. This is fortunate because the autofluorescence of rodent β-cells is not strong enough to be useful for rodent LCM.

The successful application of this technique requires careful procurement of pancreatic tissue. Pancreatic tissue obtained from heart-beating cadaveric donors (with a cold ischemia time of less than 12 h) or from surgical samples (within 20 min from the surgical procedure), snap frozen as soon as they reach the laboratory consistently yields high-quality tissue for macromolecular extraction. A straightforward protocol for human β-cell identification and tissue dehydration is available *(7)*. The use of well-established procedures for RNA extraction and amplification makes it possible to obtain the amount of RNA appropriate for gene-profiling studies. The availability of a sensitive technique for the evaluation of RNA integrity allows assessment of the quality of the RNA and determination of the appropriateness for gene-profiling studies.

2. Materials

2.1. Pancreatic Tissue Processing

1. Isopentane (2-Methylbutane) (Fisher Scientific).
2. Dry ice.
3. Ethanol 100%.
4. Cryomold (Fisher Scientific).

5. Tissue-Tek OCT medium (Sakura Finetek, Torrance, CA).
6. Frosted microscope slides (Fisher Scientific).
7. Slide box.

2.2. Tissue Dehydration and LCM

1. RNaseZap (Ambion, Foster City, CA).
2. Polypropylene conical tubes.
3. DEPC-Treated Water.
4. 70% ethanol, prepared by diluting 100% ethanol with DEPC-treated water.
5. 100% ethanol solution.
6. Xylene (Fisher Scientific).
7. PrepStrip™ Tissue Preparation Strip (Arcturus, Mountain View, CA).
8. CapSure HS LCM Caps (Arcturus).
9. PixCell® IIe Laser Capture Microdissection System (Arcturus).
10. Alignment Tray for CapSure HS LCM Caps and ExtraSure Sample Extraction Devices (Arcturus).
11. GeneAmp® Autoclaved Thin-Walled Reaction Tubes (Applied Biosystems, Foster City, CA).

2.3. RNA Extraction and Amplification

1. Guanidine isothiocyanate buffer (Buffer RLT, Qiagen, Valencia, CA).
2. 2M Sodium Acetate.
3. Phenol.
4. Chloroform-isoamyl alcohol mixture: 24:1.
5. Isopropanol.
6. 70% ethanol, prepared by diluting 100% ethanol with DEPC-treated water.
7. MessageClean Kit (GenHunter, Nashville, TN)
   (a) DNase I.
   (b) 10× DNase buffer.
8. Glycogen (GenHunter, Nashville TN).
9. RNase inhibitor (Promega, Madison, WI).
10. RiboAmp™ HS RNA Amplification Kit (Arcturus).
11. RNA 6000 Nano LabChip Kit (Agilent Technologies, Inc., Santa Clara, CA).
12. Agilent 2100 Bioanalyzer (Agilent Technologies).

3. Methods

Laser capture microdissection for β-cell gene profiling is a demanding technique, and all the precautions aimed at avoiding the activation of tissue RNases and the sample contamination by environmental RNases must be taken. For this, particular operating conditions must be followed. LCM experiments should be performed in a dedicated room that must be kept dehumidified and at a constant temperature of 15°C. The operator must avoid any biological contact with the sample, wear disposable gloves, and change them frequently. The laboratory bench surface, the microscope surface, pipettes, and any other surfaces that may come in contact with the sample must be cleaned using RnaseZap. Scissors, tweezers, and forceps must be washed with detergents and autoclaved at 120°C for 15 min before use. All the solutions and plasticware must be RNase free.

3.1. Pancreatic Tissue Processing

1. Prepare an icy chamber for freezing the pancreatic tissue. Pour isopentane into a glass beaker, cover the beaker with parafilm, and place the beaker in an appropriate plastic container filled with dry ice; the dry ice should completely surround the glass beaker.
2. Pour 100% ethanol into the dry ice. Bubbling of the dry ice will occur upon the addition of ethanol, add more dry ice and ethanol; the ethanol becomes slightly viscous. The isopentane must be chilled, which takes about 20 min. Test by immersing the cryomold with just OCT; it should turn opaque over 5-15 s (*see* **Note 1**).
3. Trim the pancreatic sample by removing any nonparenchymal tissue that might be present, in particular adipose tissue, connective tissue, vessels, and nerves. For the procedure, place the pancreas sample on a wax pad and use small scissors and tweezers. During trimming the integrity of the parenchyma should be preserved; in order to do this, separate the unwanted structures from the parenchyma with careful hand dissection. If the tissue specimen is large, it should be cut into individual segments. To facilitate sectioning, the tissue should be no larger than 7 mm in any maximum dimension.
4. Before freezing, dry the pancreatic tissue by putting the sample on a clean paper towel (*see* **Note 2**).
5. Take a cryomold and cover the bottom of it with a thin layer of OCT embedding compound, approximately 1-2 mm deep (*see* **Note 3**). Try to avoid introducing any bubbles.
6. Place the pancreatic tissue specimen onto the layer of OCT in the cryomold, so that the desired cutting surface of the tissue lies flat on the bottom. Carefully add more OCT until the specimen is completely covered and the cryomold is filled.

The tissue should be centered in the mold with a border of embedding compound surrounding the tissue. This orientation will facilitate cutting of frozen sections.

7. Without disturbing the tissue orientation, quickly transfer the mold into the cooled isopentane using forceps, and wait for the OCT to completely solidify (OCT becomes opaque); it takes about 30 s.
8. Place the processed specimen onto dry ice in a separate container so that the solvent (isopentane) evaporates to the point that the OCT looks dry; it takes about 30-60 min. Wrap the frozen specimen tightly in aluminum foil and store in a –80°C freezer until sectioning.
9. Sectioning must be performed in a cryostat at –20°C. Before sectioning preclean the internal surfaces of the cryostat, blade, object holder, and paintbrush with 100% ethanol.
10. Allow the sample, blade, and paintbrush to equilibrate to the cryostat temperature (–20°C), 15-20 min is usually adequate.
11. Fix the frozen tissue to the object holder by spreading a small amount of embedding medium on the surface of the holder, and place the sample on it. The object holder should be precooled at –20°C in the cryostat.
12. When the embedding medium is completely frozen and the tissue is firm, mount the object holder on the microtome head and bring the tissue close to the blade edge. Trim the block until the cutting plane is reached.
13. Cut 8 μm sections with a slow, smooth, and steady motion of the wheel. As the sections begin to form on the blade edge, use a paintbrush to gently guide the section down the face of the blade; this helps keep the section flat.
14. Mount the section on the middle third of a labeled, plain, uncharged slide by bringing the surface of a room-temperature slide very close to the section. The section will seem to jump onto the slide and the mounting medium will melt (*see* **Note 4**).
15. Clean the blade edge with clean dry paper.
16. Store the mounted sections inside the cryostat at –20°C or on dry ice for a short term (1-2 h) and then at –80°C for long term (until 6 months) (*see* **Notes 5** and **6**).

3.2. Tissue Dehydration and LCM

1. Prepare the reagents for the dehydration and washing of the tissue sections by placing 35 mL of each of them into the respective conical tube. The reagents consist of 70% ethanol, DEPC-treated water, 100% ethanol (two tubes), and xylene. Prepare two sets of dehydration reagents and washing solutions using polypropylene conical tubes (*see* **Note 7**).

2. Keep the slide box containing the tissue sections on dry ice during the LCM procedure (*see* **Note 8**).
3. Carry out the dehydration steps in a chemical fume hood precleaned with 100% ethanol and wipe the working surface with RnaseZap.
4. Perform the tissue dehydration immediately after removal of the slides from the slide box (*see* **Note 9**). Handle two slides at a time.
5. Fix the sections in 70% ethanol for 30 s, wash the sections with five quick dips in DEPC-treated water, and then dehydrate the tissue in 100% ethanol for 1 min and again in 100% ethanol for another minute, and in xylene for 4 min (*see* **Note 10**).
6. Dry the slides in the fume absorber for 3-5 min before commencing LCM (*see* **Note 11**). It is useful to treat the dried tissue with Tissue Preparation Strip, which facilitates the removal of any OCT residue and eventually evens any irregularity of the tissue, thus favoring the contact between the tissue and the cap surface.
7. The instructions for LCM of human β-cells assume the use of the manual system PixCell II; however, they are adaptable to other manual infrared capture systems.
8. Preclean the surface of the microscope with RnaseZap and the other parts of the microscope that can be touched by the operator with 100% ethanol.
9. Load the CapSure cap holder with HS LCM caps (*see* **Note 12**). Move the joystick of the system in the vertical position to ensure proper positioning of the cap in relation to the capture zone.
10. Focus the laser beam to obtain a bright, well-defined spot and test the laser pulse. Select the 7.5-μm spot size and adjust the laser power at 35 mW and the duration at 2.5 ms (*see* **Note 13**).
11. Perform the LCM using the blue color filter (excitation: 455-495 nm) and the 40× objective (*see* **Note 14**). Under microscopic visualization, locate the autofluorescent β-cells and direct the beam onto this location.
12. The microdissection session must not be longer than 15 min in order to preserve the RNA from degradation (*see* **Note 15**). An example of human β-cells as they appear in the dehydrated pancreatic tissue is shown in **Fig. 1**.
13. Remove the cap by lifting it from the slide, swing the placement arm away from the slide, and take away the cap using tweezers.

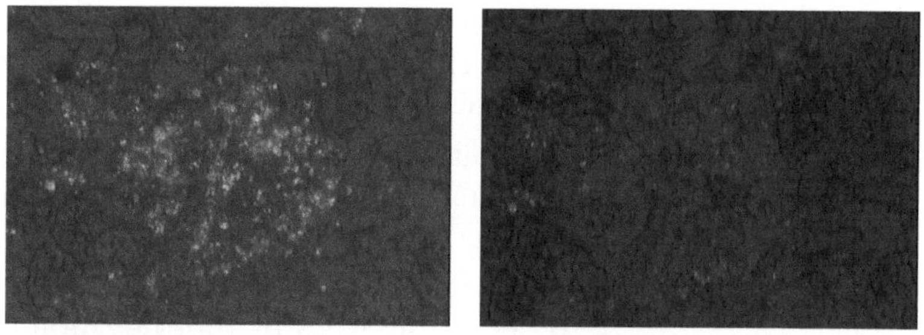

Human islet before LCM The same islet after LCM

Fig. 1. Human pancreatic tissue section dehydrated according to the described protocol and visualized using the blue color filter (excitation: 455-495 nm). The *left panel* shows an islet before the LCM, autofluorescent β-cells are noticeable as clusters. The *right panel* shows the same islet after the LCM was performed; the clusters of β-cells have been removed.

14. Remove any debris or nonspecific tissue adhesion by blotting the polymer surface with the tacky side of an adhesive note.
15. Place the cap into one spot of the Alignment Tray with the polymer end up and connect the cap with the ExtraSure device (*see* **Note 16**).
16. Place 10 μL of extraction buffer (guanidine isothiocyanate buffer) into the ExtraSure device, in contact with the dissected cells on the polymer end of the cap. Insert the ExtraSure device into the top of a thin-walled reaction tube placed upside down and incubate for 30 min at 42°C.
17. Centrifuge the tube with the ExtraSure assembly at 800 × *g* for 2 min to collect the sample in the bottom, remove the cap and the ExtraSure device, and store the sample at –80°C until the RNA extraction is performed.

3.3. RNA Extraction and Amplification

1. RNA extraction and amplification must be performed in a biosafety cabinet. We perform the RNA extraction by means of a modification of an RNA microisolation protocol *(10)* and RNA amplification using RiboAmp HS RNA Amplification Kit. However, other commercially available products may be used.
2. Combine the samples microdissected from the same pancreas into a 1.5 mL RNase-free tube in order to obtain a sample composed of at least 5,000 laser pulses (*see* **Note 15**).
3. The final volume of the sample may vary depending on the number of samples combined; in our experience it is usually less than 200 μL. In this case, in order to use the same amount of reagents for all the samples processed, it is convenient to bring the final volume of the samples to 200 μL by adding guanidinium isothiocyanate (*see* **Note 17**).

4. Add 20 μL of 2 M sodium acetate, 220 μL phenol, and 60 μL chloroform-isoamyl alcohol. Vortex vigorously and place on ice for 15 min.
5. Centrifuge at 16.1 × *g* for 30 min at 4°C to separate the aqueous and organic phases. Transfer the upper aqueous layer to a new tube; add 2 μL glycogen (10 μg/μL), 200 μL ice cold isopropanol, and place at –80°C for 1 h.
6. Pellet the RNA by centrifugation of the sample at 16.1 × *g* for 30 min at 4°C. Remove the supernatant carefully and wash the pellet with 200 μL ice cold 75% ethanol, spin at 16.1 × *g* for 5 min at 4°C; then remove ethanol and let the pellet air dry on ice to remove any residual ethanol. At this point RNA can be stored at –80°C until use.
7. For DNAse treatment resuspend the pellet in 15 μL DEPC-treated water and transfer the sample to a 500 μL tube. Add 1 μL RNase inhibitor, 2 μL 10× Reaction Buffer, and 2 μL DNase I. Incubate at 37°C for 2 h in a PCR machine.
8. For the RNA re-extraction bring the sample volume to 200 μL by adding 180 μL DEPC-treated water, place into a 1.5-mL RNase-free tube and perform the same steps described for the extraction. Add 20 μL 2 M sodium acetate, 220 μL phenol, and 60 μL chloroform-isoamyl alcohol. Vortex and place on ice for 15 min.
9. Centrifuge at 16.1 × *g* for 30 min at 4°C. Transfer upper layer to new tube; add 2 μL glycogen, 200 μL ice cold isopropanol and place at –80°C for 1 h.
10. Centrifuge at 16.1 × *g* for 30 min at 4°C to pellet the RNA. Remove the supernatant, and wash the pellet with 200 μL ice cold 75% ethanol, spin at 16.1 × *g* for 5 min at 4°C, remove the ethanol, and air dry the pellet on ice. Resuspend the pellet in 11 μL DEPC-treated water and proceed to the T7-based linear amplification of the RNA according to the protocol described by the manufacturer (*see* **Note 18**).
11. At the end of the RNA amplification, before proceeding to the RNA biotinylation and microarray analysis, assess the RNA integrity by running 100 ng of amplified RNA on Nano LabChip of Agilent 2100 Bioanalyzer (*see* **Note 19**).
12. Electropherograms, gel-like images, and RNA Integrity Numbers (RIN) of amplified RNA obtained from laser microdissected β-cells of two control and two type 2 diabetic donors are shown in **Fig. 2**.

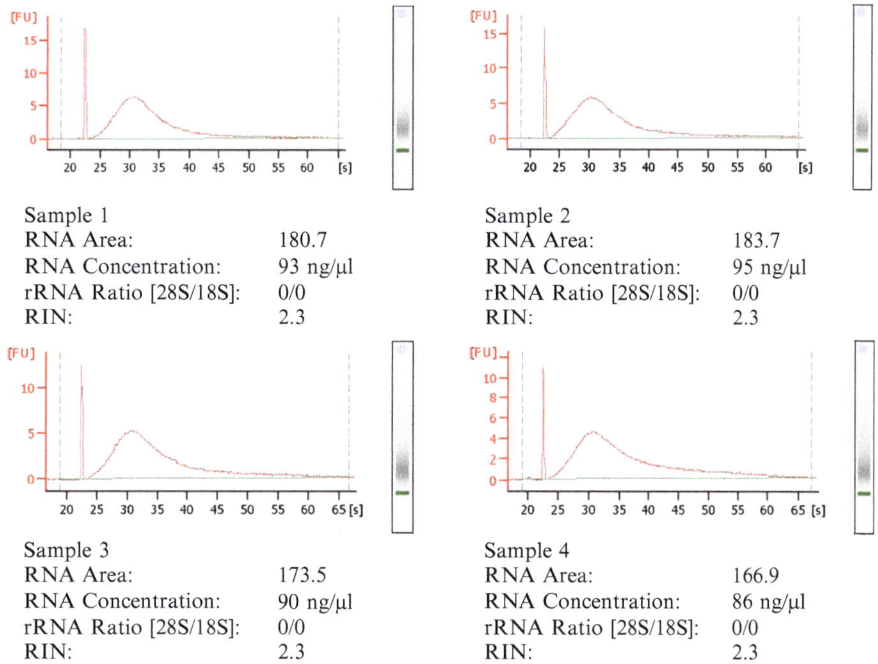

Fig. 2. Electropherograms and gel images of amplified RNA obtained from β-cells microdissected from the pancreatic tissue of two control (samples 1 and 2, *upper panel*) and two type 2 diabetic (samples 3 and 4, *lower panel*) donors. The data are representative of RNA samples obtained from six controls and six type 2 diabetic subjects. The electropherograms lose the peaks corresponding to the 18S and 28S RNA and the amplified RNA appears as a hump. On the gel-like images amplified messenger RNA appears as a smear. Extremely important and remarkable is the reproducibility of the results shown by the electropherograms, the gel images, and the RNA Integrity Numbers (RIN).

4. Notes

1. Tissue freezing should occur as soon as the specimen is procured to preserve the sample from RNA and protein degradation. The icy chamber must be prepared before the pancreatic tissue is obtained and must be ready when the tissue is provided. The freezing chamber must be maintained under a chemical fume hood until it is used for the tissue freezing.
2. The presence of nonparenchymal tissues brings a number of complexities to the LCM procedure. In particular, adipose tissue makes the sectioning procedure difficult to perform at –20°C, since the optimal sectioning temperature for adipose tissue is –30°C; this lower temperature can provoke breakage

of the tissue. Connective tissue, vessels, and nerves also affect the LCM procedure; these structures have intrinsic autofluorescence that makes identification of the autofluorescent β-cells more difficult.

3. For the tissue embedding OCT refrigerated at 4°C should be used.
4. It is important that the motion of the wheel is slow, smooth, and steady; this helps avoid breakage of the tissue and makes it possible to obtain sections without folds, which, when present, complicate the LCM procedure.
5. During the sectioning OCT may stick to the blade, making its surface uneven, and, as a consequence, lead to breakage of sections. To avoid this problem, remove the OCT by wiping down the blade using tissue paper soaked with 100% ethanol; clean the blade in an upward direction.
6. During sectioning, mark one slide of every five sections performed; keep them apart and alternatively stain them with hematoxylin/eosin (H/E) or dehydrate them using the same protocol for the LCM. The H/E staining allows evaluating the presence of islets in the tissue sections; the dehydration permits to evaluate the intensity of the autofluorescent signal. It is recommendable to draw a map of the islet distribution in the sections, which can help to quickly identify the islets and therefore the β-cells in the dehydrated sections during the LCM procedure.
7. The dehydration reagents must be prepared fresh every time and not be reused since once open ethanol absorbs water from the air, which causes reduction of the ethanol dehydration efficiency and affects the ability to perform LCM. For the same reason, in the middle of the session it can be helpful to switch to the new set of dehydration reagents and DEPC-treated water that have been prepared. The use of fresh reagents also helps avoid possible contamination by tissue RNases. The use of polypropylene conical tubes is mandatory since polypropylene is resistant to the corrosive activity of xylene.
8. Keep the box containing dry ice outside the room where the LCM experiments are performed. Dry ice sublimates into carbon dioxide gas, which displaces oxygen in the air with toxic consequences for the operator.
9. Do not allow the sections to thaw at room temperature prior to dehydration; it is critical for sections to remain frozen for successful laser microdissection.
10. Washing the sections in DEPC-treated water allows removal of OCT from the tissue, thus facilitating the adhesion of

the thermoplastic polymer film mounted on the cap, to the selected cells during the passage of the laser beam. However, for this step some precautions must be taken: the dips must be brisk and fast, since a protracted contact of the tissue with water is associated with an inexplicable decrease of β-cell autofluorescence and an increase of the autofluorescence in the pancreatic tissue, thus making the contrast between β-cells and non-β-cells faint and the identification of the β-cells difficult.

11. We have observed that keeping the slides in xylene more than 4 min dramatically decreases the β-cell autofluorescent signal. In addition, autofluorescence is very sensitive to photobleaching; therefore, in order to reduce the photobleaching and prolong the autofluorescent signal, keep the slides protected from light during the air-drying step under the fume absorber.
12. HS Caps are recommended when small spot sizes must be obtained.
13. The laser power and duration must be tested with each new pancreas sample, and, if adjustments are needed to obtain an effective laser spot, it is recommended to increase the power instead of the duration; since increasing the duration will increase spot diameter, the duration must be kept as low as possible.
14. The autofluorescence of human β-cells is more noticeable using the blue color filter, which makes the β-cells appear green.
15. The number of captured cells cannot be easily estimated since the dehydration of the tissue alters the morphology of the cells and the number of captured cells is influenced by the efficiency of the microdissection. However, a rough estimation of the quantity of captured tissue can be obtained by counting the laser pulses performed during the microdissection session. In our experience samples obtained from 5,000 laser pulses generate enough RNA for microarray.
16. The use of the Alignment Tray to connect the cap to the ExtraSure device is optional. However, we have found that its use helps to connect the cap and device firmly, thus preventing any leak of the extraction buffer.
17. For microarray experiments, it is advisable to process all the samples at the same time.
18. The RNA amplification is quite a long procedure; it requires three full days during which the protocol can be stopped overnight. Appropriate stopping points are suggested by the manufacturer. However, since cDNA is more stable than

RNA, we found it convenient to stop the procedure after the cDNA purification of round one and after cDNA purification of round two.

19. The integrity of RNA molecules is extremely important for experiments of gene profiling. The advent of microcapillary electrophoretic RNA separation provides the basis for an automated valuable approach to estimate the integrity of RNA samples in an unambiguous way.

Acknowledgments

We thank Ludger Fink and Robert Star for the help provided during the preparation of the protocol for human β-cell microdissection.

References

1. Laybutt, D.R., Kaneto, H., Hasenkamp, W., Grey, S., Jonas, J.-C., Sgroi, D.C., Groff, A., Ferran, C., Bonner-Weir, S., Sharma, A., and Weir, G.C. (2002). Increased expression of antioxidant and antiapoptotic genes in islets that may contribute to β-cell survival during chronic hyperglycemia. *Diabetes* **51**, 413–423
2. Laybutt, D.R., Sharma, A., Sgroi, D.C., Gaudet, J., Bonner-Weir, S., and Weir, G.C. (2002). Genetic regulation of metabolic pathways in β-cells disrupted by hyperglycemia. *J Biol Chem* **277**, 10912–10921
3. Gunton, J.E., Kulkarni, R.N., Yim, S., Okada, T., Hawthorne, W.J., Tseng, Y.H., Roberson, R.S., Ricordi, C., O'Connell, P.J., Gonzalez, F.J., and Kahn, C.R. (2005). Loss of ARNT/HIF1β mediates altered gene expression and pancreatic-islet dysfunction in human type 2 diabetes. *Cell* **122**, 337–349
4. Del Guerra, S., Lupi, R., Marselli, L., Masini, M., Bugliani, M., Sbrana, S., Torri, S., Pollera, M., Boggi, U., Mosca, F., Del Prato, S., and Marchetti, P. (2005). Functional and molecular defects of pancreatic islets in human type 2 diabetes. *Diabetes* **54**, 727–735
5. Bottino, R., Balamurugan, A.N., Tse, H., Thirunavukkarasu, C., Ge, X., Profozich, J., Milton, M., Ziegenfuss, A., Trucco, M., and Piganelli, J.D. (2004). Response of human islets to isolation stress and the effect of antioxidant treatment. *Diabetes* **53**, 2559–2568
6. Abdelli, S., Ansite, J., Roduit, R., Borsello, T., Matsumoto, I., Sawada, T., Allaman-Pillet, N., Henry, H., Beckmann, J.S., Hering, B.J., and Bonny, C. (2004). Intracellular stress signaling pathways activated during human islet preparation and following acute cytokine exposure. *Diabetes* **53**, 2815–2823
7. Marselli, L., Thorne, J., Ahn, Y.-B., Omer, A., Sgroi, D.C., Libermann, T., Out, H.H., Sharma, A., Bonner-Weir, S., and Weir, G.C. Gene expression of purified beta cell tissue obtained from human pancreas with laser capture microdissection. *J Clin Endocrinol Metab* **93**, 1046–1053
8. Bonner, R.F., Emmert-Buck, M., Cole, K., Pohida, T., Chuaqui, R., Goldstein, S., and Liotta, L.A. (1997). Laser capture microdissection: molecular analysis of tissue. *Science* **278**, 1481–1483
9. Fend, F., Kremer, M., and Quintanilla-Martinez, L. (2000). Laser capture microdissection: methodical aspects and applications with emphasis on Immuno-laser capture microdissection. *Pathobiology* **68**, 209–214
10. Emmert-Buck, M.R., Bonner, R.F., Smith, P.D., Chuaqui, R.F., Zhuang, Z., Goldstein, S.R., Weiss, R.A., and Liotta, L.A. (1996). Laser capture microdissection. *Science* **274**, 998–1001

Chapter 9

In Vitro Transdifferentiation of Human Hepatoma Cells into Pancreatic-Like Cells

Wan-Chun Li

Summary

Transdifferentiation is defined as an irreversible switch in postnatal life of one differentiated cell to another. Transdifferentiation from different cellular origins into pancreatic-like β-cells is of clinical significance since this approach may offer a potential cure for diabetes. In order to achieve this goal, the liver is considered as a suitable candidate due to its close developmental relationship to the pancreas, its large size and a well-documented regenerative capacity that could provide enough original tissues to initiate the transdifferentiation procedure. In this chapter, we describe a protocol to overexpress Pdx1, a master regulator essential for pancreas development in the cultured human liver cell line, HepG2.

Key words: Liver, Transdifferentiation, HepG2, Pdx1

1. Introduction

It had been generally considered that the terminally differentiated state of a cell is fixed. However, we now know this is not the case and it has become clear that the differentiation status of some cell types can be reversed *(1–3)*. The conversion between two differentiated cell types is termed "transdifferentiation." It is important to study transdifferentiation for a number of reasons. First, understanding the molecular basis of cell-type switches will enhance our knowledge of normal developmental mechanisms. Second, from a pathological point view, some metaplasias predispose to malignant cancer and may therefore reveal useful cellular or molecular information for developing treatments for these diseases. Third, perhaps of most interest at present, uncovering

C. Stocker (ed.), *Type 2 Diabetes,* Methods in Molecular Biology, vol. 560
DOI 10.1007/978-1-59745-448-3_9, © Humana Press, a part of Springer Science+Business Media, LLC 2009

the molecular and cellular mechanisms controlling transdifferentiation may improve the ability to reprogram cells for the development of therapeutic transplantation *(4, 5)*. At the molecular level, the cause of transdifferentiation is thought to reflect a change in the expression of a master regulatory (master switch) gene whose normal function is to distinguish the two tissues in normal embryonic development *(3, 6)*.

A number of cell types have been used as starting material for creating β-cells in vitro. Among them, three major tissue types, pancreatic acini *(7, 8)*, pancreatic ducts *(9, 10)* and liver cells *(11, 12)*, have been of current interest. In this chapter, we will focus on liver cells as a source of pancreatic β-cells. Although adult pancreatic insulin-secreting cells and hepatocytes possess completely different morphological and physiological functions, both tissues arise from adjacent areas of the developing germ layer - anterior foregut endoderm *(13)*. It has been proposed that a common precursor cell exists and that signals from the cardiac mesenchyme and septum transversum mesenchyme are responsible for specifying the two organs *(14)*. In the absence of these signals, the default status of the ventral foregut endoderm is to become pancreas. This close developmental relationship suggests it may be possible to convert hepatocytes to pancreatic cells by adding just one or a few transcription factors *(6)*.

Numerous transcription factors have been identified that play an important role in the specification of the different cell types in the pancreas *(15)*. One of the prime candidates for the master gene distinguishing pancreas and liver is the homeobox transcription factor, pancreatic duodenum homeobox gene 1 (Pdx1). It is expressed early in the endoderm prior to morphological development of the pancreas and has been shown to play a fundamental role in pancreatic development *(16, 17)*. In Pdx1 knockout mice, the embryonic pancreatic domain is absent and thus it is considered as a key factor for making all mature pancreatic cell types including insulin-producing cells *(18, 19)*. Several groups have overexpressed Pdx1 in liver cells *(12, 20–22)* and have shown that certain pancreatic genes including insulin were detected using real-time polymerase chain reaction (RT-PCR) analysis. However, evidence showing direct transdifferentiation from a single liver cell into insulin-producing cells is still rarely demonstrated. We have used a different approach by using a modified form of Pdx1 in which the VP16 transactivation domain from Herpes Simplex virus is fused to Pdx1 creating an activated form of the transcription factor. Transfection of the Pdx1-VP16 construct into human hepatoma cells (HepG2) induces the expression of insulin in at least some cells *(23)*.

2. Materials

2.1. Cell Culture

1. Human hepatoma cell line HepG2: HepG2 cells were obtained from the European Collection of Cell Cultures (ECACC, UK). The HepG2 cell line was derived from a liver biopsy of a male Caucasian (aged 15 years) *(24)*. It is a well-differentiated hepatocellular carcinoma and has been shown to secrete a range of liver serum proteins *(24, 25)*.
2. Culture medium for HepG2 cells: Dulbecco's Modified Eagle's Medium (with 5.5 or 25 mM glucose) containing 100 units/ml penicillin, 100 μg/ml streptomycin, 2 mM L-glutamine, 1× MEM nonessential amino acids, and 10% fetal bovine serum (FBS).
3. PBS.
4. Trypsin-EDTA solution.
5. Benchtop MSE mistral 1,000 centrifuge.
6. 0.5% (w/v) Trypan blue solution.
7. Fisherbrand 22 mm × 22 mm coverslips (Fisher Scientific, UK).
8. Sterile 35 mm cell culture dishes.
9. Freezing medium: FBS mixed with 10% (v/v) DMSO.
10. Hemocytometer.

2.2. Molecular Cloning

1. Competent bacterial cells: E coli JM109 (Promega, UK).
2. Bacteria culture medium and plates: Luria-Bertani broth and Luria-Bertani agar containing ampicillin (*see* **Note 1**).
3. T4 ligase, DNA polymerase I, large (Klenow) fragment and restriction enzymes (New England Biolabs, UK) (*see* **Note 2**).
4. DNA markers (Gibco™/Invitrogen Life Technologies).
5. DNA isolation kits: QIAEX II gel extraction kit (Qiagen, UK), Wizard Plus SV minipreps DNA purification system and Wizard Plus SV maxipreps DNA purification systems (Promega, UK) (*see* **Note 3**).

2.3. Gene Delivery: Transfection Reagent

1. GeneJuice (Novagene, USA). Store at 4°C.

2.4. Semiquantitative RT-PCR

1. TRI reagent (Sigma, UK).
2. Chloroform.
3. 2-Isopropanol.
4. Spectrophotometer.
5. RNA-Complementary DNA (cDNA) hybrid decontamination: RQ1 RNase-free DNase (Promega, UK).

Table 1
Primers used for (Semi-) quantitative PCR

Human insulin (Gene accession number: NM_000207) Forward: AGCCTTTGTGAACCAACACC Reverse: GCTGGTAGAGGGAGCAGATG
Human GLP1 receptor (GLP1R) (Gene accession number: NM_002062) Forward: GTTCCCCTGCTGTTTGTTGT Reverse: CTTGGCAAGTCTGCATTTGA
Human Prohormone convertase 1/3 (PC1/3) (Gene accession number: NM_033508) Forward: TTGGCTGAAAGAGAACGGGATACATCT Reverse: ACTTCTTTGGTGATTGCTTTGGCGGTG
Human β-actin (Gene accession number: NM_001101) Forward: AGAAAATCTGGCACCACACC Reverse: GGGGTGTTGAAGGTCTCAAA

6. cDNA synthesis: SuperScript™ First-Strand Synthesis System (Gibco™/Invitrogen Life Technologies).
7. PCR reagents (final concentration): 1× PCR buffer, 1.5 mM $MgCl_2$, 0.2 mM dNTP, 50 ng sense/antisense primers, and 1.25 units platinum Taq polymerase (Gibco™/Invitrogen Life Technologies).
8. DNA thermal cycler.
9. 1 Kb ladder marker.
10. Lightcycler system.
11. SYBR® Green Taq ReadyMix™for RT-PCR.
12. Primers: synthesized by Invitrogen (*see* **Table 1**).

2.5. Immunostaining and Image Processing

1. Fixative: 4% (w/v) paraformaldehyde (PFA) (*see* **Note 4**).
2. Permeabilizing solution: 0.1% (v/v) Triton X-100 in PBS.
3. 2% (w/v) Blocking buffer (Boehringer Mannheim, UK).
4. Stainless staining rack for coverslips (102 × 28 × 30 mm, Thermo Scientific).
5. Gel/Mount mounting medium (Biomeda, Foster City, CA).
6. Rectangular staining jar.
7. Primary antibodies (*see* **Note 5**):
   (a) Guinea pig anti-insulin antiserum (1:300 dilution; Sigma, UK).
   (b) Mouse monoclonal anti-C/EBPβ antiserum (1:100 dilution; Santa Cruz Biotechnology).
   (c) Rabbit polyclonal anti-albumin antiserum (1:300 dilution; Sigma, UK).

(d) Rabbit polyclonal anti-α1-antitrypsin antiserum (1:100 dilution; Sigma, UK).

(e) Rabbit polyclonal anti-HNF4α antiserum (1:100 dilution; Santa Cruz Biotechnology).

(f) Rabbit polyclonal anti-human C-peptide antiserum (1:100; Acris Antibodies).

8. Secondary antibodies:

(g) Goat anti-guinea pig fluorescein isothiocyanate (FITC)-conjugated IgG (1:200; Vector Laboratories).

(h) Horse anti-mouse FITC-conjugated IgG (1:200; Vector Laboratories).

(i) Goat anti-mouse FITC-conjugated IgG (1:200; Vector Laboratories).

(j) Anti-rabbit tetramethylrhodamine isothiocyanate (TRITC)-conjugated IgG (1:200, Vector Laboratories).

9. Zeiss LSM 510 confocal microscope. For the immunostainings on HepG2 cells, images are taken under 10× (eyepiece) and 40× (objective).

2.6. Glucose-Stimulated Insulin Secretion ELISA Assay

1. Centricon YM-3 centrifugal filter devices (Millipore Corporation, nominal molecular weight limit 3 kDa).
2. Bio-Rad protein reagent (Bio-Rad Laboratories).
3. Protein standard: bovine serum albumin.
4. Human insulin ELISA kit.
5. ELISA standard: recombinant human insulin.
6. Microplate ELISA Reader.

3. Methods

3.1. Preparation of HepG2 Cells for Immunostaining

1. Prior to splitting the cells, prewarm the culture medium and trypsin–EDTA solution to 37°C.
2. For each 75 cm^2 flask of HepG2 cells (at ~80% confluence), decant the culture medium and wash the cells with 10 ml of sterile PBS to remove any excess medium. Remove the PBS and add 5 ml of trypsin–EDTA solution and incubate at 37°C for 3–5 min to detach the cells from the flask.
3. Tap the side of the flask to remove any adherent cells. Add 5 ml of trypsin–EDTA solution to a 50 ml Falcon tube and add the same volume of complete medium to neutralize the activity of the trypsin. Centrifuge the cells at 120–150 × *g* in a benchtop

for 4 min at room temperature. Remove the supernatant and resuspend the cell pellet with 1 ml of fresh medium.

4. For cell maintenance, 250 μl (1:4 dilution, *see* **Note 6**) of total cell suspension is plated out into a new 75 cm^2 flask containing 15 ml of fresh complete medium. For immunostaining, plate approximately 2–5 × 10^4 living cells (examined by trypan blue exclusion, *see* **Note 7**) onto a coverslip in a sterile 35 mm plastic culture dish. Incubate the cells at 37°C, in an atmosphere of 95% air/5% CO_2 (v/v). HepG2 cells express protein characteristics of mature liver cells including albumin, α1-antitrypsin, and the liver-enriched transcription factors C/EBPβ and HNF4α. Confirm the phenotype of the HepG2 cells by immunostaining (examples are shown in **Fig. 1a**; for immunostaining protocol, see below).

3.2. Plasmid Construction and Transfection

1. The plasmid backbones are:

   (a) pCS2-pTTR-Xlhbox8VP16 *(26)*: the portion of pElastase-GFP is deleted from the pCS2-pTTR-Xlhbox8VP16;

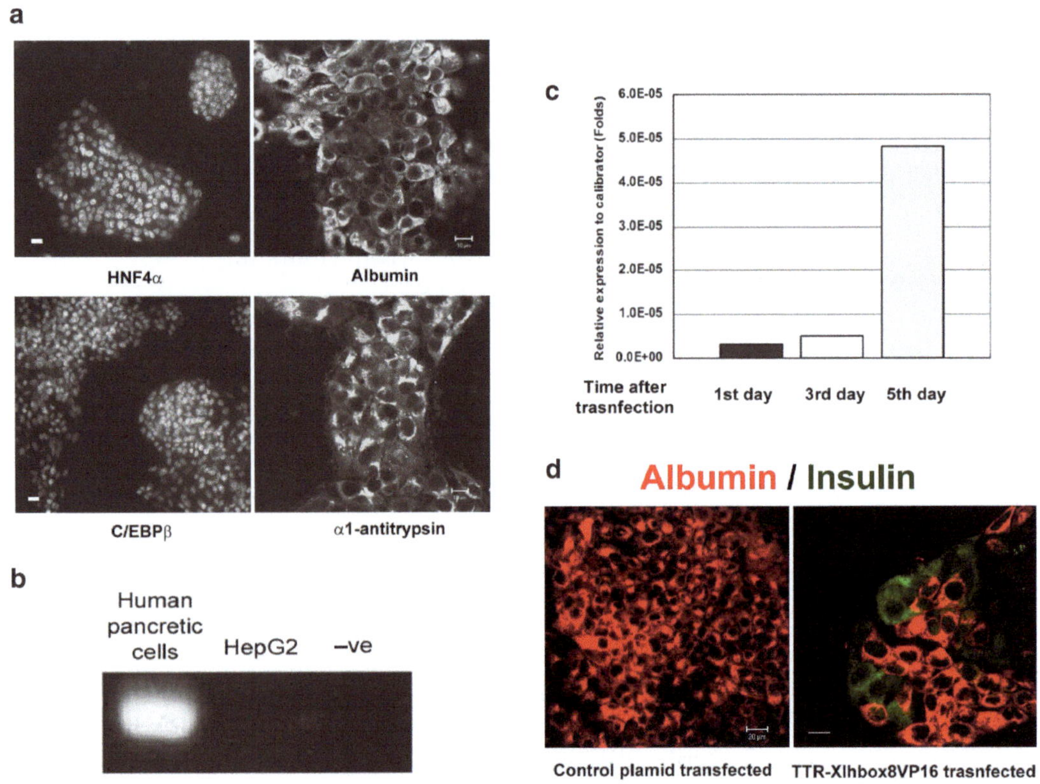

Fig. 1. Molecular changes during transdifferentiation of HepG2 cells into pancreatic-like cells. (a) Liver-specific proteins including liver-enriched transcription factors HNF4α and C/EBPβ (scale bar 50 μm) and cytoplasmic protein albumin and α1-antitrypsin (scale bar 10 μm) are detected in HepG2 cells but no insulin mRNA (b) was detected using semiquantitative RT-PCR analysis. (c) After transfection of pCS2-TTR-Xlhbox8VP16, qRT-PCR analysis shows that insulin mRNA exhibited a time-dependent increase within 5 days. Human pancreatic tissue mRNA was used as a calibrator. (d) At the protein level, some pCS2-TTR-Xlhbox8VP16 transfected HepG2 cells lost liver protein, albumin, and gained a pancreatic phenotype by the detection of insulin (scale bar 20 μm).

pElastase-GFP plasmid using *Not I* restriction digestion and relegation using T4 ligase at 20°C overnight.

(b) The control plasmid pCS2-pTTR-VP16 is generated by removing the Xlhbox8 part in pCS2-TTR-Xlhbox8VP16 with *NotI* restriction digestion and relegation using T4 ligase at 20°C overnight.

2. To confirm the accuracy of the cloning, digest the plasmid DNAs with *XbaI* restriction digestion at 37°C for 2 h.
3. Separate the digested products by electrophoresis in a 1–1.5% agarose gel. For pCS2-TTR-Xlhbox8VP16, two 4 Kb fragments can be detected and for pCS2-pTTR-VP16, one 4 Kb and one 3.2 Kb fragment will be seen.
4. Transfect the plasmids into HePG2 cells using GeneJuice transfection reagent according to the manufacturer's recommendation. Briefly, for each reaction, mix 3 μl GeneJuice reagent with 100 μl serum–free medium and allow to stand at room temperature for 5 min. Add 1–2 μg purified plasmid DNA into the GeneJuice-medium mixture and incubate for 20–30 min. Finally, evenly distribute the GeneJuice–DNA mixture over the cells. On the following day, approximately 16 h after transfection, replace the medium containing GeneJuice for fresh culture medium.
5. Replace the medium every 2 days until the desired day. Wash the cells with PBS to remove medium and fix in 4% PFA at room temperature for 20 min. The cells can be stored in PBS at 4°C long term (for up to 6 months) for further immunostaining.

3.3. Detection for Induction of Pancreatic Messenger RNA Expression in HepG2 Cells After Introduction of Active Form Pdx1

3.3.1. RNA Extraction (see Note 8)

1. Add 1 ml TRI reagent directly, using filter tips, onto each 35 mm dish to break up the cells. After pipetting up and down for several times, transfer the cells-TRI reagent mixture to a sterile 1.5 ml eppendorf.
2. For each 1 ml of TRI reagent, add 0.2 ml chloroform and vigorously vortex. Incubate the tubes at room temperature for 2-15 min and then centrifuge at 12,000 × *g* for 15 min. The total RNA is now in the upper aqueous phase.
3. Transfer the aqueous phase into a new sterile 1.5 ml eppendorf tube and add an equal volume of 2-isopropanol. Incubate the mixture at room temperature for 10 min and centrifuge at 12,000 × *g* for 10 min.
4. Remove the supernatant. The total RNA pellets may be seen transparently. Air-dry the RNA (*see* **Note 9**).
5. Add an appropriate volume of nuclease-free water and incubate at –80°C overnight to dissolve the RNA completely.
6. Perform a digestion of the total RNA with RQ1 RNase-free DNase to eliminate any contaminating genomic DNA (*see*

Note 10). Measure the concentration of the extracted RNA on a spectrophotometer. The ratio of 260 nm to 280 nm of each sample should be in the range from 1.8 to 2.0.

7. Store the isolated total RNA at –80°C.

3.3.2. Reverse Transcription

1. Messenger RNA (mRNA) is isolated from total RNA by using the SuperScript™ First–Strand Synthesis System for RT–PCR. First, isolate mRNA by incubating Oligo(dT)$_{12-18}$ oligonucleotides and 1 μl dNTP (stock concentration 10 mM) with 1 μg of the extracted total RNA. Incubate the mixture at 65°C for 5 min and cool to 4°C for at least 2 min.
2. cDNA is then prepared by SuperScript™ II reverse transcriptase treatment. For each microgram of total RNA, combine 1× Superscript first strand buffer (final concentration), 1 μl DTT (stock concentration 100 mM), 2 μl $MgCl_2$ (stock concentration 25 mM), 200 units SuperScript™ II reverse transcriptase, and 40 units of RNaseOut RNase inhibitor and incubate at 42°C for 60 min and then 70°C for 15 min followed by a chill to 4°C.
3. Incubate the cDNA reactions with two units of RNase H at 37°C for 20 min to remove the RNA-cDNA hybridized residues. The cDNA is stable at –20°C for up to 6 months for further analysis.

3.3.3. Semiquantitative PCR

1. Set up the PCR reactions containing the cDNA, 1x PCR buffer, 1.5 mM $MgCl_2$, 0.2 mM dNTP, 50 ng forward/reverse primers, and 1.25 units platinum Taq polymerase in a DNA thermal cycler using the following conditions: denaturation at 94°C for 1 min, amplification at 58°C for 1 min, and elongation at 72°C for 1 min for 30–40 cycles.
2. Analyze the samples by electrophoresis in 1–1.5% agarose using a 1 Kb ladder. The detection of insulin in human pancreatic cells and HepG2 cells is shown in **Fig. 1b**.

3.3.4. Quantitative PCR

1. To obtain more quantitative results, RT-PCR, using a Lightcycler system (Roche Applied Science) or similar, is performed. Combine cDNA from control and experimental cell extracts with 1× SYBR@ Green Taq ReadyMix™(Sigma, UK), 50 ng of forward and reverse primers and transfer into Lightcycler capillaries.
2. Set up the PCR reactions using the following conditions: denaturation at 95°C for 30 s, amplification at 58°C for 5 s followed by 72°C for 20 s for 40 cycles, and cooling at 40°C for 2 min. The fluorescence signal is detected at the same time point of each cycle. Data are presented as the normalized ratio

$$(\text{Conc.}_{[\text{target gene(experimental)}]} / \text{Conc.}_{[\text{reference gene(experimental)}]} : \text{Conc.}_{[\text{target gene(control)}]} / \text{Conc.}_{[\text{reference gene(control)}]})$$

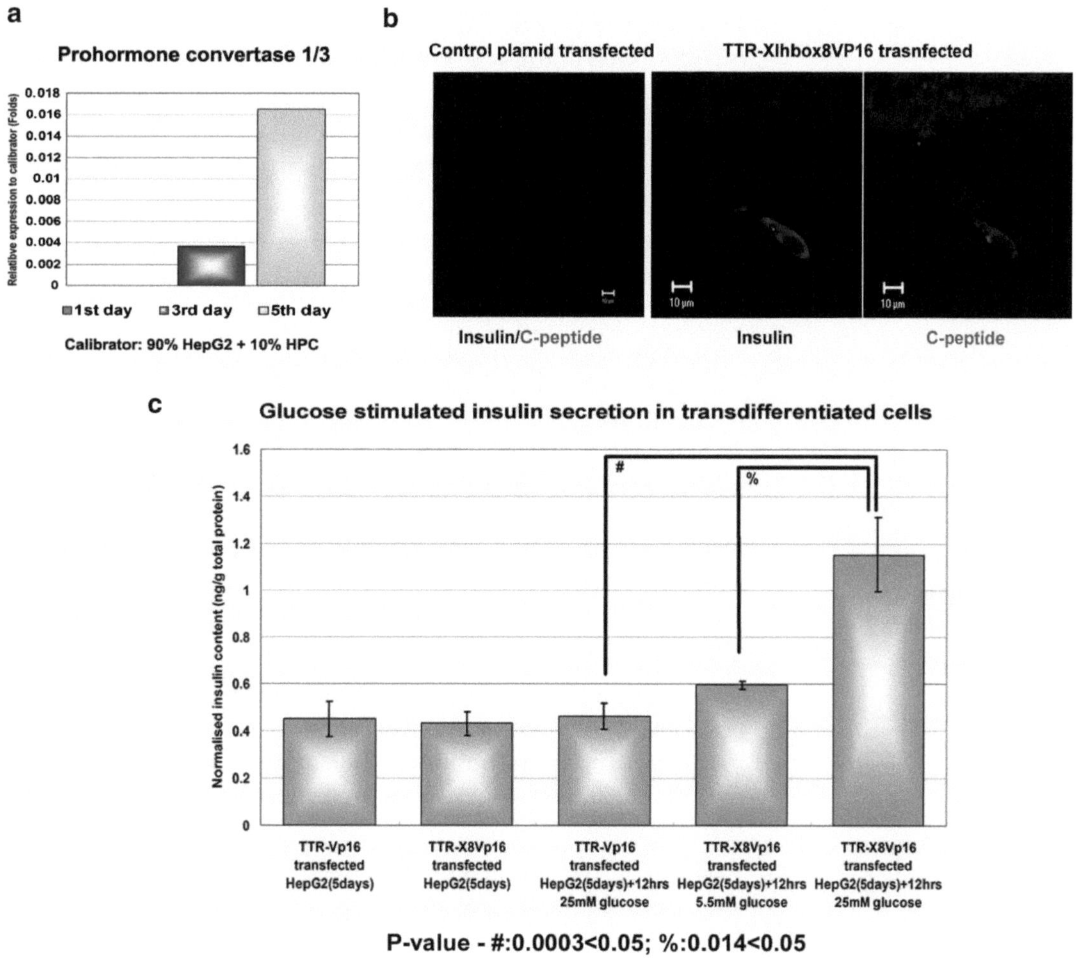

Fig. 2. Functional analysis of transdifferentiated β-like cells. (**a**) Prohormone convertase 1/3 (PC1/3) was detected in HepG2 cells following pCS2-TTR-Xlhbox8VP16 transfection. RT-PCR analysis was performed on RNA isolated from transfected cells at the time points indicated. The calibrator used is cDNA generated from the mixture of 90% HepG2 cells plus 10% human pancreatic cells. (**b**) C-peptide and insulin colocalization in transdifferentiated cells. The immunofluorescence staining showed that human C-peptide and insulin were coexpressed in transdifferentiated cells after 5 days of Xlhbox8VP16 but neither is seen in the control (TTR-VP16) transfected cells (scale bar 10 μm). (**c**) Transdifferentiated β-cells secrete insulin in response to glucose. Control cells (TTR-VP16 transfected cells and cultured for 5 days) or transdifferentiated cells (cells transfected with TTR-Xlhbox8VP16 and cultured for 5 days) were treated with physiological (5.5 mM) or higher concentrations (25 mM) of glucose for 12 h. The medium was collected and the secreted insulin was detected by ELISA. Following treatment with high concentrations of glucose, transdifferentiated cells significantly released more insulin compared with the control cells. The data are represented as mean ± SD from three independent experiments.

according to the Lightcycler Relative Quantification software. In this case, β-actin is the reference gene used. Quantitative analysis for the induced expression of insulin and PC1/3 mRNA in HepG2 cells overexpressing Xlhbox8VP16 protein is shown in **Figs. 1c** and **2a**, respectively.

3.4. Immunostaining for Pancreatic and Hepatocytes Proteins in HepG2 Cells Following Ectopic Expression of the Activated Form Pdx1

1. Permeabilize the fixed cells with 0.1% (v/v) Triton X-100 in PBS for 30 min at room temperature.

2. Incubate the cells in 2% blocking buffer for at least 1 h. Then incubate overnight at 4°C with the primary antibody.
3. On the following day, wash the cells with PBS. Add the fluorescently conjugated secondary antibodies onto the coverslips for 3 h and then wash three times with PBS for 5 min. The dilutions are given in **Subheading 2.5**.
4. If detecting more than one antigen, add the primary and secondary antibodies sequentially using the same protocol.
5. Mount the slides with Gel/Mount mounting medium or equivalent and store in the dark for later observation. The confocal image for insulin (+)/liver protein (−) cells is shown in **Fig. 1d**. The detection of colocalization of insulin and human C-peptide in single transdifferentiated cells is shown in **Fig. 2b**.

3.5. Detection of Secreted Insulin from Transdifferentiated Pancreatic Cells

3.5.1. Sample Collection

1. Transfect the cells with pCS2-TTR-VP16 or pCS2-TTR-Xlhbox8VP16 plasmids and culture for 5 days. Replace with medium containing either normal glucose (5.5 mM) or high glucose (25 mM) for 12 h.
2. Harvest the media and then concentrate using Centricon YM-3 Centrifugal Filter Devices. Around 15–20 ml medium can be applied into the sample reservoir and centrifuged at 6,500 × *g* until all medium had been filtered (*see* **Note 11**).
3. Collect the concentrated samples into retentate vials by inverting the unit and centrifuging at 1,000 × *g* for 5 min.

3.5.2. Total Protein Concentration Analysis

1. Perform a protein assay using Bio-Rad protein reagent or equivalent. Use a 1:1,000 dilution of the sample and standard (0-25 μg/μl bovine serum albumin) proteins are mixed with a 1:5 volume of assay reagent and incubated at room temperature for 5 min.
2. Measure the optical density at 595 nm using a microplate ELISA reader. Correct all samples to the blank and plot a standard curve of absorbance against total protein concentration. Determine the protein sample concentration from the standard curve.

3.5.3. Insulin ELISA Analysis

1. Measure the insulin concentration in the medium by ELISA using a human insulin assay. Dilute both the samples and recombinant human insulin standards in distilled H_2O, assay in triplicate for each experiment. Plot a standard curve of absorbance against insulin concentration and determine the insulin concentration in each sample. Represent the secreted insulin concentration in each condition as insulin (ng)/total protein (g). Sample results are shown in **Fig. 2c**.

4. Notes

1. All chemicals are dissolved in sterile distilled water unless otherwise stated.
2. For digestion of restriction enzymes, the compatible buffer needs to be used to reach maximum activity of enzymatic reaction. A detailed list can be found from New England Biolabs website at http://www.neb.uk.com
3. The protocol for the isolation of plasmid DNA from either agarose gel or cultured bacteria is according to manufacturer's instruction.
4. For the preparation of 100 ml 4% PFA, add 4 g PFA to 85 ml lukewarm PBS. Adjust the pH to 7.4 by adding 10 M NaOH and concentrated HCl. Adjust the final volume with PBS. Do not use the exact volume of PBS from the beginning due to possible need of large additions of NaOH or HCl when adjusting pH.
5. Dilute all the primary and secondary antiserum in 2% blocking buffer.
6. During the culture of HepG2 cells, ensure cells are passaged at 1:4 to retain a consistent phenotype. The use of early passages is recommended.
7. Assess cell viability using trypan blue exclusion assay in culture. Briefly, add an equal volume of cell suspension and trypan blue solution onto a hemocytometer and calculate the percentage of trypan blue negative cells, these are viable cells.
8. During all handling of RNA, prevent RNase contamination. Where possible, wipe all equipment with RNaseZap® RNase decontamination solution (Ambion, Inc.) and change gloves periodically.
9. Do not dry the RNA using a vacuum suction method as this may cause RNase contamination and can overdry the RNA pellet, which reduces the solubility of the RNA in water.
10. Set up the DNase digestion reaction as follows: mix RNA with nuclease free water to a total volume of 8 μl. Add RQ1 RNAse-free DNase 10× reaction buffer 1 μl and RQ1 RNase-free DNase 1 μl. Incubate at 37°C for 30 min. To stop the reaction, add 1 μl RQ1 DNase stop solution into the mixture and incubate at 65°C for 10 min. In general, use 1 unit of RQ1 RNase-free DNase per microgram of RNA.
11. Centrifugation of 2 ml collection medium takes around 6–8 hours. To obtain a more concentrated medium, do not change the centrifugation set between each centrifugation.

References

1. Slack, J.M., (1985). *Homoeotic transformations in man: implications for the mechanism of embryonic development and for the organization of epithelia.* J Theor Biol, **114**: 463–490
2. Slack, J.M., (1986). *Epithelial metaplasia and the second anatomy.* Lancet, **2**: 268–271
3. Tosh, D. and J.M. Slack, (2002). How cells change their phenotype. Nat Rev Mol Cell Biol, **3**: 187–194
4. Burke, Z.D. and D. Tosh, (2005). *Therapeutic potential of transdifferentiated cells.* Clin Sci (Lond), **108**: 309–321
5. Kume, S., (2005). *Stem-cell-based approaches for regenerative medicine.* Dev Growth Differ, **47**: 393–402
6. Slack, J.M. and D. Tosh, (2001). *Transdifferentiation and metaplasia - switching cell types.* Curr Opin Genet Dev, **11**: 581–586
7. Lardon, J., N. Huyens, I. Rooman, and L. Bouwens, (2004). *Exocrine cell transdifferentiation in dexamethasone-treated rat pancreas.* Virchows Arch, **444**: 61–65
8. Baeyens, L., S. De Breuck, J. Lardon, J.K. Mfopou, I. Rooman, and L. Bouwens, (2005). *In vitro generation of insulin-producing beta cells from adult exocrine pancreatic cells.* Diabetologia, **48**: 49–57
9. Bonner-Weir, S., M. Taneja, G.C. Weir, K. Tatarkiewicz, K.H. Song, A. Sharma, and J.J. O'Neil, (2000). *In vitro cultivation of human islets from expanded ductal tissue.* Proc Natl Acad Sci U S A, **97**: 7999–8004
10. Yatoh, S., R. Dodge, T. Akashi, A. Omer, A. Sharma, G.C. Weir, and S. Bonner-Weir, (2007). *Differentiation of affinity-purified human pancreatic duct cells to beta-cells.* Diabetes, **56**: 1802–1809
11. Yamada, S., Y. Yamamoto, M. Nagasawa, A. Hara, T. Kodera, and I. Kojima, (2006). *In vitro transdifferentiation of mature hepatocytes into insulin-producing cells.* Endocr J, **53**: 789–795
12. Ferber, S., A. Halkin, H. Cohen, I. Ber, Y. Einav, I. Goldberg, I. Barshack, R. Seijffers, J. Kopolovic, N. Kaiser, and A. Karasik, (2000). *Pancreatic and duodenal homeobox gene 1 induces expression of insulin genes in liver and ameliorates streptozotocin-induced hyperglycemia.* Nat Med, 6: 568–572
13. Wells, J.M. and D.A. Melton, (1999). *Vertebrate endoderm development.* Annu Rev Cell Dev Biol, **15**: 393–410
14. Jung, J., M. Zheng, M. Goldfarb, and K.S. Zaret, (1999). *Initiation of mammalian liver development from endoderm by fibroblast growth factors.* Science, **284**: 1998–2003
15. Murtaugh, L.C., (2007). *Pancreas and beta-cell development: from the actual to the possible.* Development, **134**: 427–438
16. Offield, M.F., T.L. Jetton, P.A. Labosky, M. Ray, R.W. Stein, M.A. Magnuson, B.L. Hogan, and C.V. Wright, (1996). *PDX-1 is required for pancreatic outgrowth and differentiation of the rostral duodenum.* Development, **122**: 983–995
17. Holland, A.M., L.J. Gonez, G. Naselli, R.J. Macdonald, and L.C. Harrison, (2005). *Conditional expression demonstrates the role of the homeodomain transcription factor Pdx1 in maintenance and regeneration of beta-cells in the adult pancreas.* Diabetes, **54**: 2586–2595
18. Ahlgren, U., J. Jonsson, L. Jonsson, K. Simu, and H. Edlund, (1998). *beta-cell-specific inactivation of the mouse Ipf1/Pdx1 gene results in loss of the beta-cell phenotype and maturity onset diabetes.* Genes Dev, **12**: 1763–1768
19. Jonsson, J., L. Carlsson, T. Edlund, and H. Edlund, (1994). *Insulin-promoter-factor 1 is required for pancreas development in mice.* Nature, **371**: 606–609
20. Ber, I., K. Shternhall, S. Perl, Z. Ohanuna, I. Goldberg, I. Barshack, L. Benvenisti-Zarum, I. Meivar-Levy, and S. Ferber, (2003). *Functional, persistent, and extended liver to pancreas transdifferentiation.* J Biol Chem, **278**: 31950–31957
21. Miyatsuka, T., H. Kaneto, Y. Kajimoto, S. Hirota, Y. Arakawa, Y. Fujitani, Y. Umayahara, H. Watada, Y. Yamasaki, M.A. Magnuson, J. Miyazaki, and M. Hori, (2003). *Ectopically expressed PDX-1 in liver initiates endocrine and exocrine pancreas differentiation but causes dysmorphogenesis.* Biochem Biophys Res Commun, **310**: 1017–1025
22. Tang, D.Q., L.Z. Cao, W. Chou, L. Shun, C. Farag, M.A. Atkinson, S.W. Li, L.J. Chang, and L.J. Yang, (2006). *Role of Pax4 in Pdx1-VP16-mediated liver-to-endocrine pancreas transdifferentiation.* Lab Invest, **86**: 829–841
23. Li, W.C., M.E. Horb, D. Tosh, and J.M. Slack, (2005). In vitro transdifferentiation of hepatoma cells into functional pancreatic cells. Mech Dev, **122**: 835–847
24. Aden, D.P., A. Fogel, S. Plotkin, I. Damjanov, and B.B. Knowles, (1979). *Controlled synthesis of HBsAg in a differentiated human liver carcinoma-derived cell line.* Nature, **282**: 615–616
25. Dashti, N. and G. Wolfbauer, (1987). *Secretion of lipids, apolipoproteins, and lipoproteins by human hepatoma cell line, HepG2: effects of oleic acid and insulin.* J Lipid Res, **28**: 423–436
26. Horb, M.E., C.N. Shen, D. Tosh, and J.M. Slack, (2003). Experimental Conversion of liver to pancreas. Curr Biol, **13**: 105–115

Chapter 10

The Measurement of GLUT4 Translocation in 3T3-L1 Adipocytes

Nicky Konstantopoulos and Juan Carlos Molero-Navajas

Summary

Type 2 diabetes (T2D) is one of the fastest growing threats to human health in westernised and developing countries and is associated with central obesity, atherosclerosis, dyslipidaemia, hyperinsulinaemia and hypertension. Insulin resistance, defined as a diminished response to ordinary levels of circulating insulin in one or more peripheral tissues, is an integral feature of T2D pathophysiology. This includes an impairment of insulin to inhibit hepatic glucose output and to stimulate glucose disposal into muscle and fat. While insulin is responsible for a number of specific biological responses, stimulation of glucose transport is critical for the maintenance of glucose homeostasis. The primary mechanism for insulin stimulation of glucose uptake into muscle and fat is the translocation of glucose transporter 4 (GLUT4) to the cell surface from intracellular storage vesicles within the cell. A major advantage in focussing on insulin regulation of glucose transport is that this represents the endpoint of multiple upstream signalling pathways. This chapter describes the measurement of GLUT4 translocation in cultured cells and its potential application for both mechanistic and therapeutic studies.

Key words: GLUT4, Adipocyte, Translocation assay, Plasma membrane lawns, Subcellular fractionation

1. Introduction

One of the main events of insulin action is the stimulation of glucose entry into muscle and fat cells. Glucose uptake is mediated by translocation of GLUT4 from an intracellular store to the plasma membrane (PM). In the absence of insulin, endogenous GLUT4 in adipocytes and myocytes is sequestered in intracellular tubulo-vesicular (T-V) structures that are clustered either in the trans-golgi network and/or in cytoplasm. In the presence of acute insulin, there is a marked increase in cell surface GLUT4

C. Stocker (ed.), *Type 2 Diabetes,* Methods in Molecular Biology, vol. 560
DOI 10.1007/978-1-59745-448-3_10, © Humana Press, a part of Springer Science+Business Media, LLC 2009

correlated with decreased intracellular T-V GLUT4 in endosomes and coated pits. GLUT4 then recycles from the PM in the presence of insulin *(1, 2)*.

The transport of GLUT4 into insulin-responsive cells has been described by the SNARE hypothesis. V-SNARES are membrane proteins found in the GLUT4-containing transport vesicles. T-SNARES are membrane proteins found on relevant target membranes, such as the PM. The main processes involved are highlighted below *(3)*:

1. Vesicle tethering: Rab proteins (GTPases) are responsible for tethering GLUT4-containing vesicles to the PM. This process involves the recruitment of cytosolic effector proteins for vesicle tethering to docking sites on the PM.
2. Vesicle docking: The formation of a stable complex between SNARE proteins brings GLUT4-containing vesicles and the PM into close proximity.
3. Membrane fusion: The docked GLUT4-containing vesicles fuse with the membrane and deliver their contents.

Several methodologies have been developed to measure GLUT4 movement in insulin-responsive cells. The HA-GLUT4 translocation assay can accurately quantify the amount of exogenous HA-GLUT4 exposed outside of the cell, but requires the expression of exogenous tagged GLUT4 molecules (*see* **Note 1**). Since the translocation assay quantifies the tagged GLUT4 moiety outside the PM, this assay measures 'membrane fusion' in contrast to other assays detailed here. The PM lawns technique provides a snapshot of endogenous GLUT4 translocated to the PM; however, this technique does not discern between GLUT4 molecules fused with the PM and then exposed to the exterior of the cell, and GLUT4-containing vesicles tethered to but not fused with the PM. This technique does, however, allow for the simultaneous determination of the presence and distribution of other molecules involved in GLUT4 signalling and trafficking such as SNARE proteins.

Similar to the PM lawns technique, determination of GLUT4 at the PM by differential centrifugation does not provide information about the functionality of the glucose transporters and the PM fraction is easily contaminated with membranes from other intracellular compartments. However, the subcellular fractionation technique does allow for the simultaneous analysis of post-translational modifications on GLUT4 molecules (e.g. phosphorylation and glycation) and GLUT4 interactions with GLUT4-containing vesicle resident proteins by immuno-purification. Imaging techniques such as total internal reflection fluorescence microscopy microscopy have focussed on the PM as the target, since it has been shown that insulin regulates the docking and/or fusion of GLUT4-containing vesicles with the PM. Such tools used to dissect GLUT4 trafficking are not detailed in this chapter, and the reader should refer to the following reviews *(4, 5)*. This chapter describes the detailed measurement of GLUT4 translocation in cultured 3T3-L1 adipocytes using the ELISA-based GLUT4 translocation and PM lawns techniques and their potential application for both mechanistic and therapeutic studies. A third technique is also described in this chapter, the use of subcellular fractionation to measure GLUT4 translocation, however in lesser detail. The reader should refer to the following references for thorough guidance on the latter technique *(6, 7)*.

2. Materials

2.1. Intact Cell GLUT4 Translocation Assay

2.1.1. HA-Tagged GLUT4 Mammalian Retroviral Plasmid

GLUT4 spans the PM 12 times with both its N- and C-termini located in the cytosol. This assay is based on the retroviral expression of cDNA encoding human GLUT4 with a haemagglutinin (HA1) tag inserted between amino acids 67 and 68 in the first exofacial loop, which is used as a reporter gene, so that GLUT4 translocation can be studied exclusively. The pBabe HA-GLUT4 plasmid described here was kindly provided by Prof. David James *(8)* (*see* **Notes 2** and **3**). Prepare this plasmid using Qiagen's Endofree plasmid maxi kit.

2.1.2. Gelatin Coating of 96-Well Plates

1. Black Clear Bottom 96-well Microtest™ Optilux™ plates (BD Falcon™; Becton, Dickinson and Company, UK).
2. Gelatin [1% (w/v)]: Dissolve 10 g gelatin in 1 L mH_2O, heat to 55°C for 1 h. While still warm, filter through a 0.22 μm polyethersulfone filter unit (Corning Incorporated, Corning, USA) and store at 4°C.
3. Sterile Dulbecco's phosphate-buffered saline (D-PBS) that contains no calcium or magnesium. 1× PBS pH 7.4, store at 4°C. Final concentrations 137 mM NaCl, 2.7 mM KCl, 1.5 mM KH_2PO_4 and 8.0 mM Na_2HPO_4.
4. Working solution of 0.5% glutaraldehyde: Add 1 ml 25% glutaraldehyde stock (Electron Microscopy Sciences, USA) to 50 ml sterile PBS.
5. Dulbecco's modified Eagle's cell culture medium (D-MEM), 1× liquid (high glucose) containing 4,500 mg/L D-glucose, L-glutamine and 100 mg/L sodium pyruvate.

2.1.3. Preparation of HA-GLUT4 Retrovirus Using Plat-E Packaging Cells

Cells: Platinum-E (Plat-E) cells are a potent retrovirus packaging line generated from the HEK-293T cell line *(12)*. HEK-293T or BOSC23 cells can also be used. The purpose of these packaging cell lines is to produce high and stable expression of viral structural proteins. For expression of viral structural genes (gag-pol and env), Plat-E packaging constructs use the EF1α promoter, as well as the Kozak's consensus sequence upstream of the initiation codon. This results in the high expression of virus structural proteins in Plat-E cells. To maintain high titres of retroviruses under drug selection pressure, the internal ribosome entry site sequence (IRES) has been inserted between the gene encoding gag-pol or env and the gene encoding a selectable marker in the packaging constructs (**Fig. 1**). Plat-E cells can stably produce retroviruses with an average titre of ~1×10^7/ml for at least 4 months.

Culture Medium: D-MEM supplemented with 10% foetal bovine serum (FBS), 50 IU/ml penicillin, 50 μg/ml streptomycin, 10 μg/ml blasticidin (Bsd) and 1 μg/ml puromycin (Puro).

1. Blasticidin S HCl (Invitrogen) (*see* **Note 4**). Bsd is soluble in water and acetic acid. Use sterile water to prepare stock solutions of 5–10 mg/ml. Dissolve Bsd in sterile water and filter-sterilise (0.22 μM) the solution. Aliquot the stock solution in small volumes suitable for single use only. Aqueous stock solutions are stable for 1–2 weeks at 4°C, 6–8 weeks at –20°C and indefinitely at –80°C. Do not subject stock solutions to freeze/thaw cycles. Note that the pH of aqueous solution should not exceed pH 7 to prevent inactivation of Bsd. Store D-MEM medium supplemented with Bsd at 4°C for up to 2 weeks.

2. Puromycin dihydrochloride (cell culture tested, Sigma) is soluble in water (50 mg/ml) and also in methanol (10 mg/ml). Prepare a 10 mg/ml stock in sterile water, filter-sterilise and store as 1 ml aliquots at –20°C.

Transfection reagents: Lipofectamine Reagent® and Plus® Reagent (Invitrogen) and OPTI-MEM media (Invitrogen GIBCO).

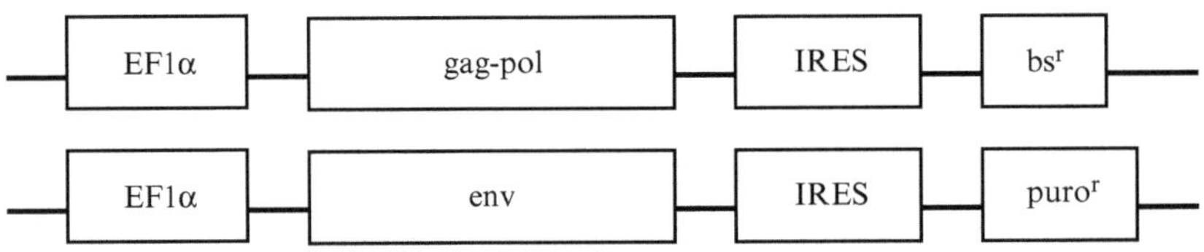

Fig. 1. Schematic diagrams of the packaging constructs pEnv-IRES-puro^r and pGag-pol-IRES-bs^r used for development of Plat-E cells. The fragments carrying the selectable marker, the blasticidin resistant gene (bs^r) or the puromycin resistant gene (puro^r), were inserted in the pMX-IRES-EGFP vector. The fragments containing the internal ribosome entry site (IRES) sequence and either of bs^r and puro^r were excised from the vector. The viral structural genes, gag-pol and env, were amplified by PCR, using the MoMuLV genome as a template. Finally, the fragment containing the viral structural genes and the fragment containing the IRES sequence and the selection marker were inserted downstream of the EF1a promoter in the pCHO vector, a derivative of pEF-BOS. Packaging constructs pEnv-IRES-puro^r and pGag-pol-IRES-bs^r were sequentially transfected into HEK293T cells using Fugene (Boehringer Mannheim, Germany) according to the manufacturer's recommendations. One day after transfection with pEnv-IRES-puro^r, HEK293T cells were selected in D-MEM containing 1 μg/ml puromycin. The selected cells were then transfected with the pGag-pol-IRES-bs^r vector, and subcloned in the presence of puromycin and blasticidin (10 μg/ml). The selected clones were tested for their potential to produce retroviruses. Figure and details reproduced from Morita et al. *(12)*.

2.1.4. Infection of 3T3-L1 Fibroblasts with HA-GLUT4 Retrovirus

1. 3T3-L1 fibroblasts: American Type Culture Collection (Rockville, USA) passaged as pre-confluent cultures.
2. Culture medium: D-MEM supplemented with 10% heat-inactivated FBS, 50 IU/ml penicillin and 50 μg/ml streptomycin (Normal Growth media).
3. Polybrene (hexadimethrine bromide, Sigma): Prepare a 10 mg/ml stock in mH_2O, filter-sterilise (0.22 μm) and store as aliquots at –20°C. Do not re-freeze after thawing. Keep at 4°C after the first thaw.
4. Puromycin: Prepare a 10 mg/ml stock in mH_2O, filter-sterilise and store as 1 ml aliquots at –20°C. Add 1 ml stock to 500 ml D-MEM for a final concentration of 2 μg/ml.

2.1.5. Translocation Assay

1. Insulin: Humulin® R (Eli Lilly, USA) is human insulin of recombinant DNA origin with a stock concentration of 100 units/ml.
2. D-MEM powder containing 4,500 mg/L D-glucose, L-glutamine and 100 mg/L sodium pyruvate but no sodium bicarbonate or Krebs Ringer phosphate (KRP) buffer (*see* **Notes 5** and **6**). Prepare D-MEM powder freshly and store at 4°C up to 1 week, with the addition of 0.2% (w/v) BSA (*see* **Note** 7) and 0.02 M HEPES, pH 7.4 prior to use. KRP buffer should be prepared prior to use.
3. Electronic multichannel pipettes are highly recommended to provide the power of pipetting in microplate formats (Matrix pipettes, Thermo Fisher Scientific, USA).
4. Sterile 1× PBS pH 7.4, store at 4°C (detailed under **Subheading 2.1.2, step 3**).
5. Three per cent(w/v) paraformaldehyde (PFA): Prepare 3% PFA in mH_2O from 16% PFA stock (10 × 10 ml, EM-grade, Electron Microscopy Sciences, USA). PFA needs to be prepared and handled in a fume hood. Prepare the PFA working solution freshly and store at 4°C for up to 1 week.
6. 0.05 M glycine: Dilute 2 M glycine stock in 1× PBS, pH 7.4. Store the stock solution at 4°C.
7. Prepare blocking reagents freshly each time:
   - Block minus saponin (**B–**): Prepare 5% normal swine serum (Normal Swine Serum; NSS, Dako Cytomation, Denmark) in 1× PBS, pH 7.4. Dilute NSS stock 1:20.
   - Block plus saponin (**B+**): Prepare 5% NSS and 0.1% saponin (latter prepared from a 10% (w/v) stock in mH_2O which has been filter-sterilised and stored at 4°C up to 2 weeks) in 1× PBS, pH 7.4. Dilute NSS stock 1:20 and saponin stock 1:100.

8. Primary antibodies: Monoclonal antibody HA.11 that recognises the influenza haemagglutinin epitope (mouse, IgG1-κ subtype, raw ascites fluid *or* purified, Covance Research Products, USA) and mouse isotype control antibody (MOPC-21, isotype IgG1-κ, purified from ascites fluid, Sigma) (*see* **Note 8**).
9. Secondary antibodies: Fluorescent antibody Alexa Fluor® 488-conjugated goat anti-mouse IgG (H + L) cross-absorbed or Alexa Fluor® 488 $F(ab')_2$ fragment of goat anti-mouse IgG (H + L) (Molecular Probes, Invitrogen).
10. Fluorescence reader with 485 nm excitation/520 nm emission wavelength specifications.

2.2. PM Lawn Assay

2.2.1. 3T3-L1 Cell Culture

1. 3T3-L1 cell culture media (detailed under **Subheading 2.1.4, step 2**). The method for 3T3-L1 adipocyte differentiation is detailed under **Subheading 3.1.3, steps 1-4**.
2. Six-well tissue culture plates.
3. Glass coverslips: Grow and differentiate 3T3-L1 fibroblasts directly onto glass coverslips and use 3T3-L1 adipocytes 8-12 days post-differentiation. Square coverslips at 22 mm are recommended, as they are easier to use when sonicating the cells in a uniform pattern. Smaller rounded coverslips can be used once the technique is proficiently performed. Use coverslips that fit into the wells of 12- and 24-well plates.

2.2.2. PM Lawn Preparation and Immunofluorescence

1. Sterile 1× PBS pH 7.4.
2. Poly-L-lysine at 0.5 mg/ml: Prepare a 1:1 solution in 1× PBS, pH 7.4 from 0.1% (w/v) stock. Place 6 ml in one 35 mm dish. Keep poly-L-lysine stock solution at 4°C.
3. PM lawn buffer: Prepare 30 mM HEPES, pH 7.2 containing 70 mM KCl, 5 mM $MgCl_2$, 3 mM EGTA (pH adjusted with KOH and store at 4°C). Add 1 mM DTT and 2 mM PMSF to PM lawn buffer with each use. Place 6 ml into two 35 mm dishes.
4. Hypotonic swelling buffer: Prepare a 1:3 dilution of PM lawn buffer in mH_2O. Place 6 ml into three 35 mm dishes.
5. Buzzing solution: Prepare PM lawn buffer supplemented with 1 mM DTT and 1 mM PMSF. Fill one 100 mm dish to the edge (~90 ml).
6. Sonicator: This protocol is optimised for a Micro Ultrasonic Cell Disrupter with a 3.2 mm probe operated with a foot pedal (Kontes). The output control is set around 15 when buzzing the cells (*see* **Note 9**).

7. PFA: Prepare a 2% solution in PM lawn buffer from a 16% solution stock (EM-grade, Electron Microscopy Sciences, USA).
8. Glycine: Prepare 150 mM glycine in 1× PBS, pH 7.4.
9. Blocking buffer: Prepare 5% (w/v) skim dry milk in 1× PBS, pH 7.4 (pH adjusted with NaOH) also known as 'blotto'.
10. GLUT4 antibody/primary antibody: Antibodies raised against the C-terminal peptide sequence produce the best results. Dilute the antibody in 1:10 blocking buffer according to the manufacturer's instructions. We recommend a starting dilution of 1:250. Before use, pulse-spin the diluted antibody to remove particulate matter, which may give background staining.
11. Fluorescent secondary antibodies: Either Alexa Fluor® 594 or 488-conjugated antibodies (Molecular Probes). Dilute the antibody in 1:10 blocking buffer. We recommend a starting dilution of 1:1,000, and as in **step 10**, spin the diluted antibody to remove particulate matter.
12. Slide mounting medium: Prepare 1% *n*-propylgallate in 50% glycerol and 50% 1× PBS, pH 7.4. Heat glycerol and PBS for 10 s in a microwave and then add *n*-propylgallate. Vortex well to dissolve, filter-sterilise and store at –20°C (*see* **Note 10**).
13. Confocal laser scanning immunofluorescence microscope.
14. Imaging software.

2.3. Subcellular Fractionation

1. 3T3-L1 cell culture media as detailed under **Subheading 2.1.4, step 2**. The method for 3T3-L1 adipocyte differentiation is detailed under **Subheading 3.1.3, steps 1-4**.
2. HES buffer: Prepare 20 mM HEPES, pH 7.4 containing 1 mM EDTA and 250 mM sucrose, adjust pH to 7.4 with NaOH and store at 4°C. Add protease inhibitors: 10 μg/ml aprotinin, 10 μg/ml leupeptin, 1 μg/ml pepstatin and 2 mM PMSF and phosphatase inhibitors: 20 mM NaF, 1 mM NaPPi and 2 mM Na_3VO_4 to HES buffer before each use.
3. Cylinder cell homogeniser.
4. Centrifuges with rotors SS-34, SS-41, Ti-80, JA-25.50, TLA-100.3 *and/or* SW-55Ti (Beckman Instruments, Inc., and Sorvall Instruments Division).
5. Sucrose cushion [32% (w/w)]: 20 mM HEPES, pH 7.4 containing 1 mM EDTA and 1.12 M sucrose.
6. Primary antibodies: GLUT4 polyclonal antibody generated against a peptide encompassing the C-terminal 19 amino

acids (clone R10, rabbit affinity purified) and fraction-specific antibodies.

7. Secondary antibodies: Horseradish peroxidase (HRP)-conjugated antibodies.
8. SDS-PAGE and Western blotting apparatus using the ECL detection system.

3. Methods

3.1. Intact Cell GLUT4 Translocation Assay

3.1.1. Gelatin Coating of 96-Well Plates

1. Label black-walled, clear-bottom tissue culture 96-well plates before coating to facilitate having the plates in the same direction. As the fluorescence reader uses bottom reading mode, avoid pipette damage to the bottom of each well.
2. Gelatin assists the differentiated adipocytes to remain attached to the wells throughout the assay. Incubate plates with 100 μl 1% (w/v) gelatin per well for 1 h at room temperature under sterile conditions. After 1 h, aspirate the gelatin.
3. Wash the plates once with 100 μl sterile PBS per well (*see* **Note 11**).
4. For glutaraldehyde-coating, fix the gelatin for 10 min with 100 μl 0.5% glutaraldehyde per well (*see* **Note 12**) and wash the plates once with 100 μl sterile PBS per well.
5. Following aspiration, add 100 μl fresh D-MEM medium (no FBS required) to each well. Repeat this wash twice more. The purpose of this wash is to remove all of the glutaraldehyde, remnants of which are toxic to the cells. Swirl the D-MEM gently so the wells are uniformly covered and do not allow the wells to sit free of solution for too long. Plates with D-MEM can be stored in a 37°C CO_2 incubator for up to 1 week.

3.1.2. Production of HA-GLUT4 Retrovirus Using Plat-E Packaging Cells

1. Maintain Plat-E packaging cells in D-MEM supplemented with 10% FBS, penicillin/streptomycin (antibiotics), 10 μg/ml blasticidin and 1 μg/ml puromycin in a 5% CO_2 environment. Passage the cells twice a week in 75 cm^2 flasks and allow the cells to reach 70% confluence. To avoid aggregation, resuspend the cells thoroughly.
2. *Transfection:* Passage Plat-E cells at 5 × 10^6 cells per 10 cm dish using D-MEM with 10% FBS but *without* antibiotics, in order to have approximately 70-80% confluence the next day. Plat-E cells *must* be a monolayer on the day of transfection with minimal clumps present. This is important in order to obtain >90% transfection efficiency (*see* **Note 13**). Cells

can be seeded into multiple 10 cm dishes to transfect at the same time.

3. Transfect each 10 cm dish with 15 μg pBabe puro HA-tagged GLUT4 retroviral expression plasmid, using Lipofectamine Reagent® and Plus® Reagent, in OPTI-MEM media for 4 h at 37°C.
   (a) Add the DNA (15 μg) and 20 μl Plus Reagent to 625 μl room temperature OPTI-MEM and incubate for 15 min at room temperature.
   (b) In a separate tube, mix 30 μl Lipofectamine Reagent and 595 μl OPTI-MEM at room temperature.
   (c) Combine the tubes from (a) and (b) and incubate for 15 min at room temperature.
   (d) During this 15 min incubation, wash the cells once with 5 ml D-MEM (no antibiotics) per 10 cm dish.
   (e) Add 5 ml OPTI-MEM (pre-warmed 37°C) and add the solution from (c) dropwise to the cells and incubate in a 37°C 5% CO_2 incubator for 4 h.
   (f) Remove the transfection media and replace with 8 ml D-MEM containing 10% FBS, no antibiotics, 1 μg/ml Puro and 10 μg/ml Bsd. Incubate in 37°C 5% CO_2 incubator for 48 h.
4. Harvest the HA-GLUT4 retrovirus by gently collecting media from all the dishes and filter (0.45 μm). Store 1 ml aliquots at –80°C (do not freeze/thaw). Alternatively, the HA-GLUT4 retrovirus supernatant can be stored at 4°C if used within 1 week.

3.1.3. Retroviral Infection

3T3-L1 Adipocyte Differentiation

1. Maintain the cells for differentiation at post-confluence for 2 days, and then induce to differentiate by the addition of D-MEM containing 10% FBS, 2 μg/ml insulin, 0.25 μM dexamethasone and 0.5 mM 3-isobutyl-1-methylxanthine.
2. After 3 days, replace the induction medium with fresh D-MEM containing 10% FBS and 2 μg/ml of insulin for a further 3-4 days. Refresh media once during this period.
3. Maintain the adipocytes in D-MEM with 5% FBS for 2 or more days thereafter. Refresh media every 2-3 days if required.
4. Use adipocytes 8-12 days after initiation of differentiation, after which time greater than 80% of fibroblasts should have differentiated into mature adipocytes.

Infection

1. One day prior to infection, seed 3T3-L1 fibroblasts into 10 cm dishes and grow to 30% confluence the next day.

2. For each 10 cm dish, prepare 4 ml infection media that contains 2 ml D-MEM with 10% FBS (normal growth media), 2 ml HA-GLUT4 retroviral stock and 12 μl polybrene that have been combined in one tube first. After removal of the normal growth media, add the infection media to the fibroblasts and incubate for 5 h in 37°C 10% CO_2 incubator. After 5 h, aspirate the infection media and replace with 10 ml normal growth media containing 2 μg/ml puromycin (selection media). Refresh selection media every 2-3 days.
3. Once the cells are confluent, differentiate as described above. At least 24-48 h prior to translocation assay, trypsinise the infected adipocytes and seed into gelatin-coated black-walled, clear-bottom 96-well plates and maintain in D-MEM containing 5% FBS (*see* **Note 14**). Once the fibroblasts are fully differentiated into mature adipocytes, there is no need to maintain the cells in selection media.

Seeding Cells into 96-Well Plates

1. Each 1 × 10 cm dish of infected 3T3-L1 adipocytes will seed 1 × 96-well plate.
2. Split and resuspend 1 × 10 cm dish of infected 3T3-L1 adipocytes into 10 ml of D-MEM with 5% FBS.
3. Resuspend the cells very well and add into a fresh 10 cm dish. Use an electronic multichannel pipette to aliquot 100 μl resuspended cells per well of a 96-well plate.
4. The cells, if seeding differentiated 3T3-L1 adipocytes into a 96-well plate (*see* **Note 14**), must not be clumped the next day. Hence, resuspending the infected adipocytes thoroughly after trypsinisation the day before is critical.

3.1.4. Translocation Assay (see Fig. 2)

1. Serum-starve the infected, differentiated 3T3-L1 adipocytes for 2 h at 37°C with either fresh KRP buffer (*see* **Note 6**) *or* serum and bicarbonate-free D-MEM containing 0.2% (w/v) BSA and 0.02 M HEPES, pH 7.4. D-MEM solution can be kept at 4°C for up to 1 week, and add BSA and HEPES prior to use and pre-warm.
2. Wash the plates twice with D-MEM buffer using 100 μl per well (using an electronic multichannel pipette from this step onwards).
3. Add 100 μl D-MEM buffer per well and leave in a 37°C water bath for 2 h with the lids reversed to prevent condensation inside the well.
4. Add insulin at 15 μl per well and incubate the plates in a 37°C water bath for the relevant incubation period (200 nM insulin for 20 min). See **Tables 1** and **2** for experimental design and *see* **Note 15**.

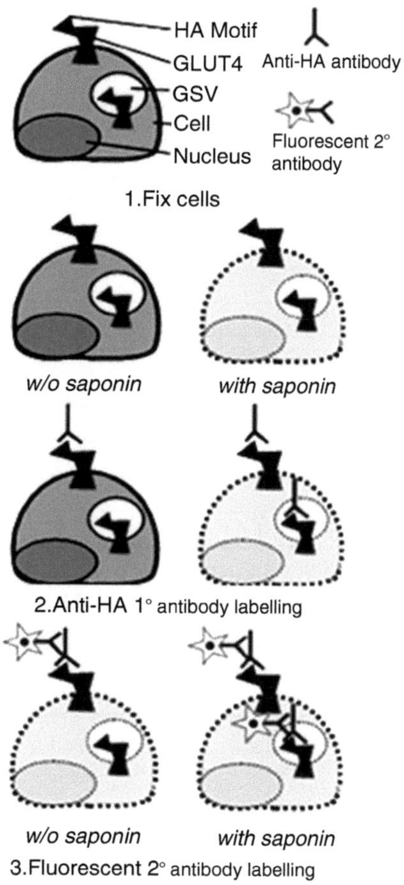

Fig. 2. Optical detection of cell surface HA-tagged GLUT4 in 3T3-L1 adipocytes. A GLUT4 reporter containing HA epitope tag in the first exofacial loop at the C-terminus was expressed in 3T3-L1 adipocytes. Insulin (and/or treatment of interest) was added at the relevant/desired time points, after which the cells were fixed in PFA. After quenching with glycine, cells were incubated in the absence or presence of saponin to analyse the amount of GLUT4 at the PM or the total cellular GLUT4 content, respectively. Cells were incubated with a saturating concentration of either an antibody directed against the HA tag or a control non-relevant antibody (i.e. MOPC-21). After extensive washing, the cells were incubated within the presence or absence of saponin to permeabilise all the cells. Cells were then incubated with saturating concentrations of a fluorescent antibody. After washing, fluorescence was measured in a fluorescence microtitre plate reader. The percentage of GLUT4 at the PM was calculated for each condition. The schematic was reproduced with permission from Dr. Cordula Hohnen-Behrens and Prof. David James, Diabetes and Obesity Research Program, Garvan Institute of Medical Research, Sydney, Australia.

5. Prepare working solutions of insulin in D-MEM buffer and lift the plate lid to wipe off condensation before pipetting.
6. Prepare treatments (insulin) in a separate 'master' plate, and add 15 μl per well using an electronic multichannel pipette. The 'master' plate is a tissue culture 96-well plate where the relevant numbers of individual wells are filled with the working solution of insulin.

Table 1
HA-GLUT4 translocation assay in 3T3-L1 adipocytes - 96-well template of an insulin-stimulated time course experiment

	1	*2*	*3*	*4*	*5*	*6*	*7*	*8*	*9*	*10*	*11*	*12*
A												
B												
C												
D												
E												
F												
G												
H												

Ins (min)	0′	0′	2′	4′	6′	8′	12′	15′	30′	30′	30′	30′
	First block minus Saponin = **B–** Primary antibody = **HA.11**									= **B+** = **HA.11**		
	First block minus Saponin = **B–** Primary antibody = **MOPC-21**									= **B+** = **MOPC-21**		

Incubate cells with 200 nM insulin over 0, 2, 4, 6, 8, 12, 15 and 30 min at 37°C

Table 2
HA-GLUT4 translocation assay in 3T3-L1 adipocytes – 96-well template of an insulin-stimulated concentration-response experiment

Ins (nM)	0	0	0.1	1	5	10	50	100	200	200	200	200
	First block minus Saponin = **B–** Primary antibody = **HA.11**									= **B+** = **HA.11**		
	First block minus Saponin = **B–** Primary antibody = **MOPC-21**									= **B+** = **MOPC-21**		

Refer to **Table 1** for 96-well template. Incubate cells with insulin for 20 min at 37°C at 0, 0.1, 1, 5, 10, 50, 100 and 200 nM

7. Put the plates on ice and wash with 3 × 100 μl per well ice-cold 1× PBS, pH 7.4 and aspirate using an electronic multichannel pipette.
8. Fix with 100 μl per well 3% PFA on ice for 15 min in a fume hood.

9. Put the plates at room temperature for a further 30 min and aspirate the PFA with an electronic multichannel pipette to remove all the PFA. Do not touch the bottom of the wells.
10. Bring 1× PBS, pH 7.4 to room temperature and wash 1 × 100 μl per well. Quench for 5 min with 100 μl per well of 0.05 M glycine followed by a wash with 1 × 100 μl per well 1× PBS, pH 7.4.
11. First block (+ or – saponin for permeabilisation) for 20 min at room temperature using 50 μl per well.
    - Block minus saponin (**B–**): 5% NSS in 1× PBS, pH 7.4. This measures only HA-GLUT4 at the PM.
    - Block plus saponin (**B+**): 5% NSS plus 0.1% saponin in 1× PBS, pH 7.4. This measures total HA-GLUT4.
12. Because of the small volumes being used, use microfuge tubes with working solutions and use an electronic multichannel pipette to dispense 50 μl.
13. Primary antibody incubation: Freshly prepare the anti-HA.11 monoclonal antibody at the optimal dilution, that is 1:600 (*see* **Note 8**) and anti-MOPC-21 antibody at a dilution comparable with the amount of HA being added to the cells, in 2% NSS diluted in 1× PBS, pH 7.4. To the designated well, add 30 μl of the primary antibody and incubate at room temperature for 45 min.
    - Negative control: Subtract the fluorescence units of the MOPC-21 wells from the fluorescence units of the HA wells in order to calculate the specific anti-HA binding.
14. Wash all wells 3-4 times with 200 μl 1× PBS, pH 7.4 per well.
15. Block for 20 min at room temperature using 50 μl per well. Carry out B+ and B– vice versa to that performed in **step 11** above in order to permeabilise all the cells so that the background labelling of the secondary antibody is similar for all wells.
    - B+ = 5% NSS plus 0.1% saponin diluted in PBS.
    - B– = 5% NSS diluted in PBS.
16. Secondary antibody incubation: Remove the blocking reagent and incubate each well for 45 min at room temperature with 30 μl per well of 1:200 Alexa Fluor® 488 antibody in 2% NSS diluted in PBS to give a detectable fluorescent signal.
17. Protect from the light during this stage.
18. Wash 5 × 100 μl per well with PBS.
19. Add 100 μl/well PBS and measure the fluorescence intensity.

20. Set the Fusion microplate reader (PerkinElmer, USA) to bottom reading mode (*see* **Note 16**). Wipe the bottom of each plate before the fluorescent intensity is measured. Use the following parameters:
    (a) Number of cycles 1
    (b) Horizontal reading
    (c) Fluorescent intensity
    (d) Excitation (λ) 485
    (e) Emission (λ) 535
    (f) Well read time 1 s
    (g) Cycle time 120
21. Fluorescent intensity is then used to calculate relative amounts of HA-GLUT4 at the PM as described below. Refer to **Tables 1** and **2** for experimental templates and **Fig. 3a, b** for experimental results.
    (a). Mean HA (B−) fluorescence units of each treatment = **1** (area A1-F1, A2-F2 and so on).
    (b). Mean of MOPC (B−) fluorescence units of all treatments together = **2** (area G1-H9).
    (c). Mean of HA (B+) fluorescence units of all treatments = **3**. This is the total cellular HA-GLUT4 (area A10-D12).
    (d). Mean of MOPC (B+) fluorescence units of all treatments = **4**. This is the total non-specific binding (area E10-H12).
    (e). Subtract 4 (mean total MOPC) from 3 (mean total HA) = **5**.
    (f). Subtract 2 (mean MOPC) from each treatment 1 (mean HA) = **6**.
    (g). Divide **6** by **5** and multiply by 100 = % of HA-GLUT4 at the PM of the treatment.
    (h). Relative fluorescent units are calculated as the percentage of the total amount of cellular HA-GLUT4 at the PM.

There are several points to consider during the HA-GLUT4 translocation assay in 3T3-L1 adipocytes. Using 200 nM insulin increases cell surface HA-GLUT4 by approximately fourfold to fivefold after 12 min of 37°C incubation and the response is maintained for 60 min. Over-expression of HA-GLUT4 in these cells, which contain endogenous GLUT4, increases non-stimulated (basal; no insulin) GLUT4, as do the transfection reagents themselves.

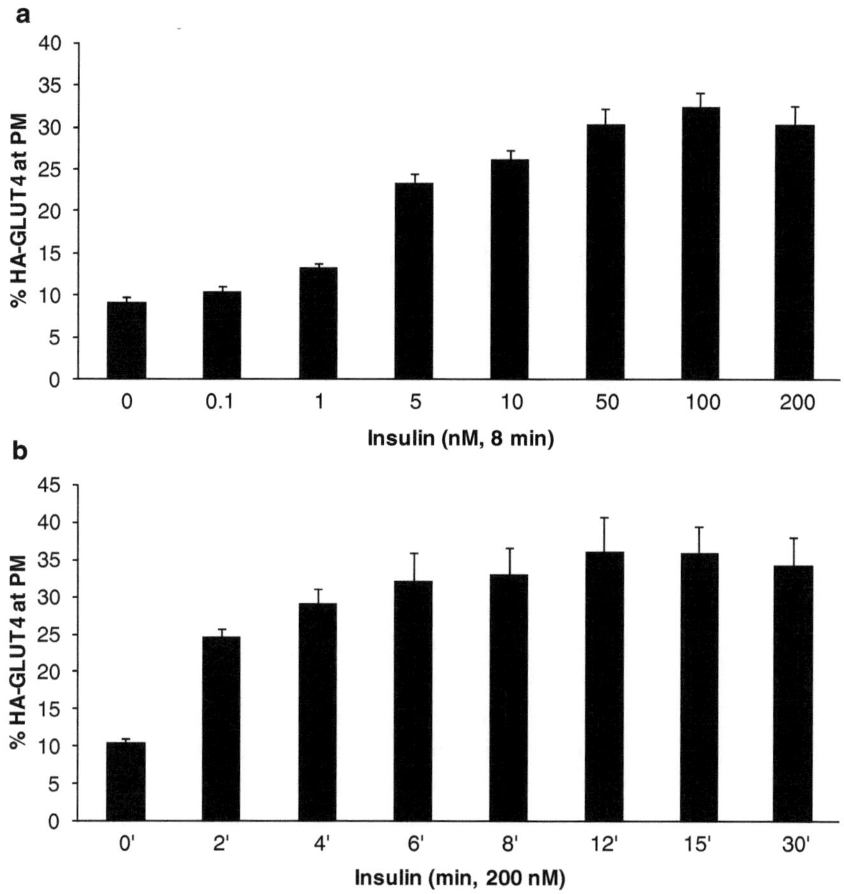

Fig. 3. Effects of insulin on HA-GLUT4 translocation in 3T3-L1 adipocytes. Following a 2-h serum starvation in $NaHCO_3$-free D-MEM containing 0.2% BSA and 0.02 M HEPES pH 7.4, 3T3-L1 adipocytes were treated with (**a**) 200 nM insulin for 0-30 min at 37°C or (**b**) 0-200 nM insulin for 8 min at 37°C. The adipocytes were then fixed with PFA, and immunofluorescence labelling assay (2 μg/ml anti-HA.11 or MOPC-21 purified antibody; 10 μg/ml Alexa Fluor® 488 $F(ab')_2$ fragment antibody) was performed as described in **Subheadings 2** and **3**. At the end of assay, the fluorescence intensity was measured and used to calculate the percentage of HA-GLUT4 present at the PM relative to total cellular amount of HA-GLUT4 (measured after detergent permeabilisation of the cells). Results are expressed as mean ± SEM of two independent experiments, whereby each measurement was performed in six replicates. Data supplied by Drs. Subhadhcha Poonsatha and Nicky Konstantopoulos, Metabolic Research Unit, Deakin University, Geelong, Australia.

3.2. PM Lawn Assay

The generation of membrane lawns provides highly purified PM fractions that allow the accurate quantification of GLUT4 present in this cellular compartment by immuno-detection *(13)*. One of the strengths of this technique is that it strips the membrane of other cell organelles but retains the different structures that constitute this heterogeneous cell compartment, for example, clathrin-coated pits or caveolae (*see* **Note 17**). This feature allows not only the quantification of the amount of GLUT4 present at the PM but also the analysis of the morphology and distribution of the glucose transporter and associated proteins simultaneously (e.g. SNAREs, exocytosis complex or signalling proteins).

3.2.1. Cell Culture

1. 3T3-L1 fibroblasts are passaged as pre-confluent cultures as described (cell culture media details under **Subheading 2.1.4, step 2**).
2. Maintain cells for differentiation at post-confluence for 2 days, and then induce to differentiate as detailed under **Subheading 3.1.3, steps 1-4**.

3.2.2. Generation of PM Lawns

1. Grow 3T3-L1 fibroblasts on glass coverslips in six-well plates and differentiate into adipocytes.
2. After 8-12 days post-differentiation, treat the adipocytes and/or serum starve as desired prior to sonication. For stimulation with acute insulin, serum-starve adipocytes in D-MEM containing 0.5% FBS (or 0.2% BSA) for 18 h prior to the addition of insulin.
3. Wash the cells twice in KRP buffer, pH 7.4 and equilibrate for 90 min at 37°C prior to the addition of insulin (100 nM).
4. Collect the coverslip with thin-tipped forceps from one corner and rinse it in ice-cold PBS for a few seconds. The coverslip must always be held from the same corner to avoid the disruption of the cell monolayer as much as possible.
5. Place the coverslip with cells side up in a 35 mm dishes with 6 ml of 0.5 mg/ml poly-L-lysine in PBS for 30 s on ice.
6. Drain off any excess poly-L-Lysine onto filter paper, and on ice, wash the coverslip briefly for 5 s successively in three 35 mm dishes each containing 6 ml of hypotonic swelling buffer. Leave the coverslip in the last dish for 30-45 s. The swelling will facilitate the cell disruption during the sonication step.
7. Fill a 100 mm dish with buzzing buffer (90 ml). Place the microprobe so that it just touches the surface of the buffer. To achieve this, place the probe 2-3 mm from the buffer. Pour a few drops of buffer on the probe so they slide down to the probe's tip forming a bridge with the buffer in the dish (*see* **Fig. 4**). Holding the coverslip with forceps, move it under the probe in a uniform pattern, slowly but without pausing and avoiding passing over the same area twice. The minimum time required to sonicate the whole coverslip is 20-30 s. The coverslip should be close enough to the probe to allow sonication but far enough away to avoid 'blasting' the cells and ripping off the PM attached to the glass (*see* **Note 18**).
8. Rinse the coverslip for a few seconds successively in two 35 mm dishes filled with PM lawn buffer on ice.

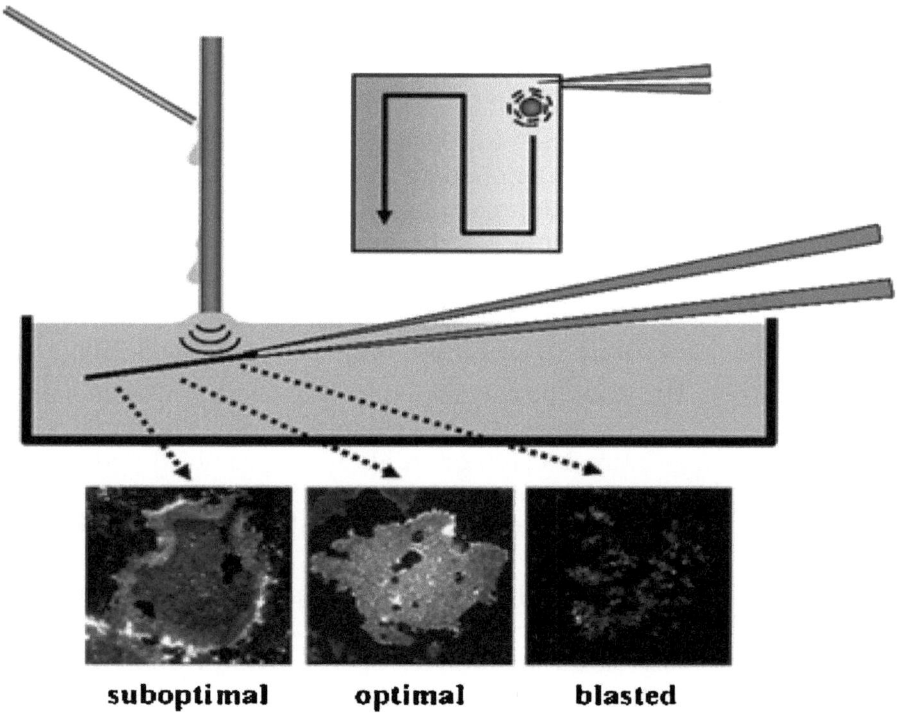

Fig. 4. Sonication of coverslip-grown 3T3-L1 adipocytes. The distance between the tip of the probe and the coverslip is modified according to the pattern described to ensure the generation of optimal PM lawns.

9. Because of the accumulation of cell debris in the buzzing buffer that could bind to the coverslip and thus increase the background of the final immunofluorescent image, change this buffer after six coverslips have been sonicated.

3.2.3. Immunofluorescence Labelling of PM Lawns

1. Place the coverslip in a dish or well containing 2% (w/v) PFA in PM lawn buffer for at least 20 min at room temperature.
2. Wash the fixed coverslips in PBS for 5 s.
3. Quench the fixative by placing the coverslips in wells containing 3 ml 150 mM glycine for 15 min at room temperature.
4. Remove the glycine and wash the coverslips three times in 3 ml PBS for 5 s.
5. Add blocking buffer to the coverslips and incubate on an orbital shaker at moderate speed for 30 min at room temperature (*see* **Note 19**).
6. Incubate the PM lawns with the GLUT4 antibody diluted in 1:10 blocking buffer for 1 h at room temperature. Alternatively, the incubation can be performed overnight at 4°C. If antibody availability is not a limiting factor, the incubation can be performed in 0.5 ml per 35 mm dish on an orbital shaker. If the amount of antibody is limiting, coverslips can

be place inverted (PM lawns facing down) on 50-100 μl diluted antibody aliquoted on parafilm.

7. Wash the coverslips three times with 3 ml PBS.
8. Incubate the PM lawns with fluorescently conjugated secondary antibodies (Alexa 488 goat anti-rabbit secondary antibody) diluted in 1:10 blotto for 1 h at room temperature. Although the antibody-bound fluorophores are stable, it is recommended to protect the coverslips from the light from this step onwards.
9. Wash the coverslips three times with 3 ml PBS.
10. Place the coverslips onto slides with 7 ml of mounting media (*see* **Note 10**) and drain the excess liquid on filter paper. The samples are now ready to be examined under the immunofluorescence microscope. The coverslips can be stored for future analysis at 4°C by sealing the edges with nail polish.

3.2.4. Microscope Imaging and Immunofluorescence Quantification

Considering that PM lawns are approximately 200 nm thick, confocal fluorescence microscopy for quantitation is recommended. Reliable quantitation can be achieved with 100 or more PM lawns per experimental condition. Images acquired with a 20× long distance lens would contain 20–30 PM lawns each. A double blind approach is strongly recommended to avoid non-arbitrary selection of PM lawns. However, random microscope fields must be selected only from the region of the coverslip containing intact PM lawns. Areas with blasted membranes or cell debris are not suitable for quantitation.

1. Determine the fluorescence intensity with one of many programs available (e.g. Axiovision, Carl Zeiss, ImageJ). Because of the irregular shape, different area size of the PM lawns and the presence of holes, we recommend to define a small region of interest, around 1-4 μm^2, within each PM lawn in the image (**Fig. 5**).
2. Examine *at least* six fields within each experiment for each condition. The confocal microscope gain settings over the period of experiments should be maintained to minimise between-experiment variability.

Cells stimulated with maximal doses of insulin (>10 nM) produce easily visible stained PM lawns, although a few insulin-insensitive cells are frequently seen as faintly-stained PM lawns. In contrast, unstimulated cells or those treated with sub-maximal doses of insulin may exhibit PM lawns with little detectable GLUT4 staining. One easy method to help visualise these low-stained PM lawns is to observe the image in full-screen mode to reduce the light coming from the monitor. Alternatively, PM lawns can be double-labelled with GLUT4 and a resident PM membrane protein (e.g. GLUT1, Clathrin or SNAP 23) labelled

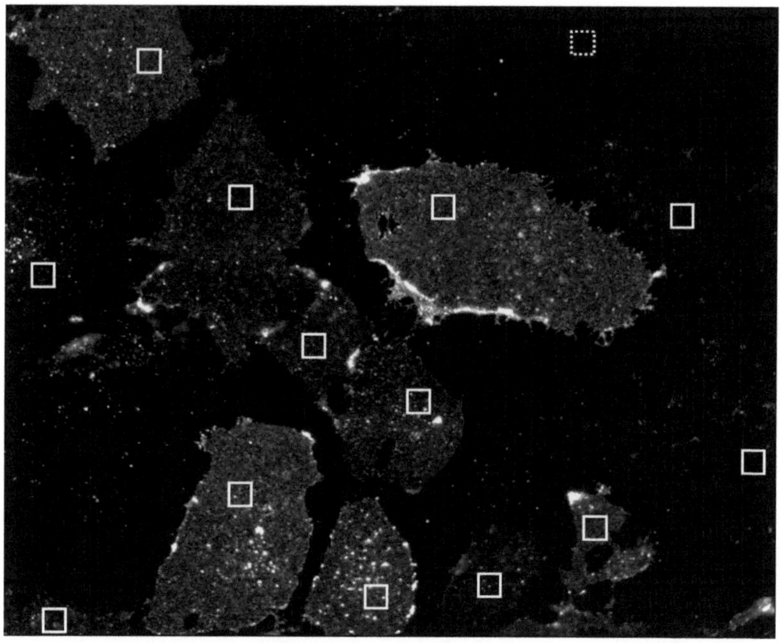

Fig. 5. Quantitation of GLUT4-specific immunofluorescence intensity on PM *lawns*. Small regions of interest of equal size are defined within the homogeneous areas of each PM lawn (*solid squares*). Another region of interest of equal size is defined outside the PM lawns as the background control (*dotted square*).

with a specific antibody raised in a different species and detected with a secondary antibody coupled to a distinct fluorophore.

3.3. Subcellular Fractionation

The basis of this technique involves the separation of cell organelles by sequential differential centrifugation. The separation depends on the size of the particles, sedimentation rates, type of the rotor used and the relative centrifugal force applied. Cell fractionation was performed essentially as described *(6, 7)*. Cytosolic fractions (CYT), low- and high-density microsomes (LDM, HDM), mitochondria (MITO), crude nuclear fraction (NUC) and PMs can be obtained. The LDM fraction is also referred to as the high-speed pellet (HSP) since it has been demonstrated that a large proportion of the protein in this fraction is not directly associated with microsomal membranes *(7)*. Protein concentrations need to be determined and 20 μg of each fraction loaded, resolved by reducing SDS-PAGE and the endogenous level of GLUT4 (or any protein of interest) in each fraction identified by Western blotting analysis.

1. Serum-starve the cells for at least 2 h to a maximum of overnight in D-MEM containing either 0.5% FBS or 0.2% BSA. Cells can then be treated in the presence or absence of acute insulin (10 or 100 nM) for 20 min at 37°C.

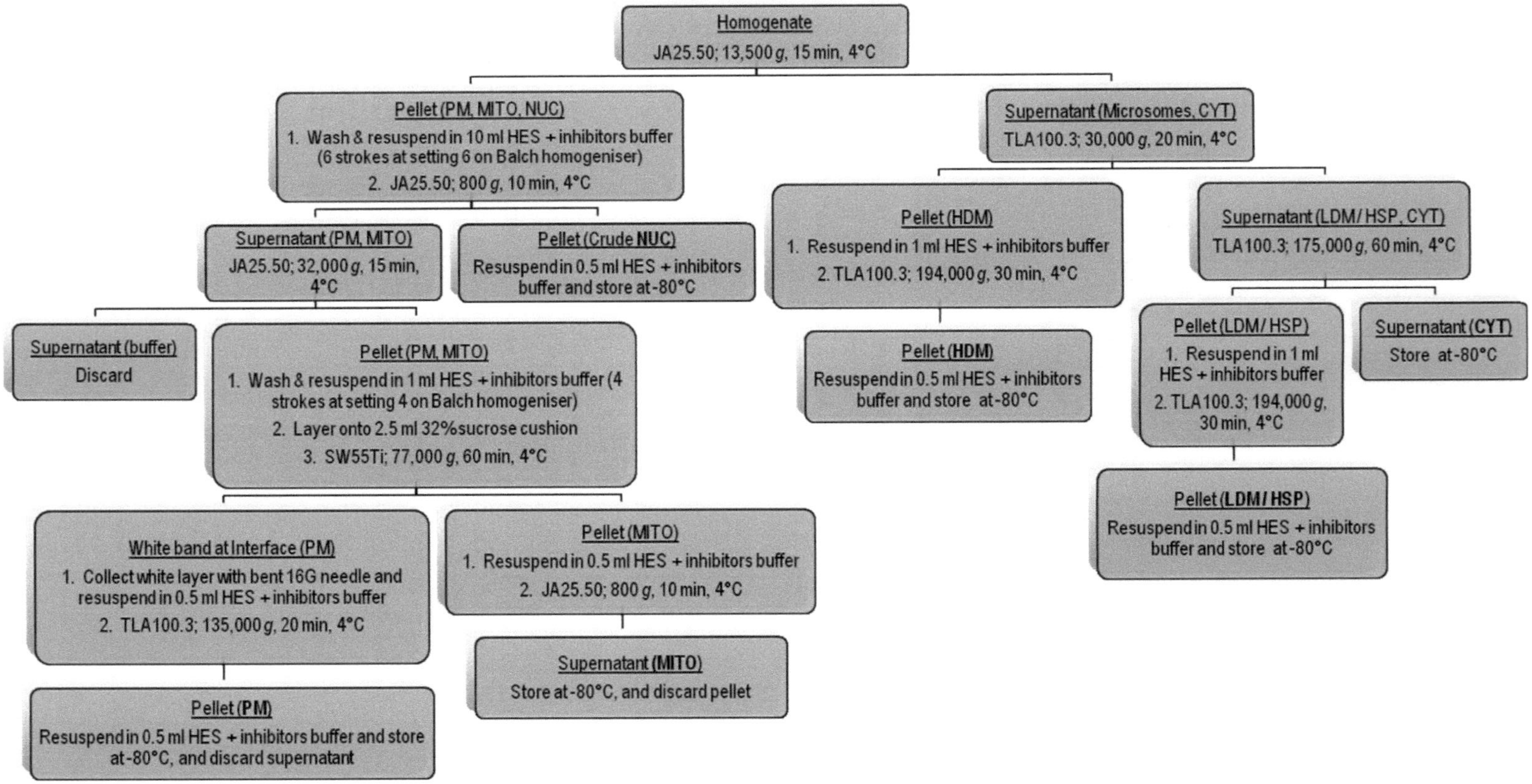

Fig. 6. Flow diagram describing purification of subcellular fractions using sequential differential centrifugation. For additional details and applications of cell fractionation, refer to Jaret *(6)*, Clark et al. *(7)*, Worrall and Olefksy *(15)*, Piper et al. *(16)* and Macaulay et al. *(17)*.

2. Wash each 10 cm dish three times with 5 ml chilled PBS or HES buffer (without protease and phosphatase inhibitors) and resuspend in chilled 1× HES buffer supplemented with the protease and phosphatase inhibitors (0.5 ml per 10 cm dish). Scrape cells from dish using a cell scraper.
3. Using an IKA-Werk homogeniser (model RW20, Janke & Kunkel, Germany) or equivalent fitted with a teflon pestle and glass vessel homogenise the cells (ten strokes at setting 10). Centrifuge the homogenate at 135,000 × *g* in a JA25.50 centrifuge (Beckman Instruments, Inc.) for 15 min at 4°C.
4. Carry out all procedures at 4°C. The centrifugation conditions are described in **Fig. 6**.
5. Further centrifuge the supernatant to obtain CYT, LDM/HSP and HDM fractions.
6. Resuspend the pellet and centrifuge to extract the NUC fraction, and finally extract the PM fraction from the MITO fraction by centrifugation on a 32% (w/w) sucrose cushion.
7. To assess the purity of the subcellular fractions, load equal amounts of protein from each subcellular fraction and using SDS-PAGE under reducing conditions and Western transfer, immuno-detect the relevant proteins. **Table 3** recommends a number of relevant proteins to assess.

Table 3
Characterisation of subcellular fraction purity by immuno-detection

Organelle	Protein
Nucleus	DNA-dependent RNA polymerase; histone
Mitochondria	Citrate synthase
Plasma membrane	5′-Nucleotidase; insulin receptor
Endoplasmic reticulum	Glucose-6-phosphatase
Golgi bodies	Galactosyltransferase
Cytosol	Lactate dehydrogenase; phosphofructose kinase; α-tubulin

The table is a guide of the relevant proteins that can be used to assess the purity of the subcellular fractions

4. Notes

1. This adds a further layer of complexity to the assay.
2. Alternative sources and expression vectors do exist and have been published - GLUT4myc *(9)* and GFP-GLUT4 or HA-GFP-GLUT4 *(10)*.
3. The reader should be aware of the difference between transient and stable over expression of c-myc or HA and/or GFP-tagged GLUT4 into L6 myotubes compared with 3T3-L1 adipocytes *(9, 11)*.
4. Prepare all solutions aseptically.
5. The constituents of KRP buffer tend to precipitate with time. KRP must be made fresh prior to use; however, 10× stocks are stable and may be kept at 4°C. Stocks (10×) are prepared (**Table 4**) and HEPES added to pH 7.4. Stocks are autoclaved and stored at 4°C. When used for the GLUT4 assay, 1× KRP buffer contains 0.2% (w/v) BSA, pH 7.4. When used for cell fractionation, KRP buffer requires 2.5 mM D-glucose (45 mg dextrose per 100 ml KRP) and 2% BSA. Note that production lots of BSA are contaminated with varying amounts of serum factors, so batch testing is required prior to use with 3T3-L1s to ensure the contaminants will not stimulate GLUT4 translocation/glucose transport. Batch test BSA with insulin-sensitive cells and use the batch that gives the lowest basal HA-GLUT4 translocation.

Table 4
Components of Krebs Ringer phosphate buffer

Chemical	Final (mM)	For 500 mL, 10× (g)	×10 Stock (mM)
HEPES	12.5	14.9	125
NaCl	120	35.1	1,200
KCl	6	2.24	60
$MgSO_4$	1.2	1.48	12
$CaCl_2$	1	0.735	10
NaH_2PO_4	0.4	0.276	4
Na_2HPO_4	0.6	0.426	6

The components of Krebs Ringer phosphate buffer precipitate with time. Therefore, KRP buffer must be made fresh prior to use. However, 10× stocks of the ingredients are stable and may be kept at 4°C. Adjust pH to 7.4 with NaOH. Prepare all solutions aseptically and for additional information, *see* **Notes 5–7**

6. D-MEM versus KRP as serum-starvation buffer. Using D-MEM appears to be more sensitive with the insulin stimulation curve shifting further to the left (translocation is faster) compared with KRP. This effect is due to the amino acids in the D-MEM, supplementation of KRP with added amino acids produces similar curves.
7. Highly recommend BSA that is essentially fatty acid free such as Sigma's RIA-grade and ≥96% fatty acid free or ICN's clinical reagent grade and 98% fatty acid free (ICN Biomedicals, USA).
8. Each new batch of primary antibody (anti-HA.11 monoclonal) must be titrated to establish its appropriate dilution. Incubate cells with 200 nM insulin for 20 min at 37°C with a range of dilutions of anti-HA.11 (1:100, 1:200, 1:400 and 1:600). Results will vary from batch to batch; hence, it is a good idea to order in a large amount of HA.11 antibody with the same batch or lot number.
9. If other sonicators with similar probes are to be used, tests must be conducted to optimise the output settings to guarantee high-quality PM lawns. It is recommended to start from a 10% output and avoid adjusting the output setting while actively sonicating the cells as it may blow the fuse.
10. Alternatively, commercially available mounting media such as the FluoroSave reagent from Calbiochem can be used.
11. Leaving the wells in PBS for prolonged periods compromises the gelatin monolayer. We do not recommend coating too many plates at any one time.
12. Glutaraldehyde is toxic and *caution* should be taken when preparing working solutions and during aspiration of plates. Aspirate using an electronic multichannel pipette and dispose of the liquid into β-iodine bottles as appropriate.
13. An excellent technique to establish the optimal transfection efficiency is to practice with a GFP-containing plasmid, where the level of transfection efficiency can readily be monitored by microscopy.
14. We have found that differentiating 3T3-L1 fibroblasts into adipocytes *evenly and to a similar extent per each well* within 96-well plates can be difficult (in contrast with differentiating fibroblasts in 48-, 24-, 12- or 6-well plates). If this is the case in your hands, then 24 h prior to the translocation assay, seed the adipocytes into gelatin-coated black-walled, clear-bottom 96-well plates. If, however, you are proficient in differentiating fibroblasts in 96-well plates, then infected fibroblasts can be seeded into 96-well plates and expect that 1 sub-confluent 10 cm dish of fibroblasts to 1 × 96-well plate produces fibroblasts that are approximately 70% confluent the next day.

15. The outside wells of a 96-well plate should not to be used solely for one treatment, that is, double up and include two basal measures or do not use the outside wells at all. It appears that the cells in the outer wells are not as well-differentiated as compared with those in inner wells. This is perhaps due to the increased evaporation of these outer perimeter wells. See template design (**Tables 1** and **2**) as to the optimal setup of experimental conditions per plate.
16. Touching the bottom of any of the wells at any stage throughout the translocation assay including treatments, washes, fixing and quenching incubations will compromise fluorescent readings.
17. PM lawns isolated from 3T3-L1 adipocytes often exhibit holes of irregular shape. These holes originate from large invaginations of the PM or 'caves' that are not in contact with the glass. These structures can intrude into the cells for several microns bringing the cell exterior in close proximity with intracellular organelles including the nucleus *(14)*.
18. To determine the optimal distance between the probe and the cells to generate good quality PM lawns, begin to sonicate the coverslip very close to the probe's tip (~1 mm) and then progressively increase the distance until no effect of sonication is observed (~1 cm). This procedure will generate a gradient from blasted to intact cells and guarantees optimal PM lawns in between. When the probe is too close to the cells it will instantaneously remove all of the cells and clear an area of glass around the probe's tip. The presence of 'caves' in the PM attached to the coverslip can make the PM lawns more susceptible to excessive sonication. Optimal PM lawns will be generated when a progressive removal of material in the shape of growing tendrils is observed ahead of the probe. Sub-optimal PM lawns generated due to an excessive distance between the probe often exhibit more intense peripheral staining because part of the lateral PM has remained attached to the glass and has folded over the basal PM (*see* **Fig. 4**).
19. Skim milk is the most effective blocking agent for PM lawns. Other agents, for example, BSA do not produce good results.

References

1. Herman, M.A., Kahn, B.B. 2006. Glucose transport and sensing in the maintenance of glucose homeostasis and metabolic harmony. *J Clin Invest* **116**: 1767–1775
2. Bryant, N.J., Govers, R., James, D.E. 2002. Regulated transport of the glucose transporter GLUT4. *Nat Rev Mol Cell Biol* **3**: 267–277
3. Larance, M., Ramm, G., James, D.E. 2008. The GLUT4 code. *Mol Endocrinol* **22**:226–233
4. Ramm, G., James, D.E. 2005. GLUT4 trafficking in a test tube. *Cell Metab* 2: 150–152
5. Watson, R.T., Pessin, J.E. 2007. GLUT4 translocation: the last 200 nanometers. *Cell Signal* **19**: 2209–2217

6. Jarett, L. 1974. Subcellular fractionation of adipocytes. *Methods Enzymol* **31**: 60–71
7. Clark, S.F., Martin, S., Carozzi, A.J., Hill, M.M., James, D.E. 1998. Intracellular localization of phosphatidylinositide 3-kinase and insulin receptor substrate-1 in adipocytes: potential involvement of a membrane skeleton. *J Cell Biol* **140**: 1211–1225
8. Govers, R., Coster, A.C., James, D.E. 2004. Insulin increases cell surface GLUT4 levels by dose dependently discharging GLUT4 into a cell surface recycling pathway. *Mol Cell Biol* **24:** 6456–6466
9. Ueyama, A., Yaworsky, K.L., Wang, Q., Ebina, Y., Klip, A. 1999. GLUT-4myc ectopic expression in L6 myoblasts generates a GLUT-4-specific pool conferring insulin sensitivity. *Am J Physiol* **277**: E572–E578
10. Bogan, J.S., McKee, A.E., Lodish, H.F. 2001. Insulin-responsive compartments containing GLUT4 in 3T3-L1 and CHO cells: regulation by amino acid concentrations. *Mol Cell Biol* **21**: 4785–4806
11. Konrad, D., Rudich, A., Bilan, P.J., Patel, N., Richardson, C., Witters, L.A., Klip, A. 2005. Troglitazone causes acute mitochondrial membrane depolarization and an AMPK-mediated increase in glucose phosphorylation in muscle cells. *Diabetologia* **48**: 954–966
12. Morita, S., Kojima, T., Kitamura, T. 2000. Plat-E: an efficient and stable system for transient packaging of retroviruses. *Gene Ther* **7**: 1063–1066
13. Robinson LJ, Pang S, Harris DS, Heuser J, James DE. 1992. Translocation of the glucose transporter (GLUT4) to the cell surface in permeabilized 3T3-L1 adipocytes: effects of ATP insulin, and GTP gamma S and localization of GLUT4 to clathrin lattices. *J Cell Biol* **117**: 1181–1196
14. Parton, R.G., Molero, J.C., Floetenmeyer, M., Green, K.M., James, D.E. 2002. Characterization of a distinct plasma membrane macrodomain in differentiated adipocytes. *J Biol Chem* **277**: 46769–46778
15. Worrall, D.S., Olefsky, J.M. 2002. The effects of intracellular calcium depletion on insulin signaling in 3T3-L1 adipocytes. *Mol Endocrinol* **16**: 378–389
16. Piper, R.C., Hess, L.J., James, D.E. 1991. Differential sorting of two glucose transporters expressed in insulin-sensitive cells. *Am J Physiol* **260**: C570–C580
17. MaCaulay, S.L., Stoichevska, V., Grusovin, J., Gough, K.H., Castelli, L.A., Ward, C.W. 2003. Insulin stimulates movement of sorting nexin 9 between cellular compartments: a putative role mediating cell surface receptor expression and insulin action. *Biochem J* **376**: 123–134

Chapter 11

Pancreatic Remodeling: Beta-Cell Apoptosis, Proliferation and Neogenesis, and the Measurement of Beta-Cell Mass and of Individual Beta-Cell Size

Eduard Montanya and Noèlia Téllez

Summary

The endocrine pancreas has a significant remodeling capacity that plays a crucial role in the maintenance of glucose homeostasis. Changes in beta-cell apoptosis, replication and size, and islet neogenesis contribute to the remodeling of the endocrine pancreas. The extent of their respective contribution varies significantly depending on the specific condition under consideration, and it is the balance among them that determines the eventual change in beta-cell mass. Thus, the study of pancreatic remodeling requires the determination of all these factors. In this chapter, we describe the quantification of beta-cell replication based on 3-bromo-2-deoxyuridine incorporation into DNA and on the expression of Ki67 antigen, of beta-cell apoptosis by the TUNEL technique and islet neogenesis by quantification of number of islets budding from pancreatic ducts, by confocal assessment of the expression of islet cell hormones in ductal cells, and by identification of small group of extra-islet beta-cells. Point counting morphometry is used to estimate beta-cell mass and planimetry to determine the cross-sectional area of individual beta-cells, a measure of beta-cell size.

Key words: BrdU, Ki67 antigen, TUNEL, Cytokeratine, IDX-1/PDX-1, Morphometry, Planimetry, Confocal microscopy, Pancreatic beta-cells, Pancreatic islets

1. Introduction

The endocrine pancreas has a significant remodeling capacity and plasticity that plays an essential role in the maintenance of glucose homeostasis. It is now well accepted that beta-cell mass is dynamic and adjusts to meet the changes in metabolic demand, both in physiological and in pathological conditions. We have

C. Stocker (ed.), *Type 2 Diabetes,* Methods in Molecular Biology, vol. 560
DOI 10.1007/978-1-59745-448-3_11, © Humana Press, a part of Springer Science+Business Media, LLC 2009

shown that beta-cell mass increases throughout life and maintains a linear correlation with body weight *(1)*, providing an insulin secretion capacity able to match the higher insulin requirements associated with increased body weight. Expanded beta-cell mass has been also shown in several other conditions characterized by increased metabolic demand, such as obesity, pregnancy, or insulin-resistance. The failure to increase beta-cell mass in response to metabolic demand results in hyperglycemia.

Beta-cell mass reduction is a central aspect in the development of both type 1 and type 2 diabetes. In type 1 diabetes, there is an absolute reduction in β-cell mass due to autoimmune destruction of β-cells *(2)*, whereas in type 2 diabetes, there is an inadequately low β-cell mass that cannot meet the increased demands generated by insulin-resistance *(3)*. The remodeling capacity of the endocrine pancreas could be used to design strategies aimed to the regeneration of beta-cell mass.

Depending on the specific condition analyzed, beta-cell apoptosis, replication, size, or neogenesis contribute differently to the remodeling of the endocrine pancreas, and it is their balance that determines whether beta-cell mass is eventually increased or reduced. Thus, the study of the pancreatic remodeling requires the determination of all these factors.

Beta-cell apoptosis and replication can be detected and quantified directly, and the methods that will be presented in this chapter are well established. In contrast, available methods to evaluated beta-cell neogenesis are indirect due to the current absence of specific markers of beta-cell neogenesis. Beta-cell mass measurement is performed by point counting morphometry, a stereological method with solid mathematical support, and beta-cell size is determined by planimetry as a mean cross-sectional area of individual beta-cells using commercially available software. Although the techniques that we will discuss have been used mostly in pancreatic sections *(1)*, they can also be applied to transplanted islets, basically with no modifications, and in cultured islets *(4-6)*.

2. Materials

2.1. Pancreas Processing

1. *Sterile saline solution*: 0.9% (w/v) NaCl.
2. *Phosphate buffer (PB) 0.1 M (500 ml)*: Prepare 250 ml of buffer A: 0.2 M $NaH_2PO_4 \cdot H_2O$ and 250 ml of buffer B: 0.2 M Na_2HPO_4. Mix 169 ml of buffer A with 81 ml buffer B and bring this final solution up to 500 ml by adding 250 ml of double distilled water (ddH_2O). Adjust pH of the solution to pH 7.2.

3. *Paraformaldehyde (PFA)*: Prepare a 4% (w/v) PFA solution in fresh 0.4 M PB. (Prepare 250 ml of buffer A: 0.8 M $NaH_2PO_4{\cdot}H_2O$ and 250 ml of buffer B: 0.8 M Na_2HPO_4. Mix 169 ml of buffer A with 81 ml buffer B and bring this final solution up to 500 ml by adding 250 ml of ddH_2O.) Adjust pH of the solution to pH 7.2. Store in the dark at 4°C (*see* **Note 1**).
4. Plastic cassettes with lid (Simport, Québec, Canada).
5. Metal moulds (Simport, Québec, Canada).
6. Cold plate (Leica, Germany).
7. Microscope slides 76 × 26 mm and microscope coverslips 24 × 32 mm (Menzel-Glaser, Braunschweig, Germany).

2.2. Beta-Cell Identification

1. Xylene, absolute ethanol, 90% ethanol, and 70% ethanol.
2. *Phosphate-buffered saline (PBS)*: 160 mM NaCl, 7 mM Na_2HPO_4, 3 mM $NaH_2PO_4{\cdot}H_2O$ (adjust to pH 7.4 with HCl if necessary).
3. *Citrate buffer*: 9.9 mM Citric acid anhydrous $C_6H_8O_7$, 43 mM sodium citrate $C_6H_5O_7Na3{\cdot}2H_2O$. Adjust to pH 6 with citric acid (when higher) or NaOH (when lower).
4. 33% Hydrogen peroxide (H_2O_2).
5. *Blocking solution*: 5% (v/v) Horse serum (Biological Industries, Kibbutz beit Haemek, Israel) in PBS.
6. *Insulin antibody*: Rabbit anti-human insulin (Santa Cruz Biotechnology, Santa Cruz, CA, USA) (dilution 1:100) (*see* **Note 2**).
7. *Secondary antibody*: Peroxidase-labeled anti-rabbit IgG (Dako, Carpinteria, CA, USA) (1:200 in PBS).
8. *Tertiary antibody*: Peroxidase-labeled antiperoxidase antibody (Dako, Carpinteria, CA, USA) (1:500 in PBS).
9. *Staining solution*: 0.05% (w/v) 3,3′-diaminobenzidine tetrahydrochloride (DAB) (Sigma, St. Louis, MO, USA) in PBS, add 0.02% (v/v) of 33% H_2O_2.
10. Harris hematoxylin (Sigma, St. Louis, MO, USA).
11. Mounting medium: DPX (Fluka).

2.3. Apoptosis

1. Proteinase K (20 μg/ml in PBS). Store at –20°C.
2. ApopTag® Peroxidase Kit (Chemicon International, Temecula, CA, USA) (*see* **Note 3**).
3. *Black staining solution*: 0.1 M PB, 0.03% (w/v) DAB (Sigma), 7 mM ammonium chloride (ClH_4N). Separately prepare 0.05 M of ammonium nickel sulfate hexahydrate ($H_8N_2NiO_8S_2$) in ddH_2O. Finally, add enough ammonium

nickel sulfate hexahydrate 0.05 M until the solution turns cloudy (6-8 ml). Filter and add 0.001% (v/v) of 33% H_2O_2.

2.4. Proliferation: BrdU

1. *BrdU solution*: Prepare a 20 mg/ml 3-bromo-2-deoxyuridine (BrdU) (Sigma) solution in PBS (*see* **Note 4**).
2. *HCl:* 2N HCl.
3. *Borax solution*: 0.1 M Borax (Sigma) in ddH_2O.
4. *Amersham Cell Proliferation Kit*: (GE Healthcare, Buckinghamshire, UK) (*see* **Note 3**).

2.5. Proliferation: Ki67

1. *Ki67 antibody*: Rabbit anti-human Ki67 from Zymed (San Francisco, CA, USA). Use diluted 1:100 in PBS (*see* **Note 5**).

2.6. Islet Neogenesis (I)

1. *Tris buffer*: 0.05 M Tris-HCl, pH 7.4, 0.16 M NaCl.
2. *Wash buffer*: Tris buffer, 1% (v/v) horse serum (Biological Industries), 0.2% (v/v) Triton, pH 7.4.
3. *CK20 antibody*: Monoclonal mouse anti-human CK20 antibody (clone K_s 20.8) from Dako. Use diluted 1:15 (*see* **Note 6**).
4. *EnVision+®System-HRP (DAB)*: From Dako, for mouse primary antibodies (*see* **Note 3**).
5. *Blocking solution*: 0.01 M Tris buffer, pH 7.4, 5% (v/v) horse serum (Biological industries), and 0.2% (v/v) Triton.
6. *Cocktail of antibodies*: Rabbit anti-human glucagon from Dako (1:500), rabbit anti-human somatostatin from Dako (1:500), rabbit anti-human pancreatic polypeptide from Chemicon (1:200), and rabbit anti-human insulin from Santa Cruz Biotechnology (1:100). Dilute all in PBS. Store them at 4°C if used within 1 month, for longer periods store at –80°C.

2.7. Islet Neogenesis (II)

1. *IDX-1/PDX-1 antibody*: Rabbit anti-human IDX-1 from Chemicon (1:250 in PBS).
2. *Secondary antibodies*: Goat anti-mouse Alexa fluor 488-labeled antibody (1:400) and goat anti-rabbit Alexa fluor 546-labeled antibody (1:400) (Molecular Probes, Invitrogen, Eugene, OR, USA). Use diluted in PBS.
3. *DRAQ5*: Red fluorescent cell-permeable DNA probe from Biostatus Limited, Leicestershire, UK (emission wavelength: 647 nm, far-red). Use diluted 1:1,000 in PBS.
4. *Mounting medium for immunofluorescence* from Dako Cytomation.

3. Methods

The measurement of beta-cell mass and individual beta-cell size requires the identification of beta-cells. This is optimally performed using an anti-insulin antibody to stain the cytosol of the beta-cells. The measurement of beta-cell apoptosis or proliferation requires a double-staining technique to identify the cells that are apoptotic or actively replicating, as well as the beta-cells. Therefore, the double immunocytochemical staining that we will describe targets the cytosol to identify the beta-cells, and the nucleus to identify the apoptotic or replicating cells.

The staining of beta-cells with an anti-insulin antibody may be weakened in several conditions, particularly when beta-cells have been exposed to high glucose concentration for a time period long enough to induce beta-cell degranulation and severe reduction of insulin content. In this condition, the insulin staining of beta-cells may appear very weak or almost negative. To overcome this limitation, a "reverse" or "negative" staining of beta-cells can be performed by staining the endocrine non-beta-cells of the islet with a cocktail of antibodies against glucagon, somatostatin, and pancreatic polypeptide *(5, 6)*. Thus, when using this technique, beta-cells are identified as the nonstained endocrine cells. It is essential to pay careful attention to the cell characteristics, in particular the nucleus shape, to exclude nonendocrine cells.

There are several reliable commercial kits available to measure apoptosis and replication. Nevertheless, apoptosis measurements are more difficult to assess and it may advisable to use a second technique. We have used, as confirmatory measurement of beta-cell apotosis, the staining with propidium iodide *(6)* and cell cytometry *(4)*.

The thymidine analogue BrdU gets incorporated into the DNA of cells in the S phase of cell cycle. Thus, BrdU staining identifies cells that have already passed the G_1-S checkpoint and that are committed to undergo cell division. The technique requires the injection of BrdU some time before harvesting the organ to allow the incorporation into the DNA of the cells. If BrdU injection is not possible (for instance, with human organs,) or has not been done, the staining with Ki67 antibody offers an alternative. Ki67 antibody stains the cells that are in G_1, S, G_2, and M phases of cell cycle, but not resting cells in G_0 phase. A caveat of the technique is that cells that may not progress beyond G_1 phase, and that will do not replicate, are also stained. Thus, Ki67 staining may be less accurate than BrdU staining in the identification of cells that really are undergoing replication.

Beta-cell neogenesis is determined using indirect indicators, such as the proximity of islet cells to pancreatic ducts, the presence of small clusters of beta-cells (extra-islet beta-cells) scattered in the exocrine pancreas, or the expression of specific islet markers in ductal cells. For bona fide colocalization of islet or beta-cell markers and ductal cell markers, confocal microscopy is required.

3.1. Pancreas Processing for Immunohistochemistry

1. The pancreas is excised, blotted, and weighed. Before weighing, the pancreas is quickly cleaned from other tissues that may have been also excised (fat, duodenum, and lymph nodes). Then the pancreas is placed in a previously weighed cassette for tissue fixation and is weighed on a scientific scale (*see* **Notes 7** and **8**).
2. Immerse the cassette in a suitable container with PFA 4% for 20-24 h at 4°C.
3. Wash the cassette containing the pancreas with PB by changing the solution three times for 5 min each.
4. Prior to paraffin embedding, the pancreas may be kept in PB solution for 2 weeks at 4°C.

3.2. Paraffin Embedding

Before embedding, the samples will need to be taken through a series of graded ethanol baths to dehydrate the tissues and then into xylene. Hot paraffin can then permeate the tissues.

1. Wash the specimen in cold run water for 5 min.
2. Immerse the specimen in 70% ethanol for 1 h.
3. Wash the specimen twice with 90% ethanol for 1 h each wash.
4. Wash the specimen three times with 100% ethanol for 1 h each wash.
5. Wash the specimen twice with xylene for 30 min each wash.
6. Wash the specimen in two changes of paraffin (65°C) for 1 h each wash (*see* **Note 9**).
7. Turn the heat block on to melt the paraffin 1 h before adding the tissue cassettes. Also warm metal block moulds on a hot plate.
8. Add hot paraffin to the mould. Use heated forceps to orient the tissues in the mould. When the tissue is in the desired orientation, add the labeled tissue cassette on top of the mould as a backing. Be sure there is enough paraffin to cover the face of the plastic cassette.
9. Slide the mould off the hot plate onto a cold plate. When the wax is completely cooled and hardened (~20 min), the paraffin block can be popped out of the mould. If the wax cracks or the tissues are not aligned well, melt them again and start over.

3.3. Tissue Sectioning

1. Turn on the water bath and check that the temperature is between 35 and 37°C.
2. Place the blocks to be sectioned face down on an ice block for 10 min.

3. Place a fresh blade on the microtome. Insert the block into the microtome chuck so the wax block faces the blade and is aligned in the vertical plane. Set the dial to cut 2–4 μm sections. The blade should angle ~10°. Face the block by cutting it down to the desired tissue plane and discard the paraffin ribbon. If the block is ribboning well (*see* **Note 10**), then cut another three sections and pick them up with a fine paintbrush and float them on the surface of the 37°C water bath. Float the sections onto the surface of clean glass slides. If the block is not ribboning well, then place it back on the ice block to cool off and firm up the wax. If the specimens fragment when placed on the water bath, then it may be too hot. Place the slides with paraffin sections in a 65°C oven for 20 min (so the wax just starts to melt) to bond the tissue to the glass. Slides can be stored overnight at room temperature.

3.4. Beta-Cell Identification: Immunohistochemistry for Insulin

1. In order to deparaffinize the tissue sections (in a coplin jar), place the slides with paraffin sections in a 65°C oven for 30 min.
2. Wash the specimen in five changes of xylene for 5 min each wash.
3. Wash the specimen in two changes of absolute ethanol for 5 min each wash.
4. Wash the specimen in two changes of 95% ethanol for 5 min each wash.
5. Wash the specimen once in 70% ethanol for 10 min.
6. Rinse the specimen once in deionized water for 2 min.
7. Wash the specimen once in PBS for 5 min.
8. For antigen retrieval prepare citrate buffer, pour it in a beaker and place it on a hotplate, turn it on full power, and wait until the solution comes to the boil (*see* **Note 11**).
9. Once boiling, transfer the slides with a slide rack from the PBS to the beaker containing the citrate buffer. Use care with hot solution - use forceps! Boil for 20 min from this point.
10. Remove the slide rack and place it under running cold tap water for 10 min.
11. In order to quench endogenous peroxidase, place slides in a coplin jar containing 3% hydrogen peroxide in PBS for 20 min at room temperature.
12. Rinse the specimen once with PBS for 5 min.
13. Place the slides in blocking solution for 15 min at room temperature.

14. Gently tap off the excess liquid and carefully blot or aspirate around the section. Apply sufficient insulin antibody (1:100) to cover specimen. Incubate overnight at 4°C.
15. Wash the specimen in three changes of PBS for 5 min each wash.
16. Wipe around the specimen and add sufficient peroxidase-labeled anti-rabbit IgG (1:200) antibody to cover the specimen. Incubate for 3 h at room temperature (*see* **Note 12**).
17. Wash the specimen in three changes of PBS for 5 min each wash.
18. Wipe around the specimen and add sufficient peroxidase-labeled antiperoxidase antibody (1:500) to cover the specimen. Incubate for 1 h at room temperature.
19. In order to develop color, immerse slides in staining solution for 1 min at room temperature.
20. In order to determine the optimal staining time, monitor the color development by looking at the section under the microscope.
21. Rinse the slides carefully under running tap water for 10 min.
22. Counterstain the specimen by immersing the slides in Harris hematoxylin for 1 min and rinse immediately with running tap water until the slides are clean.
23. Dehydrate slides by serial ethanol washing steps: twice for 2 min in 70% ethanol, twice for 2 min in 90% ethanol, and once for 5 min in 100% ethanol. Clear them by incubating in xylene and mount with DPX (*see* **Note 13**).

3.5. Apoptosis: Tunel Method

Apoptosis is a form of cell death that eliminates compromised or superfluous cells. It is controlled by multiple signaling and effector pathways that mediate active responses to external growth, survival, or death factors (*see* **Fig. 1**).

The defining characteristic of apoptosis is a complete change in cellular morphology. As observed by electron microscopy, the cell undergoes shrinkage, chromatin margination, membrane blebbing, nuclear condensation and then segmentation, and division into apoptotic bodies which may be phagocytosed. The characteristic apoptotic bodies are short-lived and minute, and can resemble other cellular constituents when viewed by bright-field microscopy. DNA fragmentation in apoptotic cells is followed by cell death and removal from the tissue, usually within several hours.

DNA fragmentation is usually associated with ultrastructural changes in cellular morphology in apoptosis. The ultimate DNA fragments are multimers of about 180 bp nucleosomal units. These multimers appear as the familiar "DNA ladder" seen on standard agarose electrophoresis gels of DNA extracted from many kinds

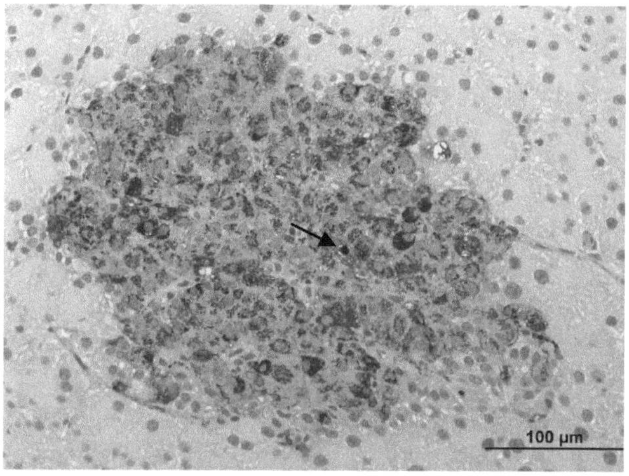

Fig. 1. Beta-cell apoptosis in a rat islet stained for TUNEL (nuclear staining) and insulin (cytoplasmic staining). *Arrow* shows the characteristic condensed nucleus stained for TUNEL in an insulin-positive cell.

of apoptotic cells. The principle of the TUNEL (TdT-mediated dUTP Nick End Labeling) method is based on the DNA strand breaks that are detected by enzymatically labeling the free 3′-OH termini with modified nucleotides. These new DNA ends that are generated upon DNA fragmentation are typically localized in morphologically identifiable nuclei and apoptotic bodies.

1. Perform tissue section deparaffinization as described in **Subheading 3.4**, steps 1–7.
2. For antigen retrieval, apply freshly diluted proteinase K (20 μg/ml) to the specimen for 15 min at room temperature in a coplin jar or directly on the slide.
3. Wash the specimen in two changes of ddH_2O in a coplin jar for 2 min each wash.
4. In order to quench endogenous peroxidase, place slides in a coplin jar containing 3% hydrogen peroxide in PBS for 20 min at room temperature.
5. Rinse the specimen once with PBS for 5 min.
6. Gently tap off excess liquid and carefully blot or aspirate around the section.
7. Immediately apply the equilibration buffer supplied in the ApopTag Peroxidase Kit directly onto the specimen. Incubate for at least 10 s at room temperature.
8. Gently tap off the excess liquid and carefully blot or aspirate around the section. Immediately pipette onto the section enough working strength TdT enzyme supplied in the ApopTag Peroxidase Kit. Incubate in a humidified chamber at 37°C for 1 h.

9. Put the specimen in a coplin jar containing working strength stop/wash buffer (supplied in the ApopTag Peroxidase Kit), agitate for 15 s, and incubate for 10 min at room temperature. (Prior to commencing next step, warm up antidigoxigenin conjugate supplied in the ApopTag Peroxidase Kit to room temperature.)
10. Wash the specimen in three changes of PBS for 1 min each wash.
11. Gently tap off the excess liquid and carefully blot or aspirate around the section.
12. Apply room temperature antidigoxignenin conjugate to the slide. Incubate in a humidified chamber for 30 min at room temperature.
13. Wash the specimen in three changes of PBS in a coplin jar for 3 min per wash at room temperature.
14. While the slides are washing, prepare the black staining solution.
15. Immerse the slides in black staining solution for 5–10 min at room temperature.
16. In order to determine the optimal staining time, monitor the color development by looking at the slide under the microscope.
17. Wash the specimen in three changes of dH_2O in a coplin jar for 5 min each wash (*see* **Note 14**).
18. Counterstain the specimen by immersing the slides in Harris hematoxylin for 1 min and rinse immediately with running tap water until the slides are clean.
19. Dehydrate, clear, and mount (as described in **Subheading 3.4**, step 23).
20. To quantify beta-cell apoptosis, visualize the slides under a brightfield microscope. Count the insulin-positive cells that are positive for TUNEL and divide by the total number of beta-cells (nucleus of insulin-positive cells) (*see* **Note 15**).

3.6. Proliferation: BrdU Incorporation

During cell proliferation, the DNA has to be replicated before the cell is divided into two daughter cells (*see* **Fig. 2**). This close association between DNA synthesis and cell doubling makes the measurement of DNA synthesis very attractive for assessing cell proliferation. If labeled DNA precursors are added to the cell culture or injected into the living animal, cells that are about to divide will incorporate the labeled nucleotide into their DNA. BrdU is a thymidine analogue that is incorporated into the DNA of proliferating cells in the S phase of cell cycle. Therefore, it can be subsequently detected by immunohistochemistry.

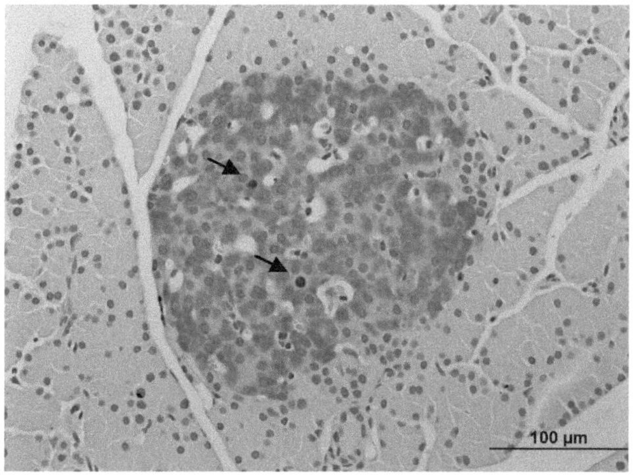

Fig. 2. Beta-cell replication (BrdU incorporation) in a rat islet stained for BrdU (nuclear staining) and insulin (cytoplasmic staining). *Arrows* show the two double-positive cells (BrdU and insulin positive). Similar images are obtained with Ki67 and insulin immunohistochemistry.

1. *BrdU injection.* 6 h before pancreas removal, administer BrdU solution at a dose of 100 mg/kg by intraperitoneal injection (*see* **Note 16**).
2. Carry out tissue section deparaffinization and endogenous peroxidase quenching as described in **Subheading 3.4**.
3. DNA denaturation and stabilization are carried out in a coplin jar. Denature DNA by immersion of slides in 2N HCl for 5 min at room temperature.
4. Wash the slides with 0.1 M borax solution for 10 min at room temperature (*see* **Note 17**).
5. Wash the specimen in three changes of PBS for 5 min each wash.
6. Block the specimen in blocking solution for 15 min at room temperature.
7. Gently tap off the excess liquid and carefully blot or aspirate around the section.
8. Apply sufficient reconstituted nuclease/anti-5-bromo-2′-deoxyuridine to cover the specimen. Incubate for 1 h at room temperature.
9. Wash the specimen in three changes of PBS for 5 min each wash.
10. Wipe around the specimen and add sufficient peroxidase anti-mouse IgG2a to cover the specimen. Incubate for 30 min at room temperature.
11. Wash the specimen in three changes of PBS for 5 min each wash.

12. Immerse the slides in staining solution for 5–10 min at room temperature.
13. In order to determine the optimal staining time, monitor the color development by looking at the slide under the microscope.
14. Rinse the slides carefully under running tap water for 10 min (*see* **Note 18**).
15. Counterstain by immersing the slides in Harris hematoxylin for 1 min and rinse immediately with running tap water until the slides are clean.
16. Dehydrate, clear, and mount (as described in **Subheading 3.4**, step 23).
17. To quantify beta-cell replication, visualize the slides under a brightfield microscope connected to a color monitor. Count the number of nuclei of insulin-positive cells that are positive for BrdU and divide by total number of beta-cells (nuclei of insulin-positive cells) (*see* **Note 15**).

3.7. Proliferation: Ki67

Ki67 is a nuclear antigen associated with cell proliferation and is present throughout the active cell cycle (G_1, S, G_2, and M phases), but absent in resting cells (G_0). Compared with BrdU staining, the advantage of Ki67 is that no antigen must be injected to identify replication. This makes Ki67 particularly useful when beta-cell replication is measured in human pancreas. However, Ki67 staining includes cells that are in G_1 phase of cell cycle and that may end up not progressing into S phase and reach mitosis.

1. Carry out tissue section deparaffinization, antigen retrieval, and endogenous peroxidase quenching as described in **Subheading 3.4**.
2. Place the slides in blocking solution for 15 min at room temperature.
3. Gently tap off the excess liquid and carefully blot or aspirate around the section. Apply sufficient Ki67 antibody (1:100) to cover the specimen. Incubate overnight at 4°C.
4. Wash the specimen in three changes of PBS for 5 min each wash.
5. Place the slides in blocking solution for 15 min at room temperature.
6. Wipe around the specimen. Add sufficient peroxidase labeled anti-rabbit IgG (1:200) antibody to cover the specimen. Incubate for 3 h at room temperature.
7. Wash the specimen in three changes of PBS for 5 min each wash.
8. Wash the specimen once with Tris buffer for 5 min.

9. Wipe around the specimen, and add sufficient peroxidase-labeled antiperoxidase antibody (1:500) to cover the specimen. Incubate for 1 h at room temperature.
10. Wash the specimen once with Tris buffer for 5 min.
11. Immerse slides in black staining solution for 1 min at room temperature.
12. In order to determine the optimal staining time, monitor the color development by looking at the slide under the microscope.
13. Rinse slides carefully under running tap water for 10 min.
14. Counterstain specimen by immersing slides in Harris hematoxylin for 1 min and rinse immediately with running tap water until the slides are clean.
15. Dehydrate, clear, and mount (as described in **Subheading 3.4**, step 23).
16. Quantify beta-cell replication (as described in **Subheading 3.6**, step 17).

3.8. Neogenesis (I): Islets Budding from Ducts – Immunohistochemistry for CK20 and Endocrine Islet Cells (Cocktail of Insulin, Glucagon, Somatostatin, and Pancreatic Polipeptide)

Beta-cell neogenesis has been reported in many experimental conditions in the adult pancreas, particularly with pancreatic injury, strongly suggesting the presence of adult stem/progenitor cells *(7)*. However, recent studies using lineage-tracing techniques have indicated that proliferation of differentiated beta-cells is the major mechanism for beta-cell formation in adult mice, with little or no contribution of beta-cell neogenesis *(8, 9)* or transdifferentiation *(10)*. Thus, the origin of new beta-cells in adult life, and the presence of neogenesis, is controversial.

The putative pancreatic stem/progenitor cell has been suggested to be located in islet, acinar, oval, and ductal cells, but it

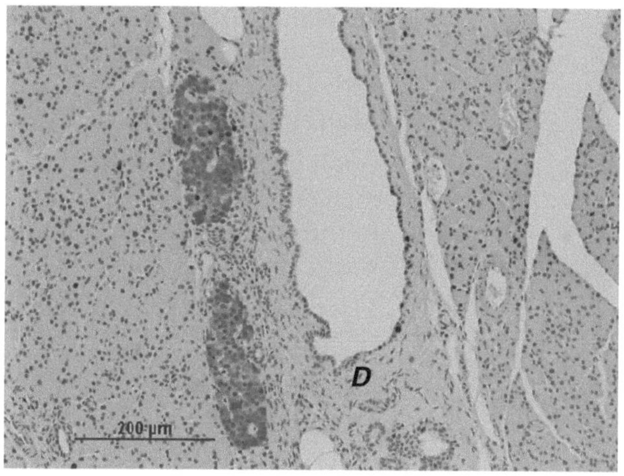

Fig. 3. Islet neogenesis (intraductal islet). The figure shows two insulin-stained islets in a pancreatic duct. *D* indicates ductal area.

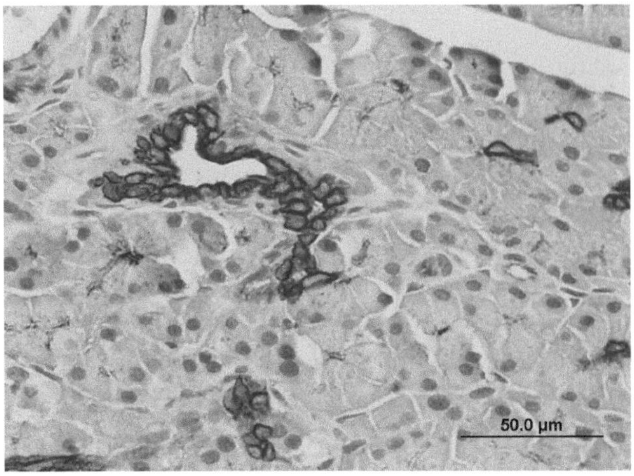

Fig. 4. Identification of pancreatic ducts of a rat pancreas stained with CK20.

has not yet been identified. The most extensive body of evidence supports the view that adult pancreatic duct cells are the main source of β-cell progenitors. The technique that we describe here is based on the consideration that islet neogenesis is defined by the presence of hormone-positive cells budding from ducts. Main duct and interlobular ducts can be easily identified on haematoxylin counterstained sections, and the presence of islet cells budding from ducts can be assessed with no specific ductal cell staining (*see* **Fig. 4**). Small interlobular ducts and intralobular or intercalated ducts are more difficult to identify, and specific staining for cytokeratine 20 (CK20) (*see* **Note 6**) antibody is needed (*see* **Fig. 3**). Islet cells are considered to be budding from ducts when they are in contact or in near contact (less than 5-8 cells apart) with ductal cells.

1. Carry out tissue section deparaffinization, antigen retrieval, and endogenous peroxidase quenching as described in **Subheading 3.4**.
2. Apply freshly diluted proteinase K (20 μg/ml) to the specimen for 40 min at 37°C in a water bath. Wash the specimen in three changes of wash buffer in a coplin jar for 5 min each wash.
3. Place the slides in blocking solution for 1 h at room temperature.
4. Gently tap off the excess liquid and carefully blot or aspirate around the section. Apply sufficient anti-CK20 antibody (1:15) to cover specimen. Incubate overnight at 4°C.
5. Wash the specimen in three changes of washing buffer for 5 min each wash.

6 . Wipe around the specimen and add sufficient anti-mouse IgG labeled polymer-HRP antibody from the EnVision+® System-HRP (DAB) kit to cover the specimen. Incubate for 1 h at room temperature.
7. Wash the specimen in three changes of Tris for 5 min each wash.
8. To develop color in peroxidase substrate, follow instructions described in **Subheading 3.4**.
9. Place the slides in blocking solution for 15 min at room temperature.
10. Gently tap off the excess liquid and carefully blot or aspirate around the section. Apply sufficient cocktail antibodies to cover the specimen. Incubate overnight at 4°C.
11. Wash the specimen in three changes of PBS for 5 min each wash.
12. Wipe around the specimen. Add sufficient peroxidase labeled anti-rabbit IgG (1:200) antibody to cover the specimen. Incubate for 3 h at room temperature.
13. Wash the specimen in three changes of PBS for 5 min each wash.
14. Wipe around the specimen. Add sufficient peroxidase labeled antiperoxidase antibody (1:500) to cover the specimen. Incubate for 1 h at room temperature.
15. Develop color as described in **Subheading 3.4**.
16. Counterstain specimen by immersing slides in Harris hematoxylin for 1 min and rinse immediately with running tap water until the slides are clean.
17. Dehydrate, clear, and mount.
18. To quantify islet neogenesis, visualize the slides under a brightfield microscope connected to a color monitor. Count the number of islets that are within the ducts (intraductal), those that are less than five cells apart from ducts (periductal), and the islets that are more than five cells distant from ducts (extraductal). Results may be expressed as percentage of intraductal, periductal, or extraductal islets. Analysis of two to three sections (150 μm apart) from each pancreas is usually needed to get a representative result.

3.9. Neogenesis (II): Confocal Immunofluorescence for PDX-1 and CK-20

The technique that we describe here is based on the consideration that colocalization of specific pancreatic endocrine cells markers and ductal cell markers in the same cell indicates islet neogenesis (*see* **Fig. 5**). Thus, expression of islet endocrine hormones in CK-20-positive ductal cells (or in acinar cells) is considered an indication of islet neogenesis. In embryonic development, the

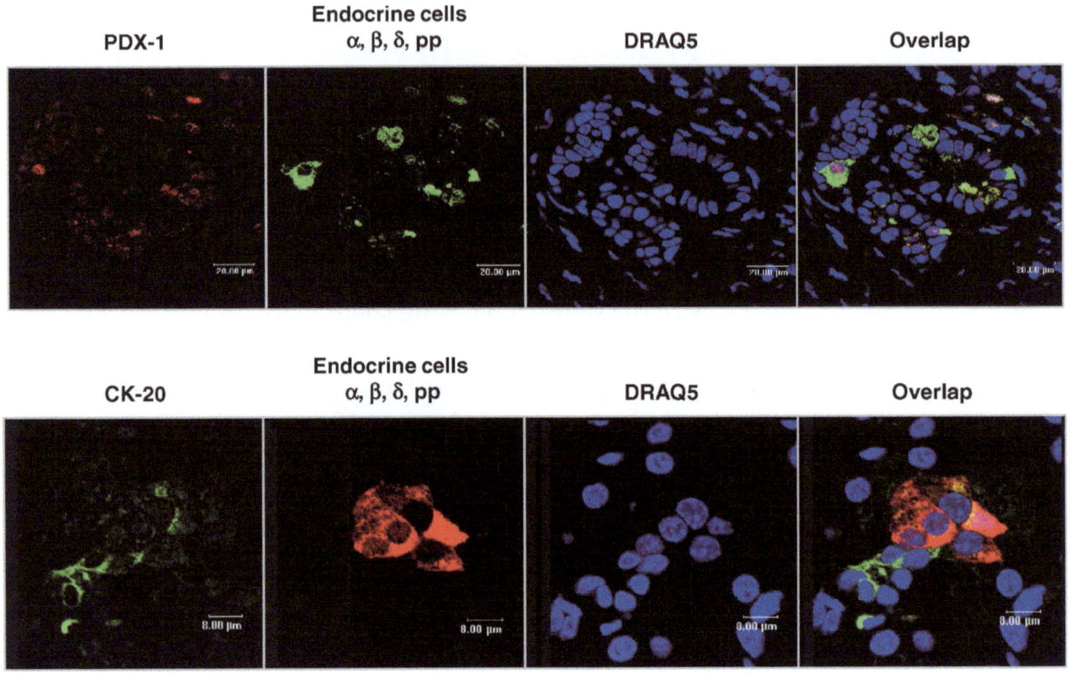

Fig. 5. Expression of endocrine markers in a ductal area of a 95% pancreatectomized rat assessed by confocal microscopy. Pancreatic remnants were stained for PDX-1 or CK-20, and a cocktail of antibodies against α, β, δ, and PP cells. *Upper panel* shows PDX-1 and endocrine costaining in ductal cells, identified by the characteristic ductal pattern shown with nuclear staining. *Lower panel* confirms expression of endocrine hormones in CK-20-positive ductal cells.

transcription factor PDX-1 is expressed in pancreatic endocrine progenitor cells. In adult life, PDX-1 is expressed and identifies beta-cells, and is not expressed in other pancreatic endocrine or exocrine cells. The expression of PDX-1 in ductal cells is considered an indication that the cell is undergoing a process of differentiation toward a beta-cell phenotype and a marker of beta-cell neogenesis.

1. Carry out tissue section deparaffinization and antigen retrieval as described in **Subheading 3.4**.
2. Apply freshly diluted DNase (10 μg/ml) to the specimen for 1 h at 37°C.
3. Wash the specimen in three changes of wash buffer in a coplin jar for 5 min each wash.
4. Place the slides in blocking solution in a coplin jar for 1 h at room temperature.
5. Gently tap off the excess liquid and carefully blot or aspirate around the section. Apply sufficient cocktail of anti-IDX (1:250) and CK20 (1:15) antibodies to cover the specimen. Incubate overnight at 4°C.

6. Wash the specimen in three changes of PBS for 5 min each wash.
7. From this step, protect slides from light. Wipe around the specimen. Add sufficient cocktail of Alexa fluor 488-labeled anti-rabbit IgG (1:400) and Alexa fluor 546 labeled-anti-mouse IgG (1:400) antibodies to cover the specimen. Incubate for 1 h at room temperature.
8. Wash the specimen in three changes of PBS for 5 min each wash.
9. Counterstain sections by applying DRAQ5 (1:1,000) to the specimens for 10 min at room temperature.
10. Mount with mounting medium for immunofluorescence (*see* **Note 19**).
11. Expression of beta-cell neogenesis is based on colocalization of PDX-1 staining in CK20-positive ductal cells on the confocal microscope. Results may be expressed as the percentage of CK20- and PDX-1-positive cells.

3.10. Neogenesis (III): Frequency of Small Groups of Extra-Islet Beta-Cells

With the normal expansion of beta-cell mass throughout life, islet size increases due to (1) the addition of new islet cells by replication of preexisting cells (beta-cell hyperplasia) and (b) the increased size of individual cells (beta-cell hypertrophy) *(1)*. It has been proposed that outside the already existing islets, new beta-cells or small new islets are formed by neogenesis from progenitor cells or by transdifferentiation from acinar cells. Thus, the presence of small clusters of insulin-positive cells is considered an indication of beta-cells neogenesis.

1. For beta-cell identification, perform immunohistochemistry for insulin as described in **Subheading 3.4**.
2. After beta-cell identification (described in **Subheading 3.4**), visualize the slides under the microscope connected to a color monitor and count the number of small clusters (<5 cells) of extra-islet insulin-positive cells. In order to standardize counting, the total pancreatic tissue area has to be measured and beta-cell neogenesis is expressed as the number of extra-islet beta-cells by square millimeter of pancreatic tissue. Analysis of two to three sections from each experimental pancreas is usually needed to get a representative result.

3.11. Beta-Cell Mass: Point Counting Morphometry

Despite recent progress *(11)*, reliable in vivo quantification of beta-cell mass is not yet feasible, and current estimation of beta-cell mass is only possible based on tissue sections. The estimation of pancreatic beta-cell mass (or any other tissue) based on microscopic study of tissue sections is a complex issue. Flat, two-dimensional sections must be related to the three-dimensional parameters that define the volume of interest, and the tissue sections provide restricted information about the distribution of the tissues of interest in the whole structure (*structure* being defined as "something made up of interdependent parts in a definite patter of organization"). Stereology, defined as "the body of mathematical methods relating three-dimensional parameters defining the structure to two-dimensional measurements obtainable on sections of the structure" *(12)*, was proposed to solve the difficulties of the spatial interpretation of sections. It provides methods by which to obtain reliable quantitative data on structure despite the restrictive nature of the information gathered by the study of tissue sections. Stereology uses a sophisticated and complex mathematical reasoning that is well beyond the scope of this chapter, to derive rather simple results in the form of formulas that can be easily applied by biologists without much knowledge about the process by which they were derived. To quantify the relative cell volume of the tissue of interest, several methods can be used, such as point counting, planimetry, or linear scanning. Systematic point counting has been reported to be the best method for estimating the volume density by stereological methods *(12)*.

To estimate the total beta-cell mass of the pancreas, it is indispensable to have the weight of pancreas and to determine the relative beta-cell volume. The pancreas weight is obtained as described in **Subheading 3.1**. The relative beta-cell volume is obtained by point counting. With these data, the absolute mass of the pancreatic beta-cells can be estimated with the equation:

Note that pancreatic weight is equated with pancreatic volume or mass based on the assumption that 1 cm^3 tissue weighs 1 g *(13)*. The same holds true for beta-cell mass.

If pancreatic weight is not available then the relative beta-cell volume, but not the absolute beta-cell mass, can be estimated. Since relative beta-cell volume depends on the number of intercepts over beta-cells *and* on other tissues (basically exocrine pancreas), a reduction in the exocrine portion of the pancreas would increase the relative beta-cell volume in the absence of changes in total beta-cell mass (that could be even reduced). Thus, increments in relative beta-cell volume do not necessarily mean that beta-cell mass is increased.

1. Pancreases have to be processed and weighed as described in **Subheading 3.1**
2. For beta-cell identification, perform immunohistochemistry for insulin as described in **Subheading 3.4**.
3. To quantify beta-cell mass, visualize the slides under a bright-field microscope (*see* **Note 20**) connected to a color monitor with an overlapped 48-point grid (*see* **Note 21**).
4. Obtain the number of intercepts over beta-cells, over endocrine non-beta-cells (if interested in endocrine non-beta-cell mass) and over other tissue (*see* **Note 22**).

5. Calculate the beta-cell relative volume by dividing the intercepts over beta-cells by intercepts over total tissue. Then estimate the beta-cell mass by multiplying beta-cell relative volume by pancreas weight using the above equation.
6. To validate the counting, a nomogram is used relating total number of points counted to volume density and expected relative standard error in percentage of the mean *(12)*. We use less than 10% as acceptable relative standard error in percentage of the mean *(14)*. Thus, the nomogram establishes the total number of intercepts needed for a representative sampling. Clearly, the number of intercepts needed for a valid counting will depend on the abundance of the specific tissue of interest in the counted section. For instance, to measure the endocrine non-beta-cell mass, the number of total intercepts needed to have a valid counting is much higher than the number of total intercepts needed to estimate beta-cell mass.

3.12. Individual Beta-Cell Size: Planimetry

The contribution of beta-cell hypertrophy or atrophy to changes in beta-cell mass is often overlooked, despite the very important impact that cell size has on the total mass of a tissue. The method that we will discuss here quantifies the mean cross-sectional area of individual beta-cells, a measure of individual beta-cell size. In essence, the beta-cell area of the pancreatic islets is measured using an image analysis program (*see* **Note 23**), and it is then divided by the number of beta-cell nuclei identified in that area. It must be taken into account that this method overestimates the size of the beta-cells because the actual number of beta-cells in the islets is higher than that counted since not all beta-cells are sectioned across their nuclei, and therefore some beta-cell nuclei are not identified.

1. For beta-cell identification, perform immunohistochemistry for insulin as described in **Subheading 3.4**.
2. To quantify the individual cell size, visualize the slides under a brightfield microscope connected to a computer and systematically capture enough images containing beta-cells (300 beta-cells from a minimum of six different islets per pancreas). Use an image analysis software with an arbitrary area measurement tool to determine the beta-cell area.
3. Calibrate the image (*see* **Note 24**).
4. Trace carefully the perimeter of the beta-cell area stained for insulin in the captured image. To exclude any other tissue or areas with no tissue (such as vasculature, ducts, and their lumen) that may lie inside the traced beta-cell area, trace also their perimeters. The program calculates the areas that have been traced. Add these areas and subtract them from the initially traced beta-cell area to obtain the final beta-cell area

in that image. Count all beta-cell nuclei located in the beta-cell area. Repeat the procedure with all capture images, and add their respective beta-cell areas and number of beta-cell nuclei.

5. Obtain the individual cross-sectional beta-cell area by dividing the total beta-cell area by the total number of beta-cell nuclei that it contains.

4. Notes

1. The solution needs to be carefully heated (use a stirring hotplate in a fume hood) to dissolve. Then cool to room temperature and store.
2. We have found this antibody to be useful for rat, mouse, and human pancreas. Numerous competitive reagents are available from other commercial sources.
3. We have found this kit to work very well in pancreas. Numerous competitive reagents are available from other commercial sources.
4. This solution needs to be carefully heated (~40°C) to dissolve.
5. We have found this antibody to work very well in human, but not in rodent pancreas.
6. CK20 is commonly used to identify ductal cells in rodents. For human pancreas, CK19 is recommended.
7. Excision of pancreas, placement in the cassette, and immersion in fixative must be done particularly quickly if apoptosis is to be measured.
8. It is advisable to place the pancreas in the cassette in a way that maintains the spatial orientation of the pancreas, so that position of head, body, and tail can be identified. This will also facilitate the identification of the main duct and other ductal structures when the pancreas is sectioned. For mouse pancreas, the whole pancreas can be placed in one cassette. For adult rats, the pancreas is sectioned into two pieces that are placed in separated cassettes.
9. Blocks can be left in paraffin at 65°C.
10. The block is "ribboning well" when you get a narrow strip of consecutive tissue sections flattened and smooth.
11. For heat-induced epitope retrieval, other methods can be used such as pressure cooker or microwave.

12. For a double immunohistochemical staining, it may be useful to use secondary antibodies labeled with alkaline phosphatase, allowing subsequent development with fast red or purple blue.
13. For a quick and reliable mounting, add a drop of DPX on the specimen when it is still wet from xylene. Turn slightly the slide allowing DPX slide down and when it reaches the edge of the slide, apply the coverslip from this edge.
14. To identify the apoptotic beta-cells after **Subheading 3.5**, proceed to **Subheading 3.4** for insulin staining method.
15. We count all islets identified in the tissue section and a minimum of 1,200 nucleus of beta-cells per sample. If this number is not reached, a second section is counted.
16. The duration G_2 phase of cell cycle in beta-cells is about 6 h *(15)*. Thus, a 6 h time period between BrdU injection and pancreas harvesting is recommended because it maximizes the number of proliferating beta-cells that will be labeled, and at the same time, it ensures that none of the labeled cells has been able to complete the G2 phase and enter into mitosis (M phase). This avoids the potential overestimation of beta-cell replication if doublets of stained beta-cells (daughters of a single beta-cell that has divided) are counted as two proliferating beta-cells.
17. HCl and Borax solutions are used to denature and stabilize DNA, respectively.
18. When beta-cell proliferation is going to be determined, after **Subheading 3.6** proceed to **Subheading 3.4** for insulin staining.
19. Several mounting media for immunofluorescence containing antifade reagents are available. Apply a drop of the mounting medium and proceed as described in **Note 13**. It is important to seal the coverslip with nail polish in order to prevent sample distortion by excessive shrinkage of the mounting medium.
20. Magnification used for counting has to be constant among samples.
21. The points must be spaced in such a manner that no more than one point can fall on the same cell.
22. If the endocrine non-beta-cell mass is not a subject of interest, then it is sufficient to count the intercepts over beta-cells and over the rest of the tissue. If there is an interest on estimating the cell mass of other pancreatic tissues (such as ductal cell mass), then count also the intercepts over those cells. For simultaneous counting of intercepts over several cell types present in the same section, we recommend the use of a cell counter.
23. There are many image analysis software available. The only essential requirement is that the software must enable the user to measure areas from a drawing.

24. Magnification and resolution of images has to be constant among samples. Note that calibration of images is critical since the measurement given by the software will depend on it. Images with higher resolution would improperly show bigger beta-cell area compared to those taken at lower.

Acknowledgments

The work discussed in this chapter has been supported by grants from Juvenile Diabetes Research Foundation International (JDRFI), Fondo the Investigaciones Sanitarias de la Seguridad Social (FISss), Instituto de Salud Carlos III, and REDIMET.

References

1. Montanya E, Nacher V, Biarnés M, Soler J. (2000). Linear correlation between beta cell mass and body weight throughout the lifespan in Lewis rats. *Diabetes* **49**:1341–1346.
2. Devendra D, Liu E, Eisenbarth GS. (2004). Type 1 diabetes: recent developments. *BMJ* 328:750–754.
3. Butler AE, Janson J, Bonner-Weir S, Ritzel R, Rizza RA, Butler PC. (2003). β-cell deficit and increased beta cell apoptosis in humans with type 2 diabetes. *Diabetes* **52**: 102–110.
4. Tellez N, Montolio M, Biarnes M, Castano E, Soler J, Montanya E. (2005). Overexpression of interleukin 1 receptor antagonist (IRAP) increases beta cell replication in rat pancreatic islets. *Gene Therapy* **12**:120–128.
5. Tellez N, Montolio M, Estilles E, Escoriza J, Soler J, Montanya E. (2007). Adenoviral Overproduction of Interleukin-1 Receptor Antagonist Protein increases beta cell replication and mass in syngeneically transplanted islets, and improves metabolic outcome. *Diabetologia* **50**:602–611.
6. Biarnés M, Montolio M, Raurell M, Nacher V, Soler J, Montanya E. (2002). β-cell death and mass in syngeneically transplanted islets exposed to short and long-term hyperglycemia. *Diabetes* **51**:66–72.
7. Bonner-Weir S, Weir GC. (2005). New sources of pancreatic beta cells. *Nat Biotechnol* **23**:857–861.
8. Dor Y, Brown J, Martinez OI, Melton DA. (2004). Adult pancreatic β-cells are formed by self-duplication rather than β-cell differentiation. *Nature* **429**:41–46.
9. Nir T, Melton DA, Dor Y. (2007). Recovery from diabetes in mice by β-cell regeneration. *J Clin Invest* **117**:2553–2561.
10. Desai BM, Oliver-Krasinski J, De Leon DD, Farzad C, Hong N, Leach SD, Stoffers DA. (2007). Preexisting pancreatic acinar cells contribute to acinar cell, but not islet beta cell, regeneration. *J Clin Invest* **117**: 971–977.
11. Evgenov NV, Medarova Z, Dai G, BonnerWeir S. Moore A. (2006). In vivo imaging of islet transplantation. *Nat Med* **12**: 144–148.
12. Weibel ER. (1979). Stereological Methods. Vol. 1. Practical Methods for Biological Morphometry. Academic Press, London.
13. Bonner-Weir S. (2001). Beta-cell turnover: its assessment and implications. *Diabetes* 50:Suppl 1:S20–S24
14. Montana E, Bonner-Weir S, Weir GC. (1993). Beta cell mass and growth after syngeneic islet cell transplantation in normal and streptozocin diabetic C57BL/6 mice. *J Clin Invest* **91**:780–787
15. Swenne I. (1982). The role of glucose in the in vitro regulation of cell cycle kinetics and proliferation of fetal pancreatic B-cells. *Diabetes* **31**:754–760.

Chapter 12

Morphology of Pancreatic Islets: A Time Course of Pre-diabetes in Zucker Fatty Rats

Petra Augstein and Eckhard Salzsieder

Summary

The Zucker fatty rat (fa/fa; ZR) is considered as a model for pre-diabetes, as characterised by a genetic defect in the leptin receptor, which results in hyperphagia, insulin resistance, hyperinsulinaemia, hyperlipoproteinaemia, and obesity. These animals become glucose intolerant but do not develop type 2 diabetes. As a consequence of increased adiposity and insulin resistance, the endocrine pancreas of ZR undergoes adaptive and compensatory changes. Measurements of the time course of the pathological changes by the histological analysis of the pancreatic islet in combination with metabolic parameters are an effective way to reveal disease progression. A loss in glucose tolerance occurs in ZR by 10 weeks of age and progressively worsens by 19 weeks of age. This process is accompanied by impaired islet histology, changes of β-cell mass, and impaired islet function. The early expression of insulin resistance and glucose intolerance in ZR results in morphological and functional changes of pancreatic islets despite their capability to maintain normoglycaemia.

Key words: Diabetes mellitus, Zucker fatty rat, Pancreatic islet, Morphology, Insulin; Glucagon, Immunofluorescence, Immunohistochemistry

1. Introduction

The development of type 2 diabetes appears to proceed via several stages *(1–3)*. Insulin resistance leading to hyperinsulinaemia, a defining feature of the development of type 2 diabetes, is accompanied by development of β-cell dysfunction mirrored by impaired islet morphology *(4–6)*. Finally, insulin resistance and decompensation of β-cell function induce the onset of the disease *(1–3)*.

C. Stocker (ed.), *Type 2 Diabetes,* Methods in Molecular Biology, vol. 560
DOI 10.1007/978-1-59745-448-3_12, © Humana Press, a part of Springer Science+Business Media, LLC 2009

Under the influence of obesity and insulin resistance, pancreatic β-cells are permanently exposed to elevated glucose concentrations as well as increased insulin levels. β-Cells adapt to these circumstances and undergo functional as well as morphological changes. Enhanced glucose levels may impose different effects on islet function and morphology as well as on β-cell survival *(1)*. The morphological correlate of insulin resistance and hyperinsulinaemia is an increased β-cell mass indicating adaptation towards increased functional demand *(1)*. Disturbed β-cell function is characterised by hypertrophy of pancreatic islets associated with increased number of immature secretory granules in the β-cells *(6)*. Prominent histopathological changes include disturbed islet architecture with invading exocrine tissue and derangement of α-cell distribution within the islet as well as islet fibrosis.

The Zucker fatty rat (fa/fa; ZR), characterised by insulin resistance and glucose intolerance, is a model for the study of prediabetes *(7-12)*. Young ZRs with near normal glucose tolerance are characterised by small islets and low volume of both islets and β-cells (**Figs. 1** and **2**). With manifestation of hyperinsulinaemia and glucose intolerance (**Table 1**), the number of small islets within the total islet population decreases (**Figs. 2** and **3**), reflecting disturbed islet function. Consequently, β-cell volume increases with progression of glucose intolerance in ZR until 19 weeks of age (**Fig. 1**, **Table 1**) *(9)*. These findings imply that islet histology of ZR reflects the progression of insulin resistance and decompensation of β-cell function *(4-6)*. Effective anti-diabetic approaches result in improved islet architecture, for example, rosiglitazone protects against pancreatic islet abnormalities in the ZR by reducing pancreatic islet hyperplasia and derangement of

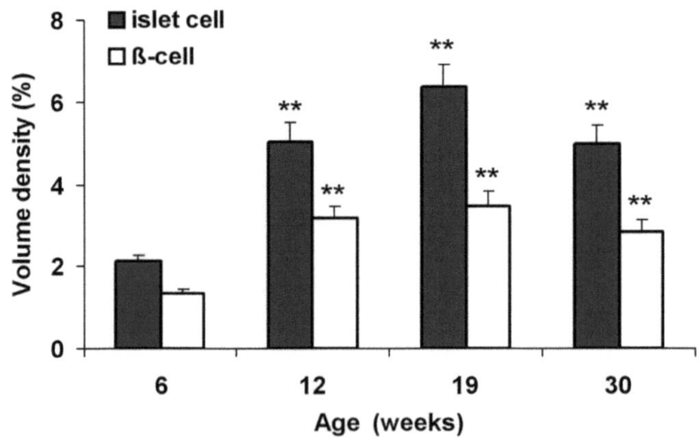

Fig. 1. Relative islet and β-cell volume density (%) in pancreata of Zucker fatty rats as a function of age. Data are mean ± SEM ($^{**}p < 0.01$ vs 6 weeks old animals).

α-cell distribution within the islet *(13)*. This chapter will outline methods for the investigation of islet histology using the Zucker rat model which have been developed at the Institute of Diabetes "Gerhardt Katsch" in Karlsburg over the last several years.

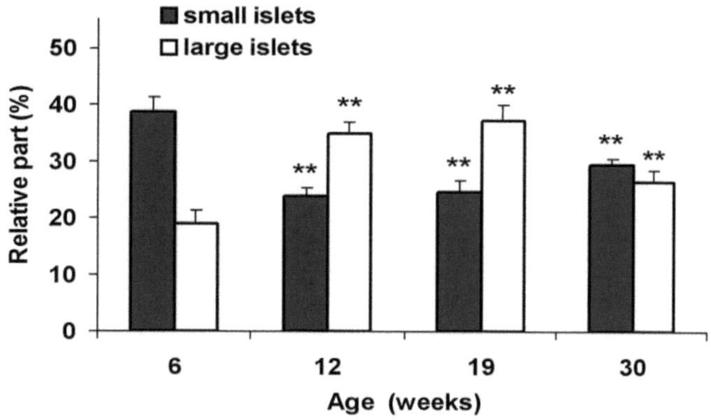

Fig. 2. Relative distribution of islet size (%) in pancreata of Zucker fatty rats as a function of age. Islet area was determined by morphometry and islets were classified according their area in small (<0.005 mm^2), medium (0.005-0.025 mm^2), and large (>0.025 mm^2) islets. Data are the relative part (%) of small and large islets. Data are mean ± SEM ($^{**}p < 0.01$ vs 6 weeks old animals).

Table 1
Characteristics of Zucker fatty rats (fa/fa) in relation to age

	Age (weeks)			
Parameter	**6 (n = 20)**	**12 (n = 19)**	**19 (n = 20)**	**30 (n = 27)**
Body weight (g)	243 ± 4	540 ± 8[a]	657 ± 11[a]	809 ± 17[a]
Blood glucose[b] (mmol/l)	5.02 ± 0.26	4.74 ± 0.15	5.65 ± 0.32	5.22 ± 0.16
Plasma insulin[b] (ng/ml)	8.44 ± 1.12	20.84 ± 3.69[a]	23.03 ± 4.09[a]	8.40 ± 1.20
G-AUC (mmol min/l)	770 ± 20	1,204 ± 44[a]	1,397 ± 66[a]	1,341 ± 48[a]
OGTT 2 h glucose (mmol/l)	4.90 ± 0.15	7.17 ± 0.37[a]	10.42 ± 0.55[a]	9.91 ± 0.46[a]
Triglycerides (mmol/l)	2.51 ± 0.20	9.93 ± 1.37[a]	18.54 ± 4.97[a]	21.07 ± 3.25[a]
Free fatty acids (mmol/l)	0.47 ± 0.02	0.82 ± 0.04[a]	1.24 ± 0.12[a]	1.18 ± 0.08[a]
Cholesterol (mmol/l)	3.70 ± 0.24	3.43 ± 0.32	7.26 ± 0.53[a]	10.55 ± 0.59[a]

Data are mean ± SEM
[a]$p < 0.01$ vs 6 weeks old animals
[b]Nonfasting

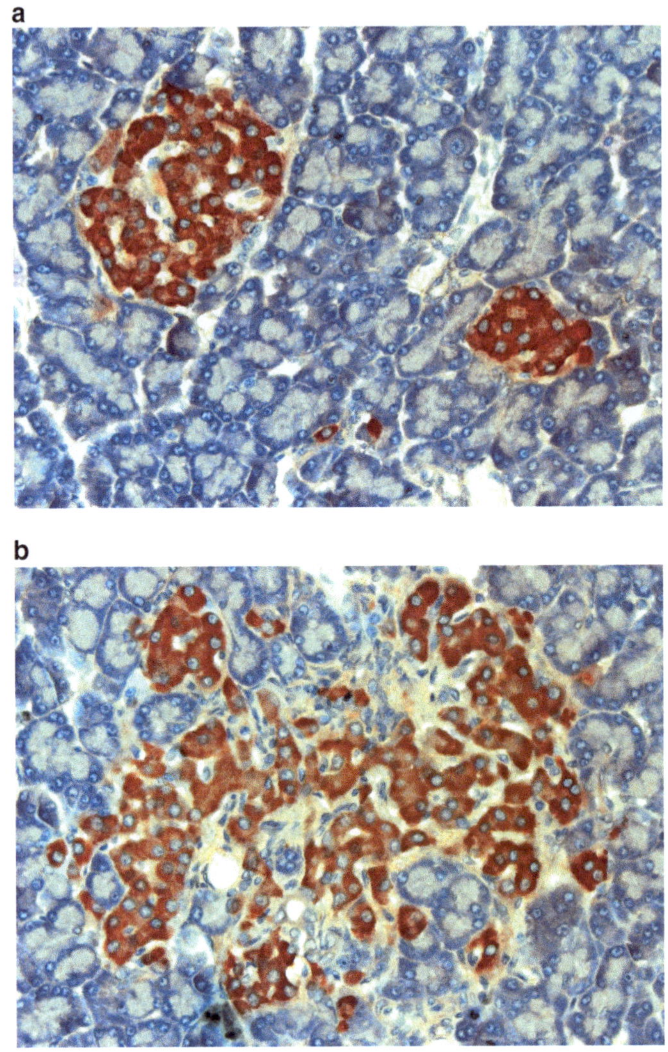

Fig. 3. Representative micrographs at 400-fold magnification demonstrating a small (**a**) and large (**b**) Zucker rat islets stained for insulin using a guinea pig anti-insulin antibody and HRP-labelled secondary antibody.

2. Materials

2.1. Preparation of Pancreatic Tissue

1. Appropriate Home Office designated preparation equipment.
2. NaCl, 0.9%.
3. Cellulose.
4. Dissection instruments.

2.2. Fixation of Pancreatic Tissue and Isolated Islets

2.2.1. Fixation of Pancreatic Tissue

Cryofixation

1. Liquid nitrogen and transport container.
2. Dry ice and transport container.
3. Optimal cutting compound (OCT; Tissue Tek, Miles Inc., Elkhart, IN, USA).
4. *N*-hexane.
5. Metal bowl.
6. Cryomoulds (Disposable Vinyl specimen moulds; Tissue Tek).
7. Plastic bags, scissors, forceps.
8. CryoTubes™ (Nalgene® Nunc™, Roskilde, Denmark).
9. –80°C freezer.

Bouin's Fluid

1. Mix components of Bouin's fixative immediately before use:

(a) Picric acid, saturated. (Caution: explosion hazard)	15 ml
(b) Formalin (37% formaldehyde)	5 ml
(c) Glacial acetic acid	1 ml

2. Aqua destillata (A. dest).
3. Ethanol, 96%, reagent grade.
4. Specimen container for fixation.
5. Plastic cassettes for tissue processing.

Paraformaldehyde

1. Phosphate-buffered saline (PBS, pH 7.2–7.4).
2. 4% (w/v) Paraformaldehyde (PFA). Weigh PFA in a fume hood wearing gloves and safety glasses, transfer to PBS and dissolve at 65°C in a water bath. Store in single use aliquots at –20°C.
3. 70% ethanol.
4. Specimen container for fixation.
5. Plastic cassettes for tissue processing.

2.2.2. Fixation of Isolated Pancreatic Islets

Cryofixation

1. Liquid nitrogen.
2. Hanks balanced salt solution.
3. Islet collection buffer with 5% (w/v) bovine serum albumin: 115.07 mM NaCl, 23.93 mM $NaHCO_3$, 5 mM KCl, 10 mM $MgCl_2{\cdot}6H_2O$, 1 mM $CaCl_2{\cdot}2H_2O$, 5 mM glucose, pH 7.4.
4. Siliconised glass pipette.
5. Centrifuge tubes, small and lockable with V-bottom.
6. Bench top centrifuge.

Bouin's Fluid

1. Bouin's fluid (*see* **Subheading 2.2.1**).
2. Ethanol.
3. **Items 2-6** listed above for cryofixation.
4. Embedding cassettes for biopsies (BioNet-Einbettungs-kassetten; Engelbrecht Medizin- und Labortechnik, Edermünde, Germany).

2.3. Embedding, Storage, and Cutting

2.3.1. Cryosections

1. OCT.
2. Dry ice or liquid nitrogen.
3. Acetone.
4. Mayer's hematoxylin (Carl Roth GmbH, Karlsruhe, Germany).
5. Specimen container for fixation.
6. SuperFrost® Plus (*see* **Note 1**) slides (Menzel-Gläser, Steinheim, Germany) or self-made silane-coated slides (*see* **Note 2**) using 3-aminopropyltriethoxy-silane (silane).
7. Cryostat.
8. Disposable blades or knife.
9. Anti-roll plate.
10. Acetone-resistant slide racks and staining dishes.
11. Slide containers.
12. –80°C freezer.

2.3.2. Embedding, Storage, and Cutting of Tissue Fixed in Bouin's Solution and PFA

1. Ethanol.
2. Xylene.
3. Paraffin, melting point 42–44°C (Merck, Darmstadt, Germany).
4. Mayer's hematoxylin.
5. Specimen container for fixation.
6. Tissue processing machine.
7. Microtome for paraffin blocks.
8. Microtome blades.
9. SuperFrost® Plus slides (Menzel–Gläser) or silane-coated slides (*see* **Subheading 2.3.1**; *see* **Note 2**).
10. Slide drying bench.
11. Water bath.
12. 60°C oven.
13. Forceps.
14. Brushes.
15. Slide containers.

2.4. Staining Procedures

1. Acetone.
2. Absolute and 96% ethanol, reagent grade.
3. Xylene or xylene substitute.
4. Methanol.
5. H_2O_2.
6. Mayer's hematoxylin.
7. Non-immune serum for blocking.
8. Primary antibody (1st Ab).
9. Isotype-matched control Ab.
10. Secondary antibody (2nd Ab).
11. Substrate for enzyme reaction.
12. Mounting medium.
13. PBS or Tris-buffered saline (TBS): 7.43 mM Tris, 43.46 mM Tris–HCl, 149.83 mM NaCl, pH 7.4 at room temperature.
14. A. dest.
15. Incubation chamber.
16. Slide racks.
17. Troughs to fit slide racks.
18. Staining dishes.
19. Dako pen (Dako, Hamburg, Germany).
20. Coverslips.
21. Microscope.

2.4.1. Detection of Pancreatic Islets

Hematoxylin and Eosin Staining

1. Mayer's hematoxylin.
2. Eosin Y (Merck). Prepare eosin Stock solution (1%); dissolve 1 g Eosin Y in 100 ml of distilled water and mix to dissolve with shaking, add 50 μl of glacial acetic acid per 100 ml.
3. Pertex® mounting medium or equivalent xylene-based or xylene substitute-based mounting medium.

Immunohistochemical Staining for Insulin

1. Anti-insulin Ab; mouse anti-insulin monoclonal Ab (mcAb) 36aC10 (IgG1; UNICUS Karlsburg OHG, Karlsburg, Germany) or guinea pig anti-insulin polyclonal (pc) Ab (Dako).
2. 2nd Ab; pc rabbit anti-mouse immunoglobulins/HRP (Ig fraction; Dako) or pc rabbit anti-guinea pig immunoglobulins/HRP (Dako).
3. AEC^+, high sensitivity substrate chromogen (3-amino-9-ethylcarbazole containing hydrogen peroxide, stabilizers, enhancers, and antimicrobial agent; Dako).
4. Aqueous-based mounting media; faramount mounting medium or Glycergel® (Dako).

5. Incubation chamber with humidified atmosphere.
6. Dako pen.

Immunohistochemical Staining for Glucagon

1. Anti-glucagon Ab; anti-glucagon mcAb 79bB10 (mouse IgG1; UNICUS Karlsburg OHG) or rabbit anti-glucagon pc Ab (Dako).
2. 2nd Ab; pc rabbit anti-mouse immunoglobulins/HRP (Ig fraction; Dako) or anti-mouse IgG/HRP (Jackson ImmunoResearch Laboratories) or pc swine anti-rabbit immunoglobulins/HRP (Dako).
3. **Items 3–6** listed above for immunohistochemical staining for insulin.

Immunofluorescence Staining for (Pro)insulin

1. Anti-(pro)insulin Ab; anti-insulin mcAb 36aC10 (mouse IgG1; UNICUS Karlsburg OHG) or anti-proinsulin mcAb K14D4 (mouse IgG1; UNICUS Karlsburg OHG).
2. 2nd Ab; FITC-labelled Ab anti-mouse IgG (Dako).
3. Fluorescence mounting medium (Dako).
4. Incubation chamber with humidified atmosphere.
5. Dako pen.
6. Fluorescence microscope.

Immunofluorescence Staining for Glucagon

1. Anti-glucagon Ab; anti-glucagon mcAb 79bB10 (mouse IgG1; UNICUS Karlsburg OHG) or rabbit anti-glucagon pcAb (Dako).
2. Fluorochrome-labelled pre-absorbed 2nd Ab; Texas Red® or Cy5 anti-species Ig (Jackson ImmunoResearch Laboratories).
3. **Items 3–6** listed above for immunofluorescence staining for (pro)insulin.

Double-Staining for Insulin and Glucagon

1. Items listed above.

2.4.2. Detection of a Fixation-Sensitive Protein

High-Level Protein Expression Detected Using Immunofluorescence

1. Acetone.
2. 1st Ab.
3. 2nd Ab FITC anti-species diluted according to the guidelines of the supplier.
4. **Items 3–6** listed above for immunofluorescence staining for (pro)insulin (*see* **Subheading 2.4.1**).

Low-Level Protein Expression Detected Using Alkaline Phosphatase Anti-Alkaline Phosphatase Technique

1. Acetone.
2. TBS.
3. Non-immune rabbit serum.

4. Mouse 1st Ab and negative control (isotype-matched control).
5. Rabbit anti-mouse IgG (Dako).
6. APAAP (alkaline phosphatase anti-alkaline phosphatase) from mouse (Sigma).
7. Naphthol AS-TR phosphate/Fast Red RC (Fast Red; Sigma).
8. Glycergel® (Dako).
9. Incubation chamber with humidified atmosphere.
10. Dako pen.
11. Microscope.

2.4.3. Detection of a Fixation-Resistant Protein

High-Level Protein Expression Detected Using Immunohistochemistry

1. 1st Ab.
2. 2nd Ab.
3. AEC^+; high sensitivity substrate chromogen (Dako).
4. 5-Bromo-4-chloro-3-indolyl phosphate/Nitro blue tetrazolium (BCIP/NPT; Fastblue, Sigma).
5. Aqueous-based mounting media (*see* **Subheading 2.4.1, items 4–6** of imunohistochemical staining for insulin).

Low-Level Protein Expression Detected by APAAP

1. *See* **Subheading 2.4.2**.

2.5. Evaluation Methods

1. Object micrometer with a 1 mm scale.
2. Eyepiece reticule, that is, ocular micrometer.
3. Microscope with an adjustable ocular.

3. Methods

Prior to investigation of pancreatic islets by immunohistochemistry, a complete understanding of the antigen(s) (Ag/Ags) of interest is essential. There are multiple means of staining pancreatic tissue and the selection of the appropriate fixation and staining techniques will yield optimum results *(14–17)*. **Figure 4** illustrates the development of an experimental strategy that will lead to the choice of an appropriate fixation and embedding procedure.

Pancreatic islets can be visualised (*see* **Subheading 3.4.1**) by staining for islet hormones as well as for islet proteins *(12–14)*. Investigation of the architecture of pancreatic islets may be accomplished by the detection of insulin and glucagon. Use of Bouin's fluid, a common fixation method, is especially suitable for

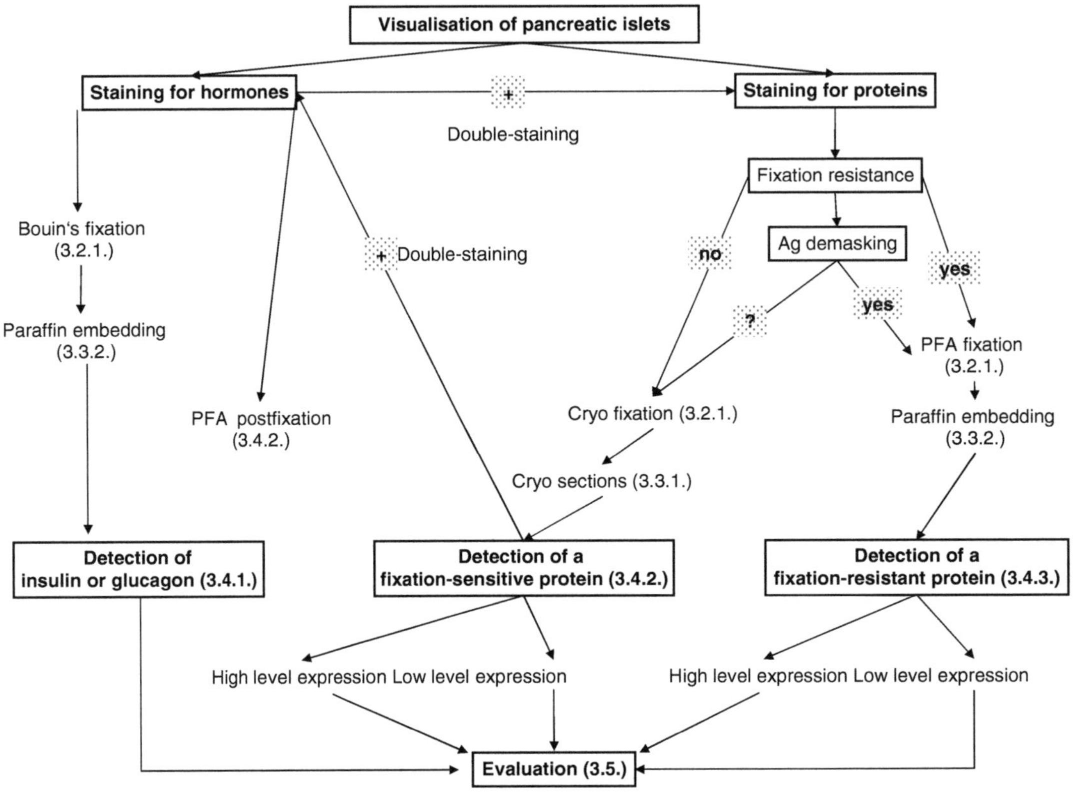

Fig. 4. Guide for developing an experimental strategy.

detection of peptide hormones (*see* **Subheadings 2.2.1** and **3.2.1**), producing a brilliant staining pattern using immunohistochemistry as well as immunofluorescence (*see* **Subheading 3.4.1**). The best procedure to examine a particular protein will be determined by its fixation resistance. This is also true for the simultaneous detection of protein and hormone expression by double-labelling (*see* **Subheadings 3.4.2** and **3.4.3**). Bouin's fixation is very often not suitable for detection of proteins due to background problems and Ag damage. If this is the case, one must determine whether the protein of interest is PFA-resistant and whether there is an Ab available that recognizes a linear epitope of the protein. If the protein is PFA-resistant, one can proceed with PFA fixation and paraffin embedding (*see* **Subheadings 3.2.1** and **3.3.2**). If it is unknown whether the protein is PFA-sensitive or whether a de-masking procedure is working reliably, the tissue may be snap frozen using liquid nitrogen (*see* **Subheadings 3.2.1** and **3.3.1**, *see* **Note 3**). If the goal is to demonstrate pancreatic islets by double-labelling for protein and hormone, a post-fixation step with 4% PFA may be performed directly on the cryostat sections (*see* **Subheading 3.4.2**).

Subsequently, a suitable detection method must be defined. This decision must take into account the level of expression of the Ag of interest, the sensitivity of selected methods, the access to immunohistochemical equipment, and possible double-labelling staining. For example, if the protein is expressed at a low level, sensitive amplification methods would improve the results. Available microscopes (light, fluorescence, and confocal) would direct the selection of the detection method (immunohistochemistry or fluorescence). If the protein of interest is expressed at a high level, the detection method can usually be established in a straightforward manner.

Finally, the evaluation method should be considered. The possibilities include (1) micrographs for demonstration of expression, (2) semi-quantitative analysis, and (3) morphometry and image analysis for co-expression studies. The evaluation method must be compatible with the detection method.

The following steps summarise a general procedure for establishing a method:

1. *Checkerboard titration experiments for establishing a new method.* Optimal dilution of 1st Abs and 2nd Abs depends on Ag expression, sample preparation, Ab affinity, amount of Ag, incubation duration, and detection system. These parameters must be determined for each method. The dilutions given in this chapter are only guidelines.
2. *Titration of the 1st Ab* on a positive control tissue with known Ag expression at the scheduled incubation time (e.g. 2 h at room temperature or overnight at 4°C.)
   (a) Start with the dilution guideline of the supplier. Always include a pre-immune serum or isotype-matched immunoglobulin as a negative control, which is handled in the same manner as the 1st Ab **(Table 2)**. The 2nd Ab is used at the lowest concentration suggested by the supplier.
   (b) Repeat the last three dilutions with convincing positive staining results on the positive control tissue and the tissue of interest.
3. *Titration of the 2nd Ab.* Test the 2nd Ab in three dilution steps similar to the dilution guidelines of the supplier. We recommend that non-specific binding of the 2nd Ab, indicated by high background on negative control sections, be dealt with by the following two approaches:
   (a) Use a pre-absorbed 2nd Ab, for example, from Jackson ImmunoResearch Laboratories (Europe Ltd., UK) according to the manufacturer's protocol.
   (b) Block sections for 10 min at room temperature with 10% (v/v) of non-immune sera of the species the 2nd Ab was

Table 2
Controls for specific staining

Slide	Control	Tissue	1st Ab	2nd Ab	Substrate
Experimental	Binding of 1st Ab	Tissue of interest	Yes	Yes	Yes
Positive control	Binding of 1st Ab	Section with known AG expression	Yes	Yes	Yes
Negative control	Binding of 2nd Ab	Tissue of interest	Non-immune serum or isotype-matched control	Yes	Yes
Negative control	Unspecific substrate reaction	Tissue of interest	Non-immune serum or isotype-matched control	Dilution buffer	Yes

raised in. For comparison of results, include one section without blocking to reveal unexpected cross-reactivities of the non-immune sera.

4. *Establishing a double-labelling method.* Repeat the above steps for the Ab recognition of the second Ag of interest. The blocking procedure must be compatible with both 2nd Abs and no cross-reactivity may occur between the 1st and 2nd Abs. The quality of the 2nd Ab is critical and preferred to apply pre-absorbed 2nd Ab. If inclusion of a blocking step is required, neonatal calf serum (NCS) is a good initial choice. However, some 2nd Abs, for example, anti-goat Ab, may cross-react with NCS.

There are several possibilities for setting up a double-labelling method. Two single-staining procedures can be performed consecutively *(17)*, Here the first staining (1st Ab 1 + 2nd Ab 1) and then the second (1st Ab 2 + 2nd Ab 2) are performed as separate steps. If these are successful, combine the incubation steps for the primary (1st Ab 1 + 1st Ab 2) and secondary antibodies (2nd Ab 1 + 2nd Ab 2).

The evaluation of double-staining may be difficult for ICH. The detection of nuclear staining by alkaline phosphatase and BCIP/NPT and cytoplasmic reactions with HRP and AEC are successful strategies *(15)*. **Table 3** provides a short overview for troubleshooting.

3.1. Preparation of Pancreatic Tissue

1. Animals are sacrificed by an appropriate Home Office method (*see* **Note 4**).
2. Pancreata must be immediately excised (*see* **Note 5**).
3. Remove the surrounding fat and lymph nodes using a black pad and wash the tissue in isotonic NaCl if necessary.

Table 3
Troubleshooting guide

Problem	Possible reasons	Action
Damaged morphology	Autolysis	Optimise preparation of tissue, improve fixation
Tissue has network appearance	Tissue was frozen improperly or frozen and thawed	Apply greater care in freezing
No staining of 1st Ab and controls	Omitted 1st Ab or 2nd Ab	Repeat staining
	Abs of bad quality	Change Abs and repeat
	Wrong handling of the chromogen solution	Repeat substrate reaction
	NaN_3-mediated inhibition of HRP	Avoid NaN_3
Tissue section come off the slide	Slides are not properly coated	Use commercially prepared slides or perform a silane coating
Weak staining of the AG	Wrong dilution	Checkerboard titration
	Reagent(s) beyond date of expiry	Change reagent(s) and repeat
	Too much serum or blocking reagent remained on the section	Repeat staining and remove excess of buffer
	Incubation too short	Repeat with longer incubation
	1st Ab has a low affinity	Exchange 1st Ab
	Tissue has been over fixed resulting in Ag masking	AG de-masking procedure or repetition with cryofixed tissue
	Problems in fixation procedure	Optimise fixation with positive control tissue
Irregular staining with diffuse background staining	Uneven fixation; unfixed tissue binds reagents unspecific	Separate tissue in pieces or use longer fixation
	Tissue contains necrotic compartments resulting in high background	Ignore necrotic areas
	Low level of AG expression	Extend incubation of the 1st Ab and apply the APAAP method
	Incorrect de-paraffination	Repeat de-paraffination
	Section dried partial during staining procedure	Avoid drying of sections
High background staining	Chromogen reaction was too long	Optimise chromogen reaction
	Cross-reactivities of 2nd Ab with tissue	Use pre-absorbed 2nd Ab
	2nd Ab too highly concentrated	Checkerboard titration
	Incorrect washing of slides	Repeat washing
	Wrong blocking serum	Use for blocking non-immune serum the 2nd Ab was raised in

(continued)

Table 3 (continued)

Problem	Possible reasons	Action
Positive cells stain with substrate reagent alone	Endogenous peroxidase reactivity present	Longer hydrogen-peroxide treatment or use of an alkaline phosphatase-labelled 2nd Ab
AEC is brown instead of red	Surplus of AEC as precipitated at the 1st Ab site	Reduce 1st Ab concentration until AEC turns red
Intense specific as well as background staining	1st Ab concentration too highly concentrated	Checkerboard titration
Focussing on a single cell layer is impossible	Section too thick	Recut thinner sections

3.2. Fixation of Pancreatic Tissue and Isolated Pancreatic Islets

3.2.1. Fixation of Pancreata

Cryofixation

1. Fix tissue in cryomoulds with OCT-embedding medium using *n*-hexane and dry ice (*see* **Note 6**). Alternatively, tissue can be snap frozen directly in liquid nitrogen after placing in CryoTubes™ (*see* **Note 7**) or aluminium foil.
2. Store the frozen blocks in sealable plastic bags or CryoTubes™ at –80°C.

Bouin's Fluid

1. Prepare Bouin's fixative immediately before use.
2. Immerse the pancreatic tissue in approximately 20-fold of the tissue volume.
3. Fix the tissue for 24 h at room temperature (*see* **Note 8**).
4. Rinse the tissue for 15 min in 50% ethanol at room temperature (*see* **Note 9**).
5. Wash 1× in 50% ethanol, transfer to 70% ethanol, change ethanol 3× (*see* **Note 10**).
6. Process through paraffin wax for embedding (*see* **Subheading 3.3.2**) or
7. Store tissue in 70% ethanol (to avoid drying out of the tissue replace the 70% ethanol every week).

PFA Fixation

1. Immerse the tissue in approximately 20-fold of the tissue volume in 4% PFA solution for 18 h at 4°C (*see* **Note 11**).
2. If the tissue cannot be paraffin embedded immediately, it can be stored in 70% ethanol *(16)*.
3. Process through paraffin wax for embedding (*see* **Subheading 3.3.2**).

3.2.2 Fixation of Isolated Pancreatic Islets

Cryofixation

1. Wash isolated islets 2× in Hanks balanced salt solution.
2. Using a siliconised glass pipette, transfer intact islets, selected by hand, under a stereomicroscope into islet collection buffer.
3. Collect 100–200 islets into a small lockable centrifuge tube.
4. Centrifugation for 1 min at 380 × g with no brake setting.
5. Freeze snap in liquid nitrogen without disturbing the pellet.

Bouin's Fluid

1. Perform **steps 1–4** as described for cryofixation of islets.
2. Remove the supernatant without disturbing the pellet.
3. Add 0.5 ml Bouin's fluid without disturbing the pellet.
4. Change the fixative twice without disturbing the pellet.
5. Fix the islets using Bouin's fluid for 4 h at room temperature.
6. Transfer the islet pellet into 70% ethanol.
7. Proceed with the embedding procedure using embedding cassettes for biopsies.

3.3. Processing of Fixed Tissue, Embedding, Storage, and Cutting

3.3.1. Cryosections, Cutting, and Storage

1. Ensure familiarity with the equipment.
2. Transfer the tissue to the cryostat using dry ice or liquid nitrogen (*see* **Note 12**).
3. Freeze the tissue on an object holder of the cryostat using OCT and the object-cooling system of the cryostat.
4. The temperature is usually set at around –20°C *(16, 17)* (*see* **Note 13**).
5. Label SuperFrost® slides with pencil or ICH-pencil.
6. Cut 5–8 µm frozen sections (*see* **Note 14**).
7. Assess the section for the presence of sufficient islets by staining with hematoxylin.
8. Air-dry the sections for at least 4 h or overnight at room temperature.
9. Fix for 10 min in acetone.
10. Store the slides at –80°C until needed in slide boxes, or proceed with staining.

3.3.2. Embedding, Storage, and Cutting of Pancreatic Tissue Fixed with Bouin's Solution or PFA

1. Place fixed tissues in embedding cassettes for dehydration and embedding procedures (*see* **Note 15**).
2. Perform dehydration *(16, 17)* and paraffin infiltration using the following regime and an automatic tissue processor (*see* **Note 16**).

(a) Ethanol 80%	1 h	40°C
(b) Ethanol 80%	1 h	40°C
(c) Ethanol 96%	1 h	40°C
(d) Ethanol 96%	1 h	40°C
(e) Ethanol 100%	1 h	40°C
(f) Ethanol 100%	1 h	40°C
(g) Xylene	30 min	40°C
(h) Xylene	1 h	40°C
(i) Xylene	1 h	40°C
(j) Paraffin	30 min	62°C
(k) Paraffin	1 h	62°C
(l) Paraffin	1 h	62°C
(m) Paraffin	1 h	62°C

3. Orientate the tissue in the long axis of the embedding mould and embed the tissue in paraffin, store paraffin blocks at room temperature.
4. Before cutting, pre-cool the paraffin block to 4°C overnight.
5. Pre-cool the paraffin block on ice and set up the microtome.
6. Trim the paraffin blocks until there is an appropriate cutting area (*see* **Note 17**).
7. Section 4–7 μm thick, check for islets by hematoxylin and eosin (HE) staining; consider the final evaluation in the cutting strategy (*see* **Note 18**).
8. Place the paraffin ribbons in a water bath at approximately 40°C to stretch them.
9. Mount the sections on SuperFrost® Plus or UltraPlus® slides. Alternatively, silane-coated slides can be prepared in advance (*see* **Note 19**). Allow sections to air-dry for 30 min at room temperature.
10. Dry the slides at 60°C on a slide drying bench or oven to remove any water beneath the tissue section and improve adherence of the section to the slide *(17)*.
11. Allow sections to cool at room temperature.
12. Store the slides in boxes at room temperature. The slides are ready to be de-paraffinised and stained.

3.4. Staining Procedure

3.4.1. Detection of Pancreatic Islets

HE Staining for Assessment of Pancreas and Islet Morphology

1. De-paraffinate and re-hydrate sections (*see* **Note 20**):

(a) Xylene or xylene substitute	5 min	Room temperature
(b) Xylene or xylene substitute	5 min	Room temperature
(c) Ethanol absolute	3 min	Room temperature
(d) Ethanol absolute	3 min	Room temperature
(e) Ethanol 96%	3 min	Room temperature
(f) Ethanol 96%	3 min	Room temperature
(g) Ethanol 90%	3 min	Room temperature
(h) Ethanol 70%	3 min	Room temperature
(i) A. dest	3min	Room temperature

2. Stain in Mayer's hematoxylin solution for 3 min.
3. Wash in running tap water for 5–10 min for blue colouration to establish.
4. Rinse in distilled water.
5. Counterstain in 1% eosin Y solution for 2–3 min.
6. Rinse in distilled water until no dye drain from the sections.
7. Dehydrate through increasing concentrations of ethanol *(16, 17)*.

(a) Ethanol 70%	3 min	Room temperature
(b) Ethanol 90%	3 min	Room temperature
(c) Ethanol 96%	3 min	Room temperature
(d) Ethanol 96%	3 min	Room temperature
(e) Ethanol absolute	3 min	Room temperature
(f) Ethanol absolute	3 min	Room temperature
(g) Xylene or xylene substitute	5 min	Room temperature
(h) Xylene or xylene substitute	5 min	Room temperature

8. Mount permanently with Pertex® mounting medium or equivalent xylene-based or xylene substitute-based mounting medium.

Immunohistochemical Staining for Insulin

1. De-paraffinise sections of pancreatic tissue fixed in Bouin's fluid as described above for HE staining.

2. Never allow the sections to dry.
3. Transfer into PBS after the last rinse in distilled water.
4. Wash 2× in PBS, 2 min each.
5. Block endogenous peroxidase using 3% H_2O_2 in methanol for 15 min at room temperature.
6. Wash 2× in PBS, 2 min each.
7. Encircle sections using a DAKO pen; this water-repelling material provides a barrier to liquids (*see* **Note 21**).
8. Block the sections with 10% non-immune serum of the species the secondary Ab was raised in. Dilute the serum in PBS and incubate sections for 10 min at room temperature.
9. Rinse in PBS.
10. Prepare an incubation chamber with humidified atmosphere (*see* **Note 22**).
11. There are two insulin Abs commercially available, both give good results (*see* **Note 23**):
    - Mouse anti-insulin mcAb 36aC10 *(18)*.
    - Guinea pig anti-insulin pcAb *(12)*.
12. Dilute Ab in PBS and incubate for 1 h at room temperature (*see* **Note 24**).
13. Wash 3× in PBS, 5 min each.
14. The Ab binding is visualised using anti-mouse/HRP and anti-guinea pig HRP, respectively, 2nd Ab diluted 1:200 for 30 min at RT.
15. Wash 3× in PBS, 5 min each.
16. Cover the sections with the ready-to-use AEC substrate-chromogen solution according to supplier's instructions (*see* **Note 25**).
17. Rinse gently in PBS.
18. Counterstain the sections with hematoxylin.
19. Coverslip with aqueous-based mounting media (*see* **Note 26**).

Immunohistochemical Staining for Glucagon

1. Perform **steps 1–10** as described above for insulin.
2. Two glucagon Abs provide excellent staining.
    - Anti-glucagon mcAb 79bB10 *(18, 19)* (*see* **Note 27**).
    - Rabbit anti-glucagon pcAb.
3. Dilute Ab in PBS and incubate for 2 h at room temperature (*see* **Note 28**).
4. Wash 3× in PBS, 5 min each.
5. The Ab binding is visualised using 2nd Ab according to the dilution guidelines provided by the suppliers (*see* **Note 28**):

   - Anti-mouse IgG/HRP.
   - Anti-rabbit/HRP.
6. Follow **steps 15–19** of previous protocol.

Immunofluorescence Staining for (Pro)insulin

1. De-paraffinise sections of pancreatic tissue as described above for HE staining.
2. Wash 2× in PBS, 2 min each.
3. Encircle the sections using a DAKO or PAP pen (*see* **Note 21**).
4. Prepare an incubation chamber with humidified atmosphere (*see* **Note 22**) and perform all incubation steps using a staining chamber.
5. Incubate sections for 2 h at room temperature with dilutions of
   - Anti-insulin mcAb 36aC10 in PBS or
   - Anti-(pro)insulin mcAb K14D4 (*see* **Note 29**).
6. Wash 3× in PBS, 5 min each.
7. Visualise the Ab binding by incubation with secondary FITC-labelled Ab anti-mouse IgG, according to the dilution guidelines provided by the suppliers, by incubation for 30 min at room temperature in darkness (*see* **Note 28**).
8. Wash 3× in PBS, 5 min each.
9. Embed in fluorescence mounting medium as this will reduce fading of immunofluorescence during microscopy.
10. Protect the slides from light.
11. Store at 4°C.
12. Take micrographs as soon as possible to avoid fading.

Immunofluorescence Staining for Glucagon

1. Follow **steps 1–4** described above.
2. Incubate sections for 2 h at room temperature in a staining chamber with (*see* **Note 27**)
   - anti-glucagon mcAb 79bB10 diluted in PBS as recommended by the supplier or
   - rabbit anti-glucagon pcAb.
3. Wash 3× in PBS, 5 min each.
4. Visualise the Ab binding by incubation with anti-species secondary fluorochrome-labelled Ab, according to the dilution guidelines provided by the suppliers, incubate for 30 min at room temperature in darkness.
5. Proceed as described above.

Double-Staining for Insulin and Glucagon

1. Perform **steps 1–4** as described above.
2. Block sections with 10% NCS in PBS for 10 min at room temperature.
3. Use one of the following combinations of 1st Abs (*see* **Note 30**):

(a) Guinea pig insulin pcAb plus anti-glucagon mcAb 79bB10.

(b) Anti-insulin mcAb 36aC10 plus rabbit anti-glucagon pcAb.

(c) Guinea pig insulin pcAb plus rabbit anti-glucagon pcAb.

4. Dilute Ab in PBS as recommended by the supplier (*see* **Note 28**).
5. Incubate combinations of 1st Abs for 2 h at room temperature in an incubation chamber.
6. Wash 3× in PBS, 5 min each.
7. Incubate sections in the dark for 30 min with a combination of fluorochrome-labelled pre-absorbed 2nd Ab against (*see* **Note 31**):

(a) Anti-guinea pig and anti-mouse 2nd Ab.

(b) Anti-mouse and anti-rabbit 2nd Ab.

(c) Anti-guinea pig and anti-rabbit 2nd Ab.

8. Wash 3× in PBS, 5 min each.
9. Embed in fluorescence mounting medium.

3.4.2. Detection of a Fixation-Sensitive Protein

High-Level Protein Expression Detected Using Immunofluorescence: Optional Detection of Endocrine Cells

1. Remove cryostat sections from −80°C.
2. Allow slides to equilibrate to room temperature (*see* **Note 32**).
3. Fix for 10 min at room temperature in acetone.
4. Air-dry the sections for 10 min.
5. Surround the sections with DAKO pen.
6. Block for 10 min with 10% NCS.
7. Wash 3× in PBS.
8. Incubate sections with 1st Ab for 2 h at room temperature or at 4°C overnight in an incubation chamber.
9. Wash 3× in PBS.
10. Incubation with 2nd Ab, FITC anti-species for 1 h at room temperature according to the dilution guidelines provided by the suppliers at darkness.
11. Wash 3× in PBS.
12. Embed in fluorescence mounting medium.

Optional, if endocrine cells are to be identified on the same or consecutive section

13. After **step 4**, perform a post-fixation up to 30 min at 4°C with 4% PFA (*see* **Note 33**).
14. Proceed after **step 9** with 1 h incubation at room temperature using anti-insulin mcAb 36aC10 or anti-glucagon mcAb 79bB10 (*see* **Note 33**).

15. Wash 3× in PBS.
16. Perform **steps 10** and **11**. Detect islet hormone using Fluorochrome (FITC or Texas Red® or Cy3)-labelled anti-mouse IgG by incubation for 30 min at room temperature in darkness (*see* **Note 31**).
17. Wash 3× in PBS.

Low-Level Protein Expression Detected Using the APAAP-Labelling System with Optional Detection of Endocrine Cells in the Consecutive Section

1. Perform **steps 1–5** as described above.
2. All washing and incubation steps are performed in TBS in an incubation chamber.
3. Block for 10 min with 10% non-immune rabbit serum in TBS.
4. Incubate the sections with a mouse Ab recognising the Ag protein of interest overnight at 4°C in an incubation chamber.

Optional, if endocrine cells are to be identified

5. The consecutive section can be simultaneously incubated with anti-insulin mcAb 36aC10 or anti-glucagon mcAb 79bB10.
6. Wash 3× in TBS, 5 min each.
7. Incubate with rabbit anti-mouse IgG diluted as recommended by the supplier at room temperature for 30 min.
8. Wash 3× in TBS, 5 min each.
9. Incubate with APAAP from mouse diluted as recommended by the supplier at room temperature for 30 min *(20)*.
10. Wash 3× in TBS, 5 min each.
11. Optional, sensitivity can be increased by repetition of **steps 6–9**; for a duration of incubation 10 min each.
12. Perform enzymatic colour reaction using Fast Red tablets.
13. Rinse in distilled water.
14. Counterstain nuclei with hematoxylin for 30 s.
15. Rinse in tap water.
16. Cover sections with a water-soluble agent.

3.4.3. Detection of a Fixation-Resistant Protein

High-Level Protein Expression Detected by Immunohistochemistry: Optional Detection of Endocrine Cells

1. De-paraffinise sections from PFA-fixed pancreatic tissue as described above for HE staining (*see* **Subheading 3.4.1**).
2. Follow **steps 2–10** as described for insulin staining on tissue fixed with Bouin's fluid.
3. Incubate with desired 1st Ab for 2 h at room temperature in a moist chamber.
4. Wash 3× in PBS, 5 min each.
5. Incubate with 2nd anti-species Ab labelled with HRP as recommended by the supplier.
6. Wash 3× in PBS, 5 min each.

7. Cover the sections with the ready-to-use AEC substrate-chromogen according to the supplier's instructions (*see* **Note 34**).
8. Rinse gently in PBS.
9. Counterstain sections with hematoxylin.
10. Coverslip with an aqueous-based mounting media.

Optional for detection of endocrine cells

11. Considering the host of the 1st Ab, incubate the consecutive section simultaneously **(step 3)** or the same section (after **step 6**) with an anti-insulin or anti-glucagon Ab.
    - Anti-glucagon mcAb 79bB10 *(18, 19)* or,
    - Guinea pig insulin pcAb or,
    - Anti-insulin mcAb 36aC10 or,
    - Rabbit anti-glucagon pcAb.
12. Wash 3× in PBS, 5 min.
13. In case of double-staining incubate with alkaline phosphatase-labelled 2nd anti-species Ab.
14. Wash 3× in PBS 5 min.
15. For double-staining the enzyme reaction is AEC$^+$ (**step 7**) a ready-to-use chromogen BCIP/NPT (*see* **Note 34**).

Low-Level Protein Expression Detected by APAAP: Optional Detection of Endocrine Cells

1. De-paraffinise sections from pancreatic tissue as described above for HE staining (*see* **Subheading 3.4.1**). Never allow the sections to dry!
2. Perform **steps 2–16** described for APAAP (*see* **Subheading 3.4.2**).

3.5. Evaluation Methods

3.5.1. Semi-Quantitative Evaluation

1. Define the evaluation criteria; 0, negative - no staining; 1, weak - faint staining; 2, clear positive - medium intensity; and 3, - strong staining (*see* **Note 35**).
2. Blind the sections before evaluation.
3. Perform the same staining experiment on at least three different days.

3.5.2. Morphometry

Calibration of an Eyepiece Reticule

1. Use an object micrometer with a 1 mm scale, the smallest distance should be 0.01 mm = 10 μm.
2. Insert the eyepiece reticule, that is ocular micrometer, into the microscope eyepiece of an adjustable ocular (*see* **Note 36**).
3. Start by focussing the eye lens on the reticle. The scale of the glass reticule disk should appear sharply focussed. Confirm the direction of the reticule to verify that the numbers of the engraved scale are not inverted. Looking through that ocular with the eyepiece only, focus the microscope. Make the adjustment for the other eye.

4. Place and centre an object micrometer in the light path.
5. Orientate eyepiece on the object micrometer so that both scales can be observed simultaneously without parallaxes. Both scales should have the same direction and overlay, at least partially.
6. Observe a longer distance of the visual field and determine the number of overlapping/congruent intercepts in both scales.
7. Determine the value of the eyepiece scale in μm adjusted to the object level using an object micrometer (*see* **Note 36**).
8. Calibrate all oculars for the desired eyepieces.

Estimation of Pancreatic Islets Area

1. Use HE-stained pancreatic sections.
2. We work with 200-fold magnification.
3. Place a calibrated eyepiece in the ocular.
4. Focus eyepiece and section.
5. Using the eyepiece determine minimal and maximal islet diameter.
6. Calculate islet area using following formula (*see* **Note 37**):

$$A = \frac{\pi\left(d_{\max} + d_{\min}\right)^2}{16}$$

Morphometric Analysis of Islet-Cell Volume Density Using Point-Counting Method

1. Use HE-stained pancreatic sections.
2. Place a square grid in the eyepiece of ocular (*see* **Note 38**).
3. According to Weibel et al. *(22)*, points that are of interest are proportional to the area and the area proportional to the volume of structure of interest.
4. Work at 200-fold magnification.
5. Evaluate six sections of each block derived from six different levels, each 200 μm apart.
6. Define the number of cross-points to be counted *(23)* according the expected volume density (**Fig. 5**); fat and connective tissue have to be excluded (*see* **Note 38**).
7. Place the grid randomly on the section. The density depends on the size of the section; however, if the nets to be counted are adjacent, it may be necessary not to count points of two edges to avoid double-counting.
8. The relative islet volume V_v is calculated using following formula:

$$\text{Relative islet volume}\,(\%) = \frac{\text{cross-points over islets} \times 100}{\text{total cross-point number}}$$

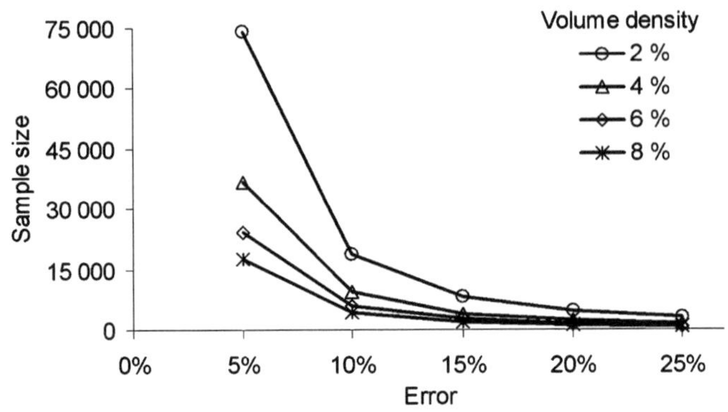

Fig. 5. Number of points counted for estimation of volume density (%) with respect confidence interval.

Morphometric Analysis of β-Cell Volume Density Using Point-Counting Method

1. Relative β-cell volume density is determined on insulin-stained sections *(21, 22, 24)*.
2. The relative β-cell volume V_v is calculated using following formula:

$$\text{Relative } \beta\text{-cell volume density (\%)} = \frac{\text{cross-points over } \beta\text{-cells} \times 100}{\text{total cross-point number}}.$$

3. By determining the pancreas weight after preparation, the absolute β-cell mass (mg) can be calculated as

$$\beta\text{-cell volume density (\%)} \times \text{pancreas weight (mg)} \;.$$

Estimation of Pancreatic Islets Number per Square Millimetre of Pancreatic Tissue

1. The number of pancreatic islets per millimetre square pancreatic tissue is assayed on sections immunostained for insulin.
2. A calibrated square grid is randomly placed ten times on each section.
3. Evaluate at least six levels per pancreas.
4. Count the number of islets hit by the eye-piece.
5. Determine the islet number per millimetre square in an area of about 25 mm^2 of each pancreas block examined and calculate the mean islet number/mm^2 *(25)*.

4. Notes

1. These are pre-treated slides with increased tissue binding, avoid use of adhesives. To perform a double-staining procedure requiring many washing steps, use SuperFrost® Plus GOLD or SuperFrost Ultra Plus®.

2. SuperFrost® slides perform well with no background or autofluorescence problems. In addition, they have frosted ends that are perfect to mark with pencil and resistant to xylene. For silane-coating load SuperFrost® slides into racks in a fume hood. Set up five dishes with solutions containing 2× acetone, 2% (v/v) 3-aminopropyltriethoxy-silane in acetone, and 2× distilled water. Rinse the slides in acetone, incubate for 5 min in 2% silane/acetone, rinse in acetone for 5 min, rinse twice in distilled water for 5 min each, and dry in oven up to 50°C. The coated slides can be stored in a covered container at room temperature for up to 6 months.
3. There are Ag de-masking procedures available, allowing the detection of PFA-sensitive proteins. Ag retrieval on paraffin sections using "Antigen Unmasking Solution" (citric acid based; VECTOR Laboratories, UK) accompanied by a microwave treatment. However, de-masking does not always work consistently and can even result in artefacts. This is especially problematical if the staining patterns of your protein are unknown; to avoid uncertainties, fix half a pancreas with liquid nitrogen and the other with PFA. For difficult protein staining, cryosections area personal preference.
4. Ensure required ethical approval is obtained.
5. To prepare the pancreas, remove the animal and place it on its back, disinfect the skin with 70% ethanol, and cut the skin horizontally near the navel without opening the peritoneal cavity. Remove the skin and open peritoneal cavity horizontally until the spleen under the left costal arch. Take the spleen with forceps, lift it slightly up. The cauda pancreatis is connected to the spleen hilus. Remove the pancreas beginning with the cauda towards the duodenum surrounding the caput pancreatis as quickly as possible as autolysis will damage the tissue. Ensure removal of non-pancreatic tissue, lymph nodes, fat, and hair.
6. We have used both methods for cryofixation successfully. For the specimen moulds (cryomoulds) and OCT, prepare a metal bowl with *n*-hexane and place it into liquid nitrogen for pre-cooling under a fume hood. After the *n*-hexane has turned white and solid, transfer the bowl in a thermobox with dry ice. Label cryomoulds in advance using a permanent ink pen. Put a layer of OCT in a cryomould of appropriate size; the tissue should require maximal two-thirds of the volume. Put the tissue on the OCT layer, orientate the tissue for an appropriate cutting area, cover with OCT. Avoid air bubbles that can cause problems with cutting later and place the cryomould on the frozen *n*-hexane. The OCT turns white upon freezing, transfer the cryomoulds to dry ice.
7. Place the tissue in a cryotube and form a compact block of pancreas. Seal the tube and snap-freeze in liquid nitrogen.

8. As reported in the literature *(16)* and from our own experience, longer fixation is not a problem. However, we standardise the fixation procedure. Preferentially, we use specimen containers with flat bottoms to ensure even fixation.
9. Rinses are done with gentle rotations, during transfer to the next ethanol bath, remove excess of fluid by short blotting onto tissue.
10. The last washing solution will not stain yellow.
11. Small pieces of tissue (<1 cm^3) can be fixed by immersion. Use fresh PFA solution from stock every time. It is important to standardise the fixation for comparable results. Use specimen containers with flat bottom to ensure even fixation. Use gloves and work in a fume hood while working with PFA as it is carcinogenic.
12. Prevent the tissue from thawing as this will destroy the Ag of interest and the morphology of the section. Always allow the tissue to adjust to the cryostat temperature for at least 30 min before sectioning.
13. Routinely cut the pancreas blocks at –21°C. Depending on the tissue consistency, a different temperature may be adopted. For example, if the pancreas is fatty, increasing the temperature may help. 'Sticky' sections indicate the temperature is too high, whereas cracked and rolling sections may be a sign that the samples are too cold.
14. To mount the tissue block on the specimen holder, add a small amount of OCT on top of the holder and put the tissue block on OCT. This will glue the tissue on the specimen holder. Prior to cutting, orientate the tissue vertically on the object holder and trim the tissue until you have an appropriate area. If your cryostat is set up with an anti-roll devise, orientate it such that it ends a small distance above the blade. If the cryostat works without an anti-roll devise, take the section using a brush. Check the knife before you start to take your sections; it should leave no scratches on the tissue. The best results are obtained with a new sharp blade which should be changed as soon as the section quality begins to decline. Cutting good quality sections requires a great deal of practice. Cut evenly by turning the wheel in a continuous uniform motion without hesitation or use the motorised modus. If the sections do not flatten or have cracks, adjust either the angle of sectioning, speed of movement, position of the knife, or position of anti-roll plate. The sections can be picked up by holding the slide just above the section at an angle so the slide touches a portion of the tissue and will float onto the slide. Static attraction will draw the section to adhere to and melt onto the warm slide. Avoid folding or stretching of the section.

15. The final wash solution will not stain yellow.
16. Before embedding in paraffin, the tissue needs to be dehydrated. There are methods for manual tissue processing *(16)*, but these are time-consuming and involve carcinogenic substances. A histological processing machine, for example, Tissue Tek® VIP™, will provide the best results and will automatically perform dehydration and paraffin impregnation of tissue. This protocol gives the procedure run with our histological processing machine. There are a variety of similar procedures, discuss the procedure with the scientist responsible for the local histological processing machine.
17. Slide preparation is standard; seek support from a histology laboratory.
18. Before cutting the tissue, the evaluation procedure should be considered. Design a cutting protocol dependent upon the scheduled micrographic, semi-quantitative, or morphometric evaluation. For micrographic or semi-quantitative analysis, cut serial sections. For morphometric analysis, obtain sections from different levels of the pancreas. Take sections from at least six levels of the pancreas, each 200 μm apart. Prepare at least four series with six sections from each level and record the sequence of sections to be able to identify β-cell or α-cells in the consecutive sections in future experiments.
19. Create a regime for following consecutive sections of a series. Mount sections onto slides by holding slides vertically in the water bath and moving sections using a brush and a water film on the slide. Try to place two sections on a slide and achieve equal orientation of the sections so that the same islet can be easily identified in both sections.
20. Use staining dishes with a slide rack to expose the slides to a large volume of solution that completely covers the slides. The solutions are re-usable; however, they must be replaced once or twice a week depending on the number of slides processed. Solutions should be changed after 50 slides *(17)*.
21. Wipe around the sections using a tissue without allowing the sections to dry. Use a DAKO or PAP pen. This pen has a water-repellent wax and creates a reservoir around the sections. Surrounding the sections with this pen permits small volumes to be applied without high risk of drying. If the Abs are very rare or expensive, the quantity for incubation can be further reduced by placing under a small coverslip on top of the pen-formed reservoir. The coverslip comes off easily during the next washing step.
22. All incubation steps are performed in the staining chamber. Cover the bottom with a layer of paper towels soaked in sterile water to maintain a moist environment. Take special

precautions to prevent slide from drying. The best practise is to change reagents on not more than four slides at a time.

23. The optimal Ab dilution depends on insulin content, sample preparation, immunoglobulin concentration, Ab affinity, amount of Ag, the incubation duration, and detection system and needs to be verified for the actual procedure and Ab *(26)*. The 36aC10 Ab recognizes a wide range of mammalian insulin species. The 36aC10 used in our protocols diluted 1:1,000 *(19, 27)* and the guinea pig pcAb at 1:750 *(12)*.
24. Depending on the area of the section, 50–100 μl of Ab dilution is required. The amount can be reduced by placing a coverslip on the section. The coverslip, together with the DAKO pen circle, forms a small reservoir. For overnight incubations, dilute the Ab in buffer substituted with 5% NCS to protect the protein.
25. Incubate with the ACE reagent for 10 min at room temperature. However, during optimisation method, check for sufficient staining under the microscope. The incubation can be extended up to 30 min. However, longer incubation may result in higher background staining.
26. Dissolve Glycergel® in a water bath (40°C). Place a small drop of Glycergel® on a coverslip, hold the slide at an angle, and place it slowly on the coverslip. Avoid air bubbles.
27. Determine your method; both glucagon Abs stain well. McAb 79bB10 at high dilutions results in brilliant staining on tissue fixed with Bouin's fluid.
28. Use the dilutions recommended by the supplier as a guideline only. Optimise dilutions in a checkerboard titration experiment. DAPI is a helpful counterstain in immunofluorescence allowing visualisation of the nuclei. It complements other fluorochromes and does not mask. Use at 0.001 mg/ml for 5 min; extensive washing is required.
29. The (pro)insulin Ab K14D4 recognizes an epitope located in one of the insulin-C-peptide junctions of the proinsulin molecule. Using ascites, the working dilution ranges from 1:400 to 1:12,800 depending on the species of the pancreatic islets *(18)*.
30. This double-immunofluorescence technique is based on the concept that two 1st Abs are from different host species. The three combinations of 1st Ab have been provided as a guideline for establishing a double-staining procedure for insulin and glucagon. The detection of the primary Abs requires highly specific secondary Abs to avoid cross-reaction. These are coupled to different fluorochromes, for example, 2nd Abs from Jackson ImmunoResearch Laboratories.

31. Traditionally, we label insulin with green fluorescence using FITC anti-species immunoglobulins (Ig) and glucagon with red fluorescence using Texas Red® or Cy3 anti-species Ig.
32. Place slides on a warm conducting metal plate and cover them by aluminium foil to avoid the appearance of condensed water.
33. Depending on the host species of the 1st Ab, the protein of interest and endocrine cells can be identified on the same (1st Ab is a non-mouse-Ig) or consecutive (1st Ab is mouse Ig) section. McAbs against glutamic acid decarboxylase 65 kD (GAD) were used to test the fixation procedure allowing detection of conformational epitopes *(14)*. Fixation up to 30 min did not affect binding of GAD Abs with fixation-sensitive epitopes, but prevented insulin leakage allowing detection by immunofluorescence. Depending on the Ag, the fixation concentration and/or time may require adaptation.
34. Perform the enzyme reaction of double-staining at the end of the whole procedure. Detect HRP first using AEC and then with BCIP/NPT. Check the necessity of counterstaining with hematoxylin.
35. Always include appropriate controls for the staining levels using tissue sections with low-, medium-, and high-expression levels of the protein of interest or use dilutions of Ab resulting in low-, medium-, and high-intensity staining patterns to exclude variation and to standardise evaluation of sections.
36. This eyepiece uses an ocular micrometer scale, that is, a scale etched on a glass disk and placed within the eyepiece. The scale is superimposed over any image seen in the microscope, allowing the user to measure any object in the field of view. To line up the ocular reticule with the object micrometer for the calibration procedure, the eyepiece can be rotated without changing focus. Calibration of an eyepiece reticule for an objective is typically conducted by using an object micrometer and holds only for the specific objective-eyepiece combination being tested. The micrometer value for objective tested can be calculated by dividing the known length of the selected part of object micrometer by the corresponding number of divisions of the eyepiece scale. There are several Web sites describing the calibration procedure. For example, Nikon microscopy provides a detailed protocol for calibration of different types of reticules (http://www.microscopyu.com/tutorials/java/reticlecalibration/index.html).
37. Note this formula is based on the calculation of the area of a circle $A = \pi d^2/4$ and the definition that the diameter of an islet is $d = (d_{max} + d_{min})/2$.

38. We used a grid with 15 × 15 squares resulting in 225 cross-points. To determine islet- and β-cell volume density for ZR, we count 15 grids per section in six different pancreas levels. **Figure 5** illustrates the sample size of points to be counted for the corresponding error.

Acknowledgement

The authors are grateful to Silke Lucke (PhD) and Klaus-Dieter Kohnert (PhD, MD) for their advice and for sharing their expertise. Our special thanks go to Peter Heinke (MSc.) for his excellent and competent support for mathematical and statistical evaluations. We acknowledge the contributions of Dieter Schröder (PhD) and Sabine Berg (MSc.). We thank Dr. Klaus-Dieter Kohnert for a critical review of the manuscript, Mrs. Cordula Rudolph and Mrs. Marlies Behm for excellent technical assistance.

References

1. Weir G. C., Laybutt D. R., Kaneto H., Bonner-Weir S., and Sharma A. (2001). Beta-cell adaptation and decompensation during the progression of diabetes. *Diabetes* **50** Suppl 1, S154–S159
2. Beck-Nielsen H. and Groop L. (1994). Metabolic and genetic characterization of prediabetic states. Sequence of events leading to non-insulin-dependent diabetes mellitus. *J. Clin. Invest.* **94**, 1714–1721
3. Ferrannini E. (1998). Insulin resistance versus insulin deficiency in non-insulin-dependent diabetes mellitus: problems and prospects. *Endocr. Rev* **19**, 477–490
4. Ritzel R. A., Butler A. E., Rizza R. A., Veldhuis J. D., and Butler P. C. (2006). Relationship between β-cell mass and fasting blood glucose concentration in humans. *Diabetes Care* **29**, 717–718
5. Clark A., Jones L., de Koning E., Hansen B. C., and Matthews D. R. (2001). Decreased insulin secretion in type 2 diabetes: a problem of cellular mass or function? *Diabetes* **50**, S169–S171
6. Chan C. B., Wright G. M., Wadowska D. W., MacPhail R. M., Ireland W. P., and Sulston K. W. (1998). Ultrastructural and secretory heterogeneity of fa/fa (Zucker) rat islets. *Mol. Cell Endocrinol.* **136**, 119–129
7. Finegood D. T., McArthur M. D., Kojwang D., Thomas M. J., Topp B. G., Leonard T. et al. (2001). Beta-cell mass dynamics in Zucker diabetic fatty rats. Rosiglitazone prevents the rise in net cell death. *Diabetes* **50**, 1021–1029
8. Tikellis C., Wookey P. J., Candido R., Andrikopoulos S., Thomas M. C., and Cooper M. E. (2004). Improved islet morphology after blockade of the renin- angiotensin system in the ZDF rat. *Diabetes* **53**, 989–997
9. Schröder D., Berg S., Altmann S., Lucke S., Augstein P., and Salzsieder E. (2006). Charakterisierung von Zucker fatty Ratten (fa/fa) - Beziehung von Stoffwechselparametern, Glukosetoleranz und Eigenschaften isolierter Langerhansscher Inseln. *Diabetologie und Stoffwechsel* **1**, 64–A-132
10. Berthiaume N., Mika A. K., and Zinker B. A. (2003). Development of insulin resistance and endothelin-1 levels in the Zucker fatty rat. *Metab. Clin. Exp.* **52**, 845–849
11. Apweiler R. and Freud P. (1993). Development of glucose intolerance in obese (fa/fa) Zucker rats. *Horm. Metab. Res.* **25**, 521–524
12. Wargent E., Stocker C., Augstein P., Heinke P., Meyer A., Hoffmann T. et al. (2005). Improvement of glucose tolerance in Zucker diabetic fatty rats by long-term treatment with the dipeptidyl peptidase inhibitor P32/98:

comparison with and combination with rosiglitazone. *Diabetes Obes. Metab.* 7, 170–181

13. Buckingham R. E., al Barazanji K. A., Toseland C. D., Slaughter M., Connor S. C., West A. et al. (1998). Peroxisome proliferator-activated receptor-gamma agonist, rosiglitazone, protects against nephropathy and pancreatic islet abnormalities in Zucker fatty rats. *Diabetes* **47**, 1326–1334
14. Augstein P., Schlosser M., Ziegler B., Hahmann J., Mauch L., and Ziegler M. (1996). Comparison of the islet cell antibody pattern of monoclonal glutamic acid decarboxylase antibodies recognizing linear and conformational epitopes. *Acta Histochem.* **98**, 229–241
15. Augstein P., Elefanty A. G., Allison J., and Harrison L. C. (1998). Apoptosis and beta-cell destruction in pancreatic islets of NOD mice with spontaneous and cyclophosphamide-accelerated diabetes. *Diabetologia* **41**, 1381–1388
16. Romeis. Mikroskopische Technik. (17th ed) (1989). München; Wien; Baltimore: Urban ' Schwarzenberg
17. Hofman F. (2002). Immunohistochemistry. In: Current Protocols in Immunology. John Wiley & Sons, Inc., New York, 21.4.1–21.4.23
18. Augstein P., Braun B., Ziegler B., Woltanski K. P., and Ziegler M. (1992). Characterization of two porcine proinsulin reactive monoclonal antibodies by immunostaining of beta-cells in pancreatic sections of different species. *Acta Histochem.* **93**, 433–440
19. Witt S., Dietz H., Ziegler B., Keilacker H., and Ziegler M. (1988). Production and use of monoclonal glucagon and insulin antibodies - reduction of pancreatic insulin in rats by treatment with complete Freund's adjuvant. *Acta Histochem.* Suppl **35**, 217–223
20. Hahn H. J., Gerdes J., Lucke S., Liepe L., Kauert C., Volk H. D. et al. (1988). Phenotypical characterization of the cells invading pancreatic islets of diabetic BB/OK rats: effect of interleukin 2 receptor-targeted immunotherapy. *Eur. J. Immunol.* **18**, 2037–2042
21. Lucke S., Ziegler B., Weidlich K., Barowski U., Besch W., and Hahn H. J. (1985). The effects of subdiabetogenic streptozotocin doses on rat beta cell volume and functions. *Biomed. Biochim. Acta* **44**, 167–171
22. Weibel E. R. (1969). Stereological principles for morphometry in electron microscopic cytology. *Int. Rev. Cytol.* **26**, 235–302
23. Lucke S. (1987) Die Bedeutung der reduzierten β-Zellmasse für die Regeneration der insulinproduzierenden Zellen im Rattenpankreas. Dissertation 1-81. Ernst-Moritz-Arndt-Universität-Greifswald
24. Kohnert K. D., Ziegler B., Falt K., Odselius R., Ziegler M., and Falkmer S. (1987). Biochemical, immunohistochemical and ultrastructural studies of the alteration of pancreatic beta cells resulting from the combined effects of complete Freund's adjuvant and non-diabetogenic doses of streptozotocin. *Exp. Clin. Endocrinol.* **89**, 259–268
25. Lucke S., Radloff E., Laube R., and Hahn H. J. (1991). Morphology of the endocrine pancreas in cyclosporine-treated glucose-intolerant Wistar rats. *Anat. Anz.* **172**, 351–358
26. Kohnert K. D., Falt K., Witt S., Ziegler B., and Ziegler M. (1988). Identification of monoclonal antibodies to pancreatic islet cells by immunoperoxidase staining. *Acta Histochem.* **83**, 159–165
27. Augstein P., Braun B., Ziegler B., Woltanski K. P., and Ziegler M. (1992). Characterization of two porcine proinsulin reactive monoclonal antibodies by immunostaining of beta-cells in pancreatic sections of different species. *Acta Histochem.* **93**, 433–440

Chapter 13

Fluorescent Immunohistochemistry and In Situ Hybridization Analysis of Pancreas

Xiuli Wang, Shundi Ge, and Gay M. Crooks

Summary

To facilitate the immunological reaction of antibodies with antigens in fixed tissues, it is necessary to unmask or retrieve the antigens through pretreatment of the specimens. However, adjustment of heat-induced antigen retrieval is always required for different tissues and antigens. Using a low-power antigen retrieval technique, with appropriate dilution of antibodies, we successfully immunostained key antigens in the pancreas such as insulin, PDX-1, glucagon, cytokeratin, and CD31, which have presented a particular challenge for investigators in the past, because of the rapid autodigestion and high nonspecific antibody binding in the tissue. Satisfactory results were obtained when immunohistochemistry and fluorescence in situ hybridization analysis were combined in the same slides.

Key words: Immunohistochemistry, Low-power antigen retrieval, Fluorescent in situ hybridization (FISH)

1. Introduction

When investigating pancreatic β-cell regeneration in type II diabetes, we experienced inherent difficulties to analyze pancreas by conventional means due to rapid autodigestion and high nonspecific antibody (Ab) binding in the tissue. We therefore developed optimal conditions that consistently work in pancreas analysis.

Fluorescence immunohistochemistry (IHC) has been proven to be a reliable and sensitive tool for morphological and functional analysis of cells in different organs, especially when it is successfully applied in paraffin-embedded tissues. Recovery of antigen in formalin-fixed, paraffin-embedded tissue sections is required prior to Ab binding and visualization. Antigen retrieval

C. Stocker (ed.), *Type 2 Diabetes,* Methods in Molecular Biology, vol. 560
DOI 10.1007/978-1-59745-448-3_13, © Humana Press, a part of Springer Science+Business Media, LLC 2009

(AR) includes a variety of methods including enzymatic digestion or heat-induced epitope retrieval through microwave irradiation, pressure cooking, or a combination of both. Enzyme digestion-related AR fails to give consistent and satisfactory immunostaining for many antigens. However, the heat-induced antigen retrieval (HIAR) technique, a method of boiling paraffin tissue sections in water or microwaving slides at 90–100° C described by Shi et al., has been widely used as a simple, effective method for unmasking the antigen in formalin-fixed tissue sections *(1)*. However, there is no single HIAR protocol that can be universally applied to various antigens *(2)*. Widespread application of IHC has raised critical issues concerning time-consuming modification of protocols for different tissue types and antigens. It would therefore be desirable to develop a technique that works well with the widest possible variety of tissue types and antigens. We developed a low-power antigen retrieval (LAR) technique and obtained satisfactory staining for all of the antigens tested in murine pancreas *(3)*. In addition, this technique was also applied to simultaneous analysis of IHC and fluorescence in situ hybridization (FISH) chromosome detection *(4)*.

2. Materials

2.1. Tissue Preparation

1. Pancreas from adult mice are dissected immediately following sacrifice to avoid autodigestion.
2. 5-Bromo-2′ deoxyuridine (BrdU) (Sigma-Aldrich, St. Louis, MO), freshly prepared in phosphate-buffered saline (PBS).
3. 10% Neutral buffered formalin, pH 6.8–7.2. Kept at 25°C.
4. 1× PBS, pH 7.4.
5. Ethanol and toluene for tissue dehydration.
6. Pancreas are embedded in paraffin following processing and sectioned on a microtome (Leica RM 2125, Leica, Nussloch, Germany, or equivalent model).
7. Superfrosted microscope slides (Fisher Scientific).
8. Slide warmer (BarnsteadLab-line, Melrose, IL).
9. Sections are deparaffinized in 100% toluene.
10. 1:100 Antigen unmasking working solution: diluted with distilled water from stock (pH 6.0, Vector Laboratories, Inc., Burlingame, CA) (*see* **Note 1**).

11. Microwave oven or equivalent with multiple power settings (Panasonic NN-S763WF, Genius Sensor 1350 W, Panasonic, NJ).

2.2. Immunohistochemistry

1. Tris-buffered saline (TBS): 100 mM Tris–HCl, 150 mM NaCl, pH 7.5.
2. TBS-T: TBS with 0.1% Tween-20.
3. Permeabilization solution: TBS with 0.1% Triton X-100.
4. Blocking solution: TBS-T supplemented with 1% BSA (IgG-free, protease-free, Jackson Immuno Research Laboratories, Inc., West Grove, PA) and 5% normal donkey serum.
5. Ab diluent: TBS-T supplemented with 1% BSA. Make in advance and store at 4°C.
6. Primary antibodies: BrdU sheep polyclonal Ab (Abcam, Inc., Cambridge, MA), platelet/endothelial cell adhesion molecule-1 (CD31) goat polyclonal Ab (Santa Cruz, CA), GFP rabbit polyclonal Ab (Novus Biologicals, Inc., Littleton, CO), insulin guinea pig polyclonal Ab (Dako Cytomation, Inc., Carpinteria, CA), pancytokeratin (PCK) mouse monoclonal Ab (Sigma, Saint Louis, MO), glucagon rabbit polyclonal Ab (Novus Biologicals, Inc.), and PDX-1 goat polyclonal Ab (Santa Cruz).
7. Secondary antibodies: anti-goat-FITC, anti-rabbit-cyanine3 (Cy3), and anti-mouse-FITC or biotin-conjugated anti-mouse, anti-guinea pig FITC, or biotin-conjugated anti-guinea pig (Jackson Immuno Research Laboratories, Inc.).
8. Vectashield mounting medium for fluorescence with 4′,6-diamidino-2-phenylindole (DAPI) (Vector Laboratories, Inc., Burlingame, CA).

2.3. Fluorescence In Situ Hybridization

1. Nonidet P-40 (Sigma) (*see* **Note 2**).
2. 20× Standard saline citrate (SSC) stock solution: 3 M NaCl, 0.3 M sodium citrate, dissolve in distilled water, adjust to pH 7.4.
3. 0.16% trypsin (Digest-All 2, Zymed, San Francisco, CA; Digest-All 2 consists of two reagents: 0.5% trypsin and diluent).
4. Probe: Cy3-conjugated mouse chromosome paint Y-specific probe (Cat. No. MCy3-02, Cambio, Cambridge, UK).
5. 4% Paraformaldehyde (4% PFA), freshly prepared in 1× PBS.
6. Hybridization buffer (Cat. No. MCy3-02, Cambio Ltd).

2.4. Imaging System

1. Leica DMRXA microscope (Bannockburn, IL) using a Plan Apo 20×/1.0 or 1.25 NA phase 3 DIC. All procedures will be using this system or equivalent model.
2. Filter sets required are DAPI, chroma 31000; fluorescein, 41001; Cy3, 41007a (Chroma technology, Rockingham, VT).
3. The microscope needs to be equipped with an LS300 W ozone-free xenon arc lamp (Sutter Instrument Co, Novato, CA) coupled to the microscope with a liquid light guide.
4. Images are acquired with an Applied Spectral Imaging Ltd SkyVision–2/VDS-1300 12-bit digital camera from Easy-FISH software (Migdal Ha'Emek, Israel).

3. Methods

It is often desirable to perform FISH and IHC on the same slide in order to see coexpression of specific chromosomes and protein, for example, to detect donor cells in sex-mismatched transplant settings. One of the primary technical concerns in these cases is that different procedures are required for FISH and IHC. We have found that unsatisfactory results of FISH staining can occur when IHC is performed prior to FISH staining, vice versa protein expression can be lost when FISH is processed first. In our studies, male pancreas was analyzed with IHC and FISH with the LAR technique. It is well known that not all the Y chromosomes can be detected in male tissues due to incomplete sampling of entire nuclei during sectioning. At best, the efficiency of Y chromosome detection in pancreas ranges from 60% to 80% with enzyme-mediated AR *(5)* and in frozen sections *(6)*. The LAR technique preserves protein expression well, for example, insulin or PCK with efficient detection of Y chromosomes. We observed 80–90% Y chromosomes in the 5 μm sections of male pancreas, with a background of 0.002% staining in negative (female pancreas) controls. LAR used here provided efficient AR for successful immunostaining of a variety of antigens under a standardized condition with low background.

3.1. Preparation of Samples

1. Following sacrifice, the pancreas are dissected immediately to avoid autodigestion.
2. To detect cycling cells in the pancreas, the experimental mouse is administered with BrdU 25 mg/kg by intraperitoneal injection. Pancreas tissues are harvested 2 h later.

3. Fix the pancreas in 10% neutral buffered formalin for 6 h at room temperature. We experienced a better morphology following 6 h fixation than overnight (*see* **Note 3**).
4. Following this, rinse the tissue twice with 1× PBS and dehydrate in graded concentrations of ethanol from 50% and then 70% for 30 min for each at room temperature (*see* **Note 4**).
5. Dehydrate tissue for a further 30 min in 100% toluene and repeat this step once.
6. Incubate the tissue in melted paraffin for 30 min at 62°C. Replace with new paraffin and incubate overnight at 62°C. Embed the tissue into paraffin blocks for 30 min at room temperature or 15 min at 4°C.
7. Following embedding, cut 5 μm series section using the microtome and float the paraffin ribbon into a 40°C water bath (Boekel 14792, Boekel Scientific, Feasterville, PA) (*see* **Note 5**).
8. Mount the sections onto Superfrosted microscope slides and allow the sections to dry for 1 h on a slide warmer, then bake overnight in a 37°C oven (*see* **Note 6**).
9. When ready to process, deparaffinize the sections in 2 Tissue tek® slide staining dishes (Electron Microscopy Sciences, Hatfield, PA) containing 100% toluene for 5 min and repeat once with 10 min incubation.
10. Rehydrate the slides through 100, 80, and 50% ethanol and distilled water for 3 min each in Tissue tek ® slide staining dishes.

3.2. LAR Prior to Fluorescence IHC Staining

1. Fill the Tissue tek® slide staining dish with 275 ml antigen unmasking working solution, keeping the lid off. Place all eight slides into a 24-slide holder (Electron Microscopy Sciences) and immerse the slide holder into the staining dish.
2. Put two staining dishes (one dish with experimental slides, another dish filled up with distilled water to balance the humidity) on the center of turnable plate, heat for 4 min at power level 4, break for 1 min, and repeat for two more times (*see* **Note 7**).
3. Let the staining dish cool down on the bench at room temperature for 30 min and carefully circle the sections with super PAP pen (liquid blocker, Ted Pella, Inc., Redding CA) after absorbing excess unmasking buffer with Kim wipes tissue.
4. Permeabilize the sections with 1× TBS containing 0.1% Triton X-100 for 20 min at room temperature.

3.3. Blocking Nonspecific Binding

Any nonspecific binding is blocked with the addition of 250–300 μl blocking solution for at least 30 min (*see* **Note 8**).

3.4. Ab Staining

1. Reconstitute all the antibodies according to the manufacturer's suggestion and store them in aliquots at –20°C avoiding repeated freeze thaw cycles.
2. Titrate the Abs with Ab diluent within a range of 100–800.
3. The effective working dilutions for each Ab as optimized is shown in **Table 1** to give the strongest specific antigen staining with the lowest nonspecific background.
4. Apply 200 μl primary antibodies on the section and incubate overnight at 4°C.
5. Wash with TBS-T for two times for 5 min each.
6. Apply diluted secondary antibodies and incubate for 30 min followed by three washes with TBS-T.
7. If IHC is to be carried out, stop at this stage and apply the coverslip with DAPI: Slides are mounted with Vectashield mounting medium for fluorescence with DAPI (*see* **Note 9**).

3.5. Fluorescence In Situ Hybridization

The regulation of gene expression is of fundamental importance for the understanding of normal and disregulated cell biology. It is always a challenge to address such questions at the single cell level as both molecular and cytological information due to the lack of reliable approach regarding the use of a combination of

Table 1
Optimal conditions of immunohistochemistry analysis of murine pancreas using low-power antibody retrieval

Abs	Primary host	Staining dilution	Secondary Abs	Staining dilution
GFP	Rabbit	1:800	Cyanine3	1:400
Pancytokeratin (PCK-26)	Mouse	1:300	Biotinylated	1:500
PECAM	Goat	1:100	Fluorescein	1:200
Insulin	Guinea pig	1:200	Fluorescein	1:200
Glucagon	Rabbit	1:100	Cyanine3	1:200
PDX1	Goat	1:50	Cyanine3	1:200
BrdU	Sheep	1:100	Cyanine3	1:200

Reconstitute all the antibodies (Abs) according to the manufacture's suggestion and store them in aliquots at –20°C, avoiding repeated freeze thaw cycles. Titrate the Abs with Ab diluent within a range of 100–C800. The effective working dilutions for each Ab are optimized as shown in the table to give the strongest specific antigen staining with the lowest nonspecific background

FISH and IHC analysis. One of the primary technical concerns in these cases is that different procedures are required for FISH and IHC. Some tissue pretreatments essential to IHC may irreversibly destroy cellular DNA/RNA molecule. Vice versa, protein expression can be lost when FISH is processed first. We have developed an optimized protocol, with which genes can be reproducibly detected with high efficiency while protein expression and morphology is well preserved.

Day 1

1. Antigen unmasking: slides are processed with LAR as described in above sections.
2. Then replace unmasking buffer with TBS.
3. Wash all slides with TBS for 5 min and absorb excess buffer with Kimä wipes tissue and air-dry for 5 min.
4. To ensure complete digestion, incubate sections with 0.16% trypsin for 10 min at 37°C (*see* **Note 10**) and wash the slides with TBS twice for 5 min, each followed by a TBS-T wash for 5 min.
5. Block the sections with TBS-T supplemented with 1% BSA and 5% normal donkey serum for at least 30 min. Incubate the sections with 200 μl diluted primary antibodies, for example, mouse PCK and guinea pig insulin in TBS-T with 1% BSA overnight at 4°C.

Day 2

6. Wash the slides for 5 min in TBS-T at room temperature and repeat this step once.
7. Incubate the sections with 200 μl diluted biotin-conjugated anti-mouse Ab in TBS-T with 1% BSA for 30 min at room temperature and then with 200 μl diluted (1:400) fluorescein DTAF-conjugated streptavidin for 30 min at room temperature.
8. Following this, incubate the sections with 200 μl diluted biotin-conjugated anti-guinea pig Ab in TBS-T with 1% BSA for 30 min at room temperature.
9. Then incubate with 200 μl diluted (1:400) Cy5.5-conjugated streptavidin for 30 min at room temperature (*see* **Note 11**).
10. Wash in TBS-T for 5 min and repeat this step once.
11. Wash the slides for 5 min once in TBS and then mount with DAPI mounting medium and view results of the dual staining and acquire some images. Continue next day if satisfactory protein staining is achieved.

Day 3

12. Soak PCK and insulin-stained slides in TBS and remove the coverslip gently. Then wash the slides in TBS for 5 min, repeating this wash step once.
13. Postfix the slides in fresh 4% PFA solution for 2 min at room temperature.
14. Wash the slides for 5 min in 1× PBS and repeat this step twice.
15. The slides are then dehydrated for 1 min each in 70, 90, and 100% ethanol and allowed air-dry for 10 min in darkness. They are then transferred into slide boxes until the probe is ready to apply.
16. Probe mixture: bring Cy3-conjugated mouse chromosome paint Y-specific probe out of –20°C and warm it at 37°C, vortex, and centrifuge for 1–3 s. Mix well 1 μl mouse paints chromosome Y probe with 2 μl distilled water and 7 μl hybridization buffer and keep it warm at 37°C before using (*see* **Note 12**). During this time, set up the slide warmer at 42–45°C.
17. Apply 10 μl paint Y probe to the center of a prewarmed (42–45°C) glass coverslip.
18. Prewarm the slides for 2 min at 42–45°C, and then gently press the slides onto the glass coverslip with the section facing the probe, remove as many air bubbles as possible from around the sections and seal edge of glass coverslip with rubber cement. Dry them in the dark.
19. Codenature sealed slides for 10 min at 65°C in a moisturized container (prewarm the container in the water bath prior to denaturation).
20. Cool down the container (slides inside) for 3 min, place the slides horizontally onto the slide staining rack in a humidified staining dishes, cover with a light-tight cover, and then hybridize them overnight in an incubator at 37°C.

Day 4

21. Carefully peel off the rubber cement and soak the slides in a 50 ml coupling jar filled with 2× SSC buffer for a few minutes and then remove the glass coverslip gently from the sections.
22. Wash the slides for 3 min in a coupling jar containing 0.4× SSC in distilled water and then 0.3% NP-40 at 62°C.
23. Wash the slides for a further 2 min in 2× SSC, 0.1% NP-40 at room temperature, and repeat this step once.
24. Mount the slides with Vectashield DAPI mounting medium.

3.6. Fluorescence In Situ Hybridization for Frozen and Cytospin Sections

1. Fix either frozen tissue sections or cytospin slides for 10 min in 4% PFA at room temperature.
2. Wash three times with 1× PBS for 5 min each and then continue with the FISH procedure as described above, starting from **step 14** above.

3.7. Microscopy

1. Images were viewed with a Leica DMRXA microscope (Bannockburn) using a Plan Apo 20×/1.0 or 1.25 NA phase 3 DIC. The most effective filter sets are DAPI, chroma 31000; Fluorescein, 41001; Cy3, 41007a (Chroma technology).
2. The microscope should be equipped with a LS300 W ozone-free xenon arc lamp or equivalent (Sutter Instrument Co) coupled to the microscope with a liquid light guide.

Images should be acquired with an Applied Spectral Imaging Ltd SkyVision-2/VDS-1300 12-bit digital camera from EasyFISH software (Migdal Ha'Emek). To compare the sensitivity and specificity of the signals (of interest) after low-power and conventional power treatment, identical exposure time and intensity parameters must be used **(Fig. 1)**.

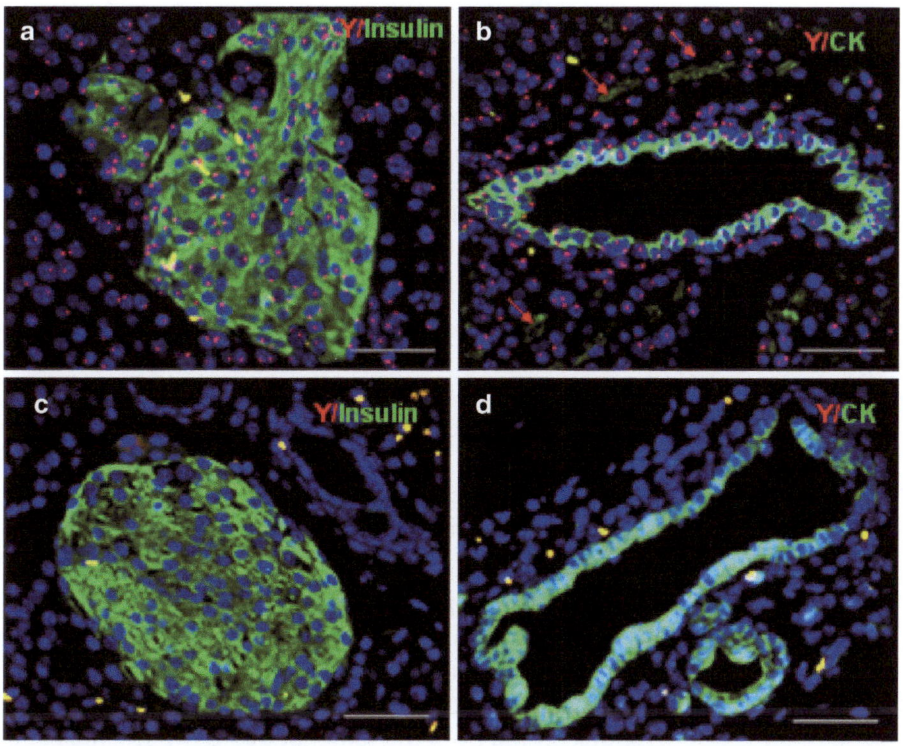

Fig. 1. Efficient detection of Y chromosome in murine pancreas. Dual staining of insulin (*green*) (**a**) or CK (*green*) (**b**) and Y chromosome (*red*) in the pancreas sections from male Nod/Scid B2 M null mice was performed using low-power antigen retrieval technique. The high sensitivity of the staining allowed detecting very small ducts (*arrows* in **b**). Pancreas sections from female animals as negative controls (**c**) and (**d**). *Yellow dots* represent autofluorescence of red blood cells (scale bars, 50 μm). Reproduced, with permission from ref. (4).

4. Notes

1. It is very important to shake this well before preparing the antigen unmasking working solution.
2. Please note that Triton X-100, Tween-20, and Nonidet P-40 are very viscous, so slow pipetting is essential.
3. Unlike the human pancreas, the mouse pancreatic tissues may appear similar to connective tissue or fat. We have found that fixing pancreas in its natural position without folding or twisting is required for good tissue morphology. For this reason, the pancreas is placed in a cassette in a supporting carrier and then dropped into the fixative solution container.
4. If the tissue cannot be processed immediately in toluene on the same day, leave the tissue in 100% ethanol at –20°C until it is convenient to proceed to the next step.
5. Between 6 and 24 sections of pancreatic tissue can be obtained from each mouse and analyzed by fluorescence microscopy. These sections are derived from the 10th, 20th, 30th, 40th, 50th, 60th, and 70th 5-μm sections spanning the length of the pancreas, thus providing representative analysis of the entire organ.
6. Generally speaking, the paraffin block can be kept for years without protein degradation at room temperature. Sectioned slides can be kept at 4°C for several months. However, PDX-1 Ab works better on fresh embedded and microtome cut sections.
7. Process one dish each time. Although the temperature reaches 100°C in the jar, ensure there was no bubbling or overflow so maintaining the buffer level in the dish throughout the whole process allowing even treatment of all the slides in the dish. If slides are treated with a conventional power level of 10 (100%), the buffer would need to be replenished in each cycle due to the loss of fluid by overflow. Caution should be taken during this step as high energy delivered by power may degenerate the antigens and cause failure of IHC staining.
8. All secondary antibodies used here are raised from donkey. Therefore, 5% normal donkey serum is used to block nonspecific binding from host of secondary Ab before incubation with primary Ab on the tissue sections. In general, normal serum should come from the same species as the secondary Ab.
9. Ab-labeled slides can be kept for 1 month at –20°C.
10. Prepare 0.16% trypsin from stock with the diluent provided with the kit.

11. We recommend using biotin–streptavidin complex signal amplification to keep the brightest labeling and fluorescence quenchless. You can incubate PCK and insulin primary Ab overnight simultaneously at 4°C. The next day, apply biotinylated anti-mouse IgG followed by fluorescein DTAF-conjugated streptavidin, and then add the second biotinylated anti-guinea pig followed by Cy5.5-conjugated streptavidin. Wash twice for 5 min after each incubation with antibodies.
12. Generally, 10 μl of probe mixture is sufficient for a 22× 22 mm glass coverslip. Total of 22.5 μl of probe mixture could be used for 22× 40 mm glass coverslip if there are three sections mounted on the same slide.

Acknowledgments

Fluorescence microscopy was performed in the Congressman Julian Dixon Cellular Imaging Core of the Saban Research Institute, CHLA. This work was generously supported by grants from the Seaver Institute and NIH (R01-DK68719).

References

1. Shi, S.R., Key, M.E., and Kalra, K.L. (1991). Antigen retrieval in formalin-fixed, paraffin-embedded tissues: an enhancement method for immunohistochemical staining based on microwave oven heating of tissue sections. *J Histochem Cytochem.* **39**, 741–748.
2. Shi, S.R., Cote, R.J., and Taylor, C.R. (1997). Antigen retrieval immunohistochemistry: past, present, and future. *J Histochem Cytochem.* **45**, 327–343.
3. Wang, X., Ge, S., Gonzalez, I., McNamara, G., Rountree, B.C., Xi, K.K., Huang, G., Bhushan, A., and Crooks, G.M. (2006). Formation of pancreatic duct epithelium from bone marrow during neonatal development. *Stem Cells.* **24**, 307–314.
4. Ge, S., Crooks, G.M., McNamara, G., and Wang, X. (2006). Fluorescent immunohistochemistry and in situ hybridization analysis of mouse pancreas using low-power antigen-retrieval technique. *J Histochem Cytochem.* **54**, 843–847.
5. Lechner, A., Yang, Y.G., Blacken, R.A., Wang, L., Nolan, A.L., and Habener, J.F. (2004). No evidence for significant transdifferentiation of bone marrow into pancreatic beta-cells in vivo. *Diabetes.* **53**, 616–623.
6. Kodama, S., Kuhtreiber, W., Fujimura, S., Dale, E.A., and Faustman, D.L. (2003). Islet regeneration during the reversal of autoimmune diabetes in NOD mice. *Science.* **302**, 1223–1227.

Chapter 14

The Measurement of Insulin Secretion Using Pancreas Perfusion in the Rodent

Edward T. Wargent

Summary

Under in vivo conditions, the study of physiological and pharmacological functions of an organ is difficult due to whole-body interactions with the organ. Thus, an *in vitro* technique for the perfusion of isolated pancreata was developed for physiologic and response studies including the investigation of endocrine function and secretory responsiveness under a variety of diabetes-associated conditions. The pancreas is isolated from the connecting spleen, stomach, and duodenum and transferred to a pre-warmed chamber, where it is perfused in isolation from all other organs. A detailed description of the isolation and perfusion apparatus is described as well as the measurement of glucose-stimulated insulin secretion using an in-house-developed radioimmunoassay.

Key words: Pancreas, Perfusion, Insulin, Radioimmunoassay

1. Introduction

In vivo, the study of physiological and pharmacological functions of an organ is difficult due to whole-body interactions with the organ. However, during perfusion, the respective organ is isolated from these interactions and placed under relatively simple experimental conditions, approximating the normal state, thereby facilitating physiological measurements. The pancreas perfusion method is therefore ideally suited for mechanistic studies examining the effects of secretagogues and pharmacological agents.

In contrast to studies looking at secretagogue responses in isolated islet preparations, the isolated whole pancreas perfusion method allows for the study of both endocrine and exocrine tissue function simultaneously as this procedure maintains cellular

C. Stocker (ed.), *Type 2 Diabetes*, Methods in Molecular Biology, vol. 560
DOI 10.1007/978-1-59745-448-3_14, © Humana Press, a part of Springer Science+Business Media, LLC 2009

integrity. There is also the possibility of a control and experimental period of study in the same pancreas preparation. Such control in other in vitro settings requires multiple incubations. The perfused pancreas can be used to evaluate the effects of drugs and secretagogues that effect pancreatic function. For example, amylin, a protein secreted by the pancreas and a major constituent of islet amyloid, deposits in patients with type 2 diabetes, while having no effect on glucose-stimulated insulin secretion, significantly inhibits arginine-stimulated insulin secretion.

The rodent is anesthetized by an appropriate means and both a lateral and midline incision made to expose the stomach, intestines, and mesenteric blood vessels. The pancreas is carefully separated from the overlaying colon, spleen, and connective tissues. The jejunum and its blood supply are ligated so that this distal section can then be removed. All other attachments of the pancreas to the descending colon are then ligated and cut, as are the splenic vessels. Once the mesenteric artery and celiac axis have been identified, the stomach is moved aside and the exposed esophagus and gastric artery are also ligated. The pancreas is isolated from the stomach following ligation of the duodenum and the vascular connections on the posterior wall exposed, which can then be ligated subsequently. By careful dissection, the aorta can be exposed, cleared from the inferior vena cava between the renal artery and superior mesenteric artery, and ligated. Loose ligatures are placed around the hepatic portal vein where it leaves the pancreas for the liver. Once the celiac and mesenteric branches have been identified along the aorta, the aorta can be freed from the vena cava to the ligature below the renal artery. Loose ligatures are positioned around the aorta just below the diaphragm preserving the origin of the celiac artery, which holds the inlet cannula, while the outlet cannula is placed in the portal vein. Once the abdominal aortic ligature is tightened, the pancreatic circulation can be completely isolated by tightening the ligature around the lower vena cava and perfusion can commence.

Based on the original apparatus used *(1)*, perfusate is pumped from a reservoir by means of a peristaltic pump into an enclosed organ perfusion chamber, and enters the pancreatic circulation through the celiac arterial cannula. The pancreas is kept moist with normal saline and perfused using a modified Krebs-Ringer bicarbonate-buffered solution containing glucose and bovine serum albumin. The production of insulin by the preparation is a reflection of its responsiveness to glucose and other secretagogues and can be collected by means of perfusate via the portal vein.

This methodology has been applied to a range of investigations studying pancreatic function with relation to diabetes covering physiological functionality in response to endogenous compounds such as nutrients (e.g., glucose-induced insulin, somatostatin, and orexin-A secretion) or the effects of fatty acids or hormones (e.g., amylin, GLP-1, and orexin-A) on the stimulation of insulin release, the inhibition of glucagon secretion or the leptin inhibition of basal insulin release *(2–5)*. The pre-diabetic state or diabetic state may be investigated using rodent models such as the Zucker fatty (*fa/fa*) or Zucker diabetic fatty (ZDF) rats. Furthermore, the isolated perfused pancreas is also a useful method for investigating potential therapeutic candidates, most notably those designed to enhance insulin secretion, such as the GLP-1 receptor antagonists *(6)*.

This chapter describes in detail the in vitro perfusion technique for the rodent pancreas. It presents a detailed description of the perfusion technique, a study of some of the functions of the preparation, and an observation of the pancreatic response to glucose as an example of secretagogue stimulation of insulin secretion. The development of sensitive radioimmunoassays of biological fluids has enabled the quantitative measurement of hormone secretion using pancreas perfusion techniques. This chapter will also describe the important salient features and optimization stages required to develop an in-house radioimmunoassay for use with this methodology.

2. Materials

2.1. Pancreas Excision

1. Anesthetic and analgesic regime capable of maintaining a level of anesthesia suitable for major surgery for 40 min, e.g., fentanyl citrate: fluanisone (0.315 mg/mL: 10 mg/mL) combined with midazolam (5 mg/mL) (*see* **Note 1**).
2. Blunt-nosed straight dissecting scissors 14–15 cm in length (FST, cat. #14000-14) (*see* **Note 2**).
3. Standard pattern forceps 14–15 cm in length (FST cat. #11000-14).
4. Blunt-nosed curved dissecting scissors 14–15 cm in length (FST cat. #14003-14).
5. Straight hemostat 14 cm (FST cat. #13004-14).
6. Saline: 0.9% $NaCl_{(aq)}$.
7. Black cotton thread cut into approximately 10 cm lengths.
8. Pair of curved eye dressing forceps 10 cm in length (FST cat. #11051-10).
9. Blunt-nosed straight dissecting scissors 10 cm in length (FST cat. #14078-10).
10. Cotton buds.

11. Pair of serrefines 35 mm length (FST cat. #18051-35).
12. Sharp straight spring scissors 10 cm in length (FST cat. #15024-10).
13. Polyethylene tubing with a bore of 0.5 mm, wall 25 mm (800/100/160, Scientific Laboratory Supplies, Nottingham, UK, cat. #TUB3660).
14. 2.5 mL syringe and needle.

2.2. Pancreas Perfusion

1. Perfusion tank (*see* **Fig. 1**).
2. 20 mL glass scintillation vials and silicon caps.
3. Water bath.
4. Silicone tubing (Scientific Laboratory Supplies, Nottingham, UK).
5. Three-way male lock stopcocks (Cole-Palmer, Illinois, USA).
6. Water heater/pump.
7. Peristaltic pump.
8. Manometer.
9. Sample collector.
10. Electronic thermometer.
11. Oxygen:carbon dioxide (95:5) cylinder.
12. Perfusion buffer (5.7 mM KCl, 1.5 mM KH_2PO_4, 113 mM NaCl, 1.2 mM $MgSO_4$, 2.3 mM calcium gluconate, 25 mM $NaHCO_3$, 3% (w/v) dextran T40, and 1% human albumin,

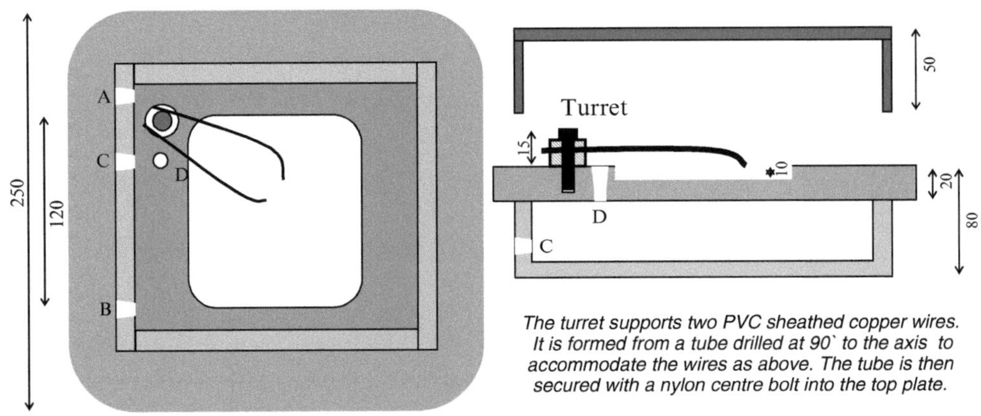

Fig. 1. Perfusion tank setup. The sheathed copper wires are attached to the two cannulae that are connected to the celiac artery and hepatic portal vein. The pancreas is housed in the central pool surrounded by perfusion buffer. (A) Inlet and (B) outlet for heated water keeps the central pool at 38°C. (C) Inlet and (D) outlet for tubing transporting the perfusate travels through the heated water re-heating it to perfusion temperature. All dimensions are expressed in millimeters.

pH 7.4). The buffer should be filtered and oxygenated steadily for 30 min before adjusting the pH to 7.4.

13. Glucose.
14. Arginine.
15. Millex HA 0.45 μm filter (Millipore, Massachusetts, USA).

2.3. Insulin Radioimmunoassay

1. Polystyrene round-base test tubes capable of holding 2 mL (e.g., 64 mm × 11 mm) (*see* **Note 3**).
2. Gamma counter, for example, Perkin-Elmer (Waltham, MA, USA).
3. [^{125}I]-insulin (diluted 10,000 cpm per 100 μL assay buffer).
4. Rat insulin standard.
5. Rat insulin antiserum.
6. Secondary antiserum (type determined by the species used to generate the insulin antisera).
7. 15% polyethylene glycol, MW 8000 (PEG-8000): This separates bound from unbound antigen by precipitating the antibody-antigen complex (*see* **Note 4**).
8. Assay buffer (50 mM NaH_2PO_4, 150 mM NaCl, 0.5% BSA (RIA grade), and 15 mM NaN_3, pH 7.4). Sera and PEG should be prepared in this buffer whilst standards should be prepared in the perfusion buffer.

3. Methods

The purpose of this surgical procedure is to create an enclosed system containing an intact pancreas with one inlet (the celiac artery) and one outlet (the hepatic portal vein) for perfusion, with all other blood vessels ligated to prevent leakage. For ease of operation, the stomach and spleen are excised with the pancreas, but are then excluded from the perfusion system by ligation of the connecting blood vessels. Prior to excision, the pancreas is perfused with saline and perfusion buffer to flush out the blood so that clots do not form which would compromise the system. An anticoagulant, such as heparin, may be introduced into the blood system after laparotomy to achieve this, in which case all the following surgical steps relating to the cannulation of the aorta should be omitted. This perfusion method is preferred unless the procedure is taking longer than 30 min or is performed on smaller rodents such as mice (*see* **Note 5**).

3.1. Pancreas Excision

1. Anesthetize the rat with an anesthetic regimen capable of providing a degree of surgical anesthesia and analgesia for 40 min. The fentanyl/fluanisone and midazolam combination described is sufficient and has low strain variability in duration of anesthesia.
2. During the surgical period, keep the rat warm by means of a heated pad or heated operating table.
3. Perform a laparotomy using blunt-nosed dissecting scissors (14–15 cm length is the optimal length for most users). First make an incision in the skin large enough for the same scissors to be inserted between the skin and abdominal wall, and then using the scissors tease apart the skin from the abdominal wall so that the skin can be cut from pubis to sternum along the mid-central line. Separate the skin and abdominal wall down the sides (a curved pair of scissors of similar size would be suited to this task) and cut the skin laterally, avoiding blood vessels as much as possible. Lift the abdominal wall with forceps and cut along the mid-central line between the pubis and xiphoid process being careful not to nick the organs below. Cut down each side of the abdominal wall after having occluded the blood vessels with the use of a hemostat (cauterizing works equally well).
4. Place pieces of saline-soaked tissue paper immediately to the left of the subject, and place the intestines carefully on top of these. Pour saline over the organs of the abdomen, and repeat periodically to prevent the organs from drying. At this point an anticoagulant, such as heparin, may be utilized by means of injection via the inferior vena cava.
5. Doubly ligate the descending colon and cut between the ligatures.
6. Use the upper ligature to raise the colon and cut the fascia underneath up to the transverse colon.
7. Tease away the top layer of fascia connecting the intestines and pancreas using a blunt tool being careful not to damage the pancreas (fingers are ideal for this task).
8. The bottom layer of fascia contains jejunal blood vessels that will need to be ligated. First remove the fascia between the vessels and ligate the vessels to the right of the transverse colon and then those of the mesenteric radix.
9. Ligate the duodenum adjacent to the ligature on the mesenteric radix and cut the intestines below the ligatures (*see* **Note 6**). The lower intestines can now be discarded.
10. Tease apart the fascia linking the pancreas, stomach, and spleen and cut the vessels connecting the stomach and spleen after double ligation.

11. Remove the fascia connecting the stomach, liver, and esophagus to expose the esophagus and esophageal artery. Doubly ligate these and cut.
12. Isolate the pancreas from the stomach by ligating the duodenum adjacent to the pylorus.
13. Remove the fat from around the descending aorta between the diaphragm and aortic bifurcation so that the aorta, caudal vena cava, and any branching vessels are clearly exposed (*see* **Note 7**).
14. Using blunt-ended forceps, separate the entire exposed length of the aorta from the body wall as well as the initial centimeter of the celiac, superior mesenteric, and renal arteries (*see* **Note 8**).
15. Separate a section of aorta from the vena cava between the renal and iliac arteries using blunt-ended forceps (*see* **Note 9**).
16. Lift the liver to the right and clear the hepatic portal vein of any connective tissue. Place an untied ligature around the vein and replace the liver exposing the celiac trunk.
17. Place untied ligatures around the aorta superior to the celiac artery, inferior to the superior mesenteric artery, and between the renal and iliac arteries. Leave several millimeters between the celiac artery and the ligature for ease of manipulation of the inlet cannula and also to avoid risk of cutting the celiac when severing the aorta.
18. Place untied ligatures around the celiac, mesenteric, and renal arteries (*see* **Note 10**).
19. Place a serrefine (*see* **Note 11**) across the aorta immediately inferior to the renal arteries and another at the aortic bifurcation. Using spring scissors make a cut into the aorta halfway between the serrefines.
20. Insert a cannula for connection to a saline-containing syringe into the aorta up to the superior serrefine and secure by tying the ligature.
21. Remove the superior serrefine and tie the ligatures around the renal and mesenteric arteries.
22. Tie the uppermost ligature around the aorta and immediately perfuse the system with 2.5 mL saline over a period of about 20–30 s. Replace the saline syringe with one containing the perfusion buffer and perfuse with 2.5 mL over 20–30 s. Immediately tie the remaining aortic ligature followed by the hepatic portal ligature. Tie the latter ligature as close to the liver as possible.

23. Cut the hepatic portal vein on the liver side of the ligature and cut the aorta on the celiac trunk side of both the top two ligatures. Lift out the section of abdominal organs, cutting any remaining underlying connective tissue, and transfer to the perfusion tank (*see* **Note 12**).
24. Dispose of rest of carcass by an appropriate means.

3.2. Ex vivo Preparation for Pancreas Perfusion

1. Locate the ligatures around the celiac artery and hepatic portal vein, lift and replace in the centre of the tank with the two blood vessels exposed.
2. Maneuver the inlet cannula next to the celiac trunk so that it is as almost horizontal. Holding the opening of the aorta adjacent to the celiac artery, but on the opposite wall, slip the cannula into the celiac trunk so that the cannula enters the celiac artery via the aorta. Secure in place by tying the ligature around the celiac artery and the cannula.
3. Maneuver the outlet cannula vertically next to the hepatic portal vein. Lift the vein by the ligature and make an incision into the vein as close to the ligature as possible (*see* **Note 13**). Holding the thread of the ligature in one hand and the lip of the aperture in the vein with forceps, slide the cannula into the vein by almost a centimeter. Tape the ligature threads to the cannula holder so that the vein does not slip off and secure a ligature around both the vein and the cannula (*see* **Note 14**).
4. Perfuse the pancreas at a rate of 2 mL/min until the perfusate begins to flow out and then perfuse at 4 mL/min for 20 min to flush out any secretagogues released into the system during the setup period (*see* **Note 15**).

3.3. Pancreas Perfusion

1. Set the perfusion equipment up as shown in **Fig. 2**. The temperature of the water bath and water heater/pump must maintain the perfusion buffer and perfusion tank temperature at 38°C. Check the perfusion tank temperature prior to surgery and monitor throughout the experiment (*see* **Note 16**).
2. Glucose is required in the perfusion buffer to maintain the integrity of the pancreas. The perfusion system can detect an increase in insulin secretion at 4.4 mM glucose. 2.8 mM glucose is used to maintain a basal level of insulin secretion and pancreas function. 5.6 mM glucose represents the normal level of glucose exposure to the pancreas in a free-fed state. Diabetes is defined when glucose appears in the urine and occurs when blood concentrations rise above 11 mM. Concentrations higher than this are important to include when looking at the diabetic state.

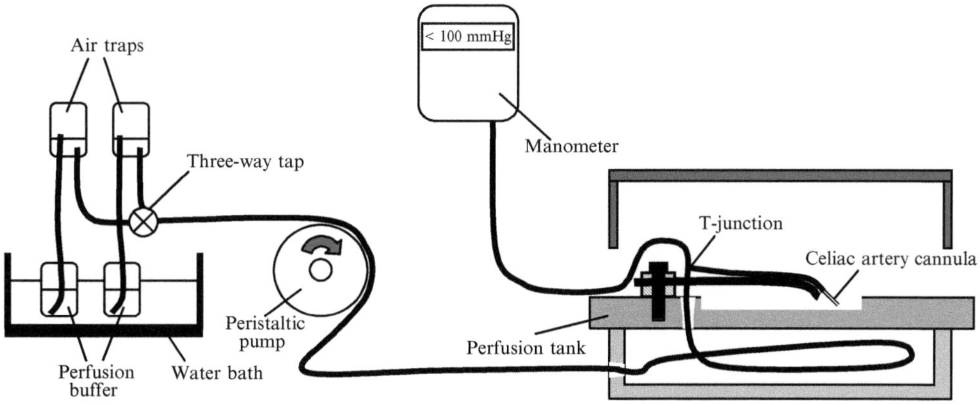

Fig. 2. Perfusion apparatus. The perfusion buffers are heated in a water bath and connected to air traps. Tubing connects the air traps to a tap, the number and type depending upon the number of different perfusates to be analyzed. The system powered by a peristaltic pump; immediately after which the perfusion tank is connected. A T-junction separates the perfusate into two tubes. One is attached to the cannula inserted into the celiac artery and the other connected to a manometer.

3. Arginine stimulates insulin secretion by a mechanism independent from that induced by glucose. Use 20 mM to demonstrate integrity of the system when investigating mechanisms where glucose-induced insulin secretion maybe impaired.
4. The sample collector should be set to collect samples over a 1 min period for most experiments. Whilst the perfusion is in progress, the samples already collected can be aliquoted in triplicate into tubes ready for radioimmunoassay.
5. Avoid designing perfusions exceeding 100 min in length, though this will not include the initial 20 min "flush-out" period.
6. Check the pH of the perfusion buffer at the end of the perfusion as pH 7.4 is outside the optimal buffering capacity of bicarbonate buffers (pH 5.1–7.1).
7. Monitor the pressure in the perfusion system continuously with the manometer. A pressure rise above 100 mmHg is indicative of a blockage in the pancreas resulting in swelling followed by leakage. Should this occur the perfusion should be terminated and the collected perfusate discarded.

3.4. Insulin Radioimmunoassay

In a radioimmunoassay, a fixed concentration of labeled tracer antigen is incubated with a constant amount of specific antiserum such that the concentration of antigen binding is limiting. If unlabeled antigen is added, there is a competition between labeled tracer and unlabeled antigen, so that the amount of tracer bound to the antibody will decrease as the concentration of unlabeled antigen increases. This can be measured after separating antibody bound from free tracer and counting the bound fraction, free fraction, or both.

Inter-assay controls are included in each assay system. These samples should be of identical composition to the material being assayed, from the same species and medium. These are used to validate the assay and to measure the variation within and between assays. The number of these required should be determined statistically during the method evaluation. The inter-assay drift must be determined from assay tubes containing identical amounts of reagents (sample, primary antibody, tracer, and secondary antibody). Duplicate sample pools should be placed at the beginning and end of the assay to determine if drift is a problem.

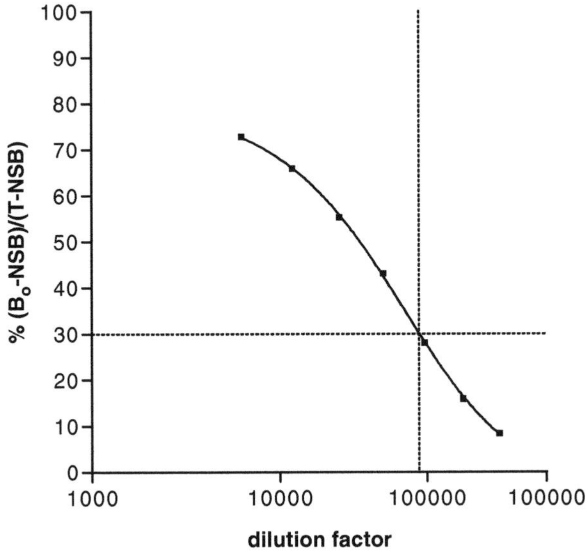

1st Ab dilution factor = 1 in 86,955

Fig. 3. Primary antibody titer test. The primary antibody will bind to the hormone of interest as well as the labeled tracer and standard. The bound fraction of the assay is that part of the labeled and unlabeled antigen specifically bound to the primary antibody and counted in the gamma counter. The primary antibody titer test is a preliminary radioimmunoassay to determine what concentration of primary antibody should be used. The amounts of tracer and secondary antibody remain constant between groups of NSBs and 100% tubes, while only the primary antibody concentration in the total tubes varies. Typically three totals, three NSBs, and three 100%s for each concentration of primary antibody are tested. The concentration selected depends on the sensitivity desired in the assay. The least primary antibody used the lower the standard curve doses can be reliable. In this example, the final dilution of primary antisera corresponds to the dilution of the original stock that precipitates 30% of hot antigen added to the tubes (minus non-specific precipitation). Here this corresponds to a final dilution of 1:86,955 of the original stock solution. Note that the primary incubation contains 100 μL of the standard/sample, 100 μL of label, and 100 μL of the primary antibody so, in this example, the primary antibody would be diluted 1:28,985 dilution (final dilution 1:86,955).

3.4.1. Setting up an In-House Radioimmunoassay

1. Determine the primary antibody dilution required. Set up three tubes each for total counts (T), non-specific binding (NSB), and at each dilution of primary antibody binding (B_0, a range of 1,000- to 1,000,000-fold is usually ample (*see* **Note 17**)). Proceed with **Subheading 3.4.2** from **step 3**. Plot the data as % ((B_0-NSB)/(T-NSB)) versus primary antibody dilution factor ($\log_{10}$ scale) using a sigmoidal curve-fit **(Fig. 3)**. The primary antibody dilution required corresponds to 30% ((B_0-NSB)/(T-NSB)) (*see* **Note 18**).
2. Determine the secondary antibody titer by setting up three tubes each for total counts, NSB, and each dilution of secondary antibody. Proceed with **Subheading 3.4.2**. Plot the data as % ((B_0-NSB)/(T-NSB)) versus secondary antibody dilution factor ($\log_{10}$ scale) using a sigmoidal curve-fit **(Fig. 4)**. The secondary antibody dilution required is the lowest that gives maximal precipitation (*see* **Note 19**).

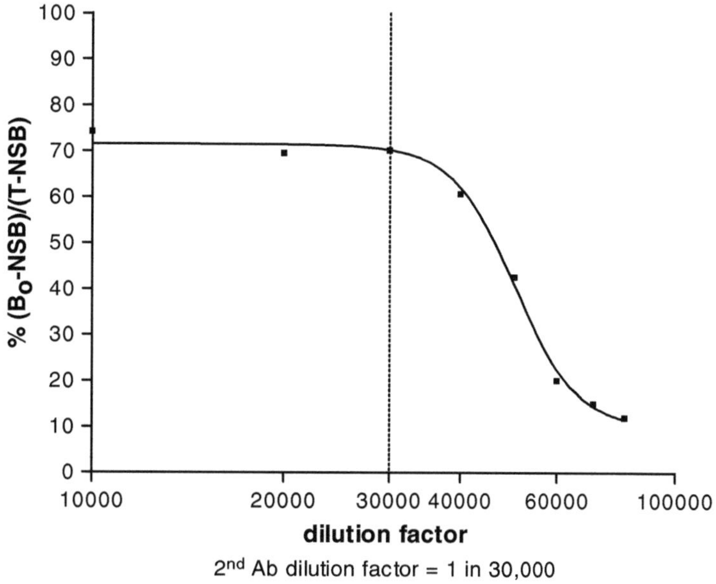

Fig. 4. Secondary antibody titer test. The secondary antibody binds to the primary antibody-antigen complex (bound fraction), and after centrifugation it is precipitated. After the free supernatant is decanted, the assay tube and precipitate are counted in the gamma counter. A secondary antibody titer test is a preliminary radioimmunoassay to determine what concentration of secondary antibody maximally precipitates the bound fraction of the primary antibody–antigen complex. In this test, the amount of tracer and primary antibody remain constant, while only the secondary antibody concentration varies. Typically three total count tubes, and for each different amount of secondary antibody, three NSBs, and three 100% tubes. In this example, the final dilution of secondary antisera corresponding to the lowest concentration that will still maximally precipitate the label is 1:30,000 would be used.

3. Validate the assay with a serial dilution of perfusate containing insulin. Either concentrate the perfusate or add enough rat insulin to make a 10 nM solution and serially dilute for a range from 1 pM to 10 nM. Perform **Subheading 3.4.2** from **step 3**, and compare the range to the standard curve. Express the concentrations relative to the top concentration or stock solution to ascertain whether the regression curves are vertically parallel. If the dilution curves are parallel then the assay is valid to analyze insulin secretion **(Fig. 5)**.

3.4.2. Radioimmunoassay Protocol

1. Generate radioimmunoassay standard curves from nine concentrations in quadruplicate. Ensure three standards fall on the steep part of the curve, and three standards at or near both the top and the bottom of the curve. When analyzing insulin secretions from the pancreas perfusion use the following concentrations: 0.02, 0.05, 0.1, 0.2, 0.5, 1, 2, 5, and 10 nM (*see* **Fig. 6**). Add 100 μL of standard to the appropriate tubes.
2. In addition to the samples and standards include: total counts (T), NSB, maximum binding (B_0), and variance determinants (*see* **Note 20**). Set up at least 20 variance tubes, ten at the start and end of the assay. Set up all other three groups in quadruplicate.
3. Add 100 μL [^{125}I]-insulin solution to all tubes and mix by vortexing.

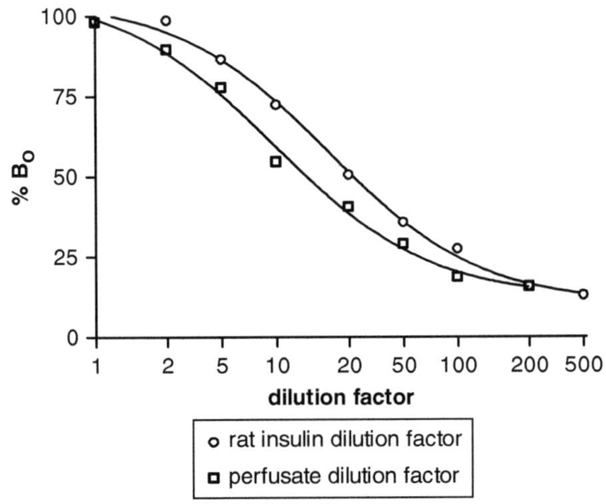

Fig. 5. The parallelism test. The parallelism test is performed to validate the assay or sample material. A serial dilution of a pooled sample is compared to varying standard curve doses within the same assay. Lines of equal slope demonstrate no significant proportional analytical error within these ranges. This allows the assay of unknown samples with the confidence that the dose estimate per mL will not have a significant error. This is important when unknowns are run in the same assay at different volumes.

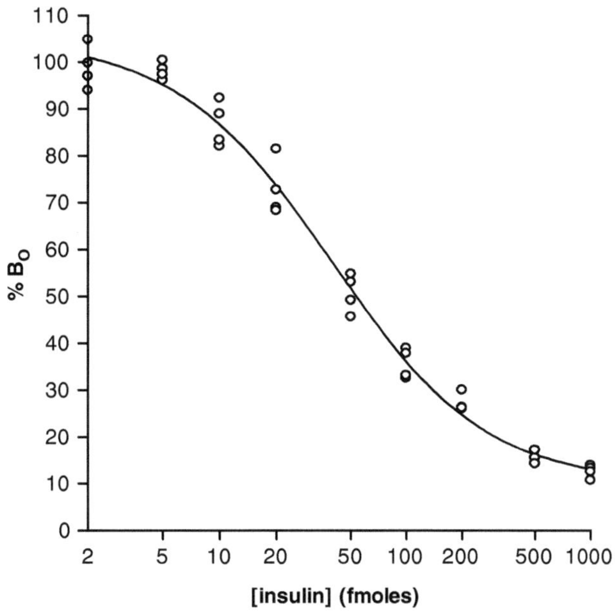

Fig. 6. Standard curve for the insulin radioimmunoassay. A calibration or standard curve is set up with increasing amounts of known antigen, and from this curve the amount of antigen in the unknown samples can be calculated. The four basic necessities for a radioimmunoassay are an antiserum to the compound to be measured, the availability of a radioactively labeled form of the compound, a method whereby antibody-bound tracer can be separated from unbound tracer, and a standard unlabeled material. Each *circle* represents a single data point and a sigmoidal regression line generated.

4. Add 100 μL of primary antisera to all tubes except T and NSB (add 100 μL assay buffer to these) and mix thoroughly (*see* **Note 21**).
5. Cover and incubate at 4°C for 24 h.
6. Add 100 μL of secondary antisera and incubate for 2–24 h.
7. Add 100 μL of PEG solution (*see* **Note 22**).
8. Add 1 mL distilled water at 4°C to each tube, mix and leave for 10 min.
9. Centrifuge all tubes for 10 min at 3,000 × *g*.
10. Remove the supernatant and count each tube for a minimum of 1 min with a gamma counter (*see* **Fig. 7**).

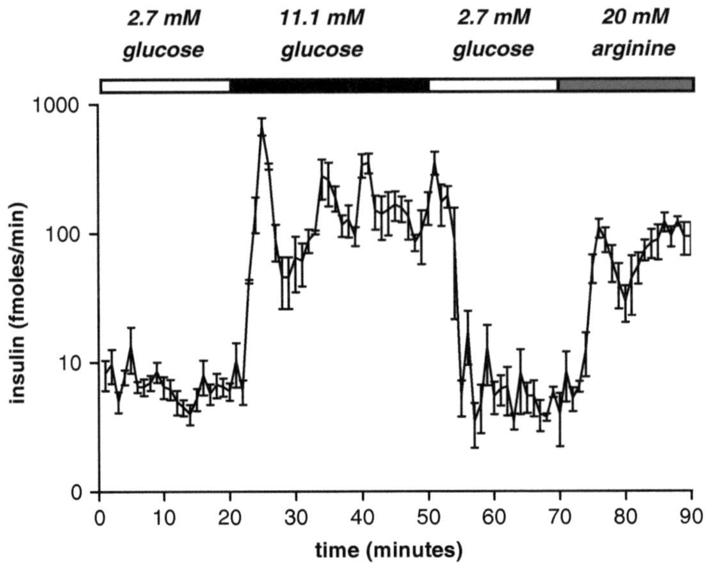

Fig. 7. Typical insulin secretion profile from a perfused pancreas from Wistar rats (n = 6). Basal insulin secretion was measured with 2.7 mM glucose in the perfusate and secretagogue-stimulated insulin secretion was measured with 11.1 mM glucose or 20 mM arginine in the perfusate.

4. Notes

1. The appropriate anesthetic regime will vary with strain and species. The regime detailed will be fine for commonly used strains such as Wistar and Sprague–Dawley rats.
2. All surgical tools described may be obtained from Fine Science Tools and the catalogue numbers are listed (website www.finescience.com).
3. Borosilicate tubes should be used for radioimmunoassays where peptides stick to tubes made from polystyrene or polypropylene, for example, GLP-1. Borosilicate tubes should also be used if the pellet formation is inadequate.
4. Some commercial products are a combination of secondary antibody and precipitating agent making this step quicker and easier. If a commercial secondary antibody/precipitator mix is used, then follow the manufacturer's instructions.
5. This technique is applicable to smaller rodents although the majority of the parameters, including the equipment and perfusion rates, will need to be appropriately scaled down with respect to the species used. For rodents smaller than rats, it is advisable to use the anticoagulant method to prevent clotting rather than pre-perfusion via the aorta. Also the perfusion should be performed in situ with the whole

animal in the perfusion tank rather than excising the isolated pancreas.

6. A double ligature is preferable here as an incomplete ligation at this site is the most common cause of leakage during the perfusion stage.
7. The left gastric and lineic arteries are easily disrupted and so the area must be cleared with care. Cotton buds are useful in exposing this area, but the entire length of these arteries need not be exposed as long as the celiac trunk is cleared of fat and connective tissue.
8. The right renal artery may prove difficult to access, if so this ligation may be missed, but it will minimally affect the initial perfusion step. In some strains of rat, the left and right renal artery arise from the same junction of the aorta and may be ligated together.
9. The connective tissue between the aorta and vena cava may be difficult to remove but do not be tempted to use sharp implements as the vena cava is easily disrupted. Should the vena cava be pierced quickly clamp both the aorta and the vena cava where the aorta would be clamped in **step 17**, remove traces of blood, and proceed as rapidly as possible to the initial perfusion step. In this way, blood clots in the pancreas may possibly be avoided.
10. Ensure that all loose ends of all untied ligatures are untangled and easily identified as minimal delay is optimal to prevent clots occurring in the pancreas.
11. A serrefine is a small spring forceps used to close an artery during surgery.
12. The section of excised organs will include the pancreas, spleen, stomach, and part of the intestines, although only the pancreas will be perfused in this system.
13. A small volume of blood will have drawn back into the portal vein due to the lack of valves in the hepatic portal system. This actually aids the insertion of the cannula as when the internal solution is translucent the hole in the vein can be difficult to locate.
14. The tape is unnecessary if there is a second person available to tie the ligature around the portal vein and cannula whilst the operator is holding it in place.
15. Perfusate collected during this period may be used to help validate and assess the variability of the secretagogue assays.
16. Setting up the perfusion equipment in a temperature-controlled room helps achieve a consistent perfusion tank temperature with little or no adjustment of water bath and water heater/pump temperature.

17. This dilution represents the final dilution, i.e., after the label and cold/blank solution has been added.
18. The lower the concentration of primary antisera used, the higher the sensitivity of the assay and the more reliable the lower end of the standard curve. A primary antibody dilution giving 30% of maximum amount of label precipitated is usually ideal.
19. When performing the primary antibody titer test for the first time, an excess of secondary antisera may be used. When the secondary antibody titer test has been carried out, the primary test should be repeated with the newly calculated secondary antibody dilution. The manufacturer of the secondary antibody will recommend a workable dilution factor. This value should be the middle point dilution in the second antibody titer test.
20. The total counts (T) are used to confirm that the label is in excess to the antibody (% B_0/T should be about 30%). This can also be used to estimate gamma counter efficiency (% cpm/dpm). NSB tubes contain no primary antibody and represent the proportion of non-bound label precipitated. This amount should be subtracted from all other values before any further calculations. It represents 0% binding. Maximum binding (B_0) tubes contain no added cold insulin and effectively all binding sites are occupied by hot insulin. These tubes should have the highest counts (apart from T tubes) and represent 100% binding. All standards and samples are expressed as a percentage of this value. Intra-assay and inter-assay variance are determined using the same stock of insulin for all assays used in the experiment (this has to be at an insulin concentration not used to generate the standard curve). Intra-assay variance is expressed as a % standard deviation of variance tubes/mean of variance tubes, and should be less than 10%. Inter-assay variance is expressed as a % standard deviation of the mean of intra-assay means/mean of intra-assay means, and should be less than 15%.
21. Incubating with primary antisera before addition of the label saturates the binding sites with cold antigen. A shortened incubation time following addition of the hot antigen prevents equilibrium being achieved and results in a more sensitive radioimmunoassay. If a lack of sensitivity is seen try incubating with primary antisera for 12 h prior to the 8–12 h incubation with hot antigen.
22. A final concentration of 3% PEG has been found to give the greatest percentage of specific binding and the lowest percentage of NSB in double antibody radioimmunoassays *(7)*.

References

1. Sussman, K.E., Vaughan, G.D., and Timmer, R.F. (1966). An in vitro method for studying insulin secretion in the perfused isolated rat pancreas. *Metabolism* **15**: 466–476.
2. Emilsson, V., Liu, Y.L., Cawthorne, M.A., Morton, N.M., and Davenport, M. (1997). Expression of the functional leptin receptor mRNA in pancreatic islets and direct inhibitory action of leptin on insulin secretion. *Diabetes* **46**: 313–316.
3. de Heer, J., Rasmussen, C., Coy, D.H., and Holst, J.J. (2008). Glucagon-like peptide-1, but not glucose-dependent insulinotropic peptide, inhibits glucagon secretion via somatostatin (receptor subtype 2) in the perfused rat pancreas. *Diabetologia* **51**: 2263–2270.
4. Göncz, E., Strowski, M.Z., Grötzinger, C., Nowak, K.W., Kaczmarek, P., Sassek, M., Mergler, S., El-Zayat, B.F., Theodoropoulou, M., Stalla, G.K., Wiedenmann, B., and Plöckinger, U. (2008). Orexin-A inhibits glucagon secretion and gene expression through a Foxo1-dependent pathway. *Endocrinology* **149**: 1618–1626.
5. Egido, E.M., Hernández, R., Marco, J., and Silvestre, R.A. (2009). Effect of obestatin on insulin, glucagon and somatostatin secretion in the perfused rat pancreas. *Regul Pept* **152**: 61–66.
6. Tseng, C.-C., Zhang, X.-Y., and Wolfe, M.M. (1999). Effect of GIP and GLP-1 antagonists on insulin release in the rat. *Am J Physiol Endocrinol Metab* **276**: E1049–E1054.
7. Eisenman, J.R., and Chew, B.P. (1983). Polyethylene Glycol in conjunction with a secondary antibody for 24 hour radioimmunoassay of bovine prolactin and growth hormone. *J Dairy Sci* **66**: 1174–1179.

Chapter 15

Hyperinsulinemic–Euglycemic Clamp to Assess Insulin Sensitivity In Vivo

Jason K. Kim

Summary

Insulin resistance, the impaired ability of insulin to stimulate glucose utilization, is a major characteristic of type 2 diabetes. Insulin sensitivity can be measured using a variety of techniques that are commonly employed in diabetes research and care. Of these, hyperinsulinemic-euglycemic clamp is the gold-standard method to assess insulin sensitivity. The euglycemic clamp is widely used in clinics and laboratories to measure insulin action on glucose utilization in humans and animals for clinical and basic science research. Incorporation of radioactive-labeled glucose during euglycemic clamps makes it possible to measure glucose metabolism in individual organs. In recent years, euglycemic clamps have been actively performed in transgenic animal models of obesity, diabetes, and its complications, and have significantly advanced our understanding on the etiology and pathogenesis of type 2 diabetes. This chapter describes our standardized methods of the euglycemic clamp and associated surgical and biochemical procedures to measure insulin sensitivity in conscious rodents.

Key words: Insulin resistance, Type 2 diabetes, Insulin action, Glucose metabolism, Euglycemic clamp, Transgenic animal models

1. Introduction

Insulin resistance is a major characteristic of numerous metabolic disorders including diabetes, obesity, and HIV-associated lipodystrophy, and plays a primary role in the development of type 2 diabetes *(1-3)*. Since insulin resistance is an early event in the progression of metabolic abnormalities ("metabolic syndrome") to type 2 diabetes (onset of hyperglycemia), insulin sensitivity is commonly assessed to predict the risk and evaluate the management of type 2 diabetes in clinical and research settings.

C. Stocker (ed.), *Type 2 Diabetes,* Methods in Molecular Biology, vol. 560
DOI 10.1007/978-1-59745-448-3_15, © Humana Press, a part of Springer Science+Business Media, LLC 2009

There are several methods to measure insulin action that differ in sensitivity, limitation, and sophistication of technical procedures. A glucose tolerance test (GTT) examines the effects of exogenous glucose delivered via oral, intraperitoneal, or intravenous administration on the systemic clearance of glucose *(4)*. While glucose tolerance directly correlates with insulin sensitivity in most states, it does not account for endogenous insulin secretion and therefore is limited in subjects with altered pancreatic function. An insulin tolerance test (ITT) examines the effects of intraperitoneal administration of insulin on systemic glucose clearance, and insulin tolerance also correlates with insulin sensitivity. However, ITT often induces severe hypoglycemia, and its results may be affected by systemic counterregulatory responses. Despite these limitations, both GTT and ITT are the most widely used methods to assess insulin sensitivity, largely because of their ease of use and the minimally invasive nature of these procedures.

The hyperinsulinemic-euglycemic clamp ("euglycemic clamp") is considered the gold-standard method to assess insulin sensitivity in vivo and addresses the limitations associated with GTT/ITT *(5, 6)*. Intravenous administration of insulin at a constant rate raises and maintains systemic insulin levels ("hyperinsulinemic") during euglycemic clamps. Glucose is intravenously infused at variable rates to maintain "euglycemia" during euglycemic clamps, and the steady-state rate of glucose infusion directly correlates with insulin sensitivity. Incorporation of radioactive-labeled glucose during euglycemic clamps further measures glucose metabolism in individual organs. Despite the wealth of information provided by the euglycemic clamp, the sophisticated and technical nature of this procedure has limited its use.

Insulin regulates glucose homeostasis by increasing glucose utilization in peripheral organs (skeletal muscle and adipose tissue) and suppressing hepatic glucose production (HGP) *(1)*. Insulin binds to a cell surface receptor that activates a cascade of intracellular signaling proteins (insulin signaling) and increases glucose transport into cells *(7, 8)*. Transgenic mice with muscle-specific deletion of insulin receptor (MIRKO) were generated to determine the role of insulin receptors in glucose metabolism *(9)*. Despite more than a 95% reduction in muscle insulin receptors, MIRKO mice were normoglycemic and showed normal response during GTT and ITT *(9)*. However, the euglycemic clamp study showed that MIRKO mice are insulin resistant. Insulin-stimulated glucose metabolism was significantly reduced in skeletal muscle of MIRKO mice, but glucose uptake into white adipose tissue was increased due to hyperinsulinemia in these mice (**Fig. 1**)*(10)*.

This study revealed two important aspects of the euglycemic clamp: it is a more sensitive measure of insulin action and assesses

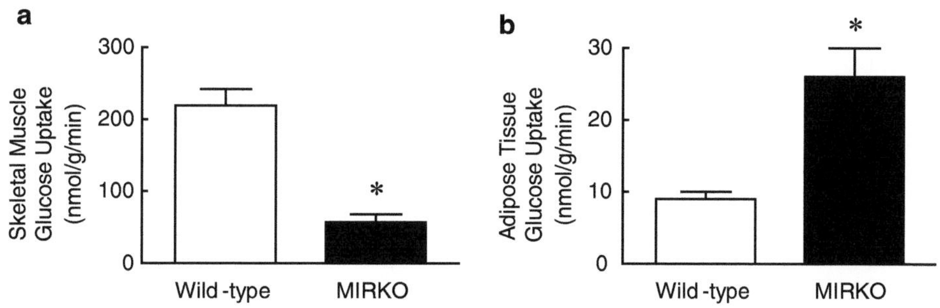

Fig. 1. Insulin sensitivity was measured using hyperinsulinemic-euglycemic clamps in conscious mice. Insulin-stimulated glucose uptake in skeletal muscle was reduced in MIRKO (muscle-specific insulin receptor knockout) mice, but glucose uptake in white adipose tissue was increased in MIRKO mice as compared with wild-type littermates. $*p < 0.05$ versus wild-type mice.

insulin sensitivity in individual organs. Since glucose metabolism was differentially altered in MIRKO mice, systemic glucose tolerance was not altered *(10)*. This is a major limitation of GTT/ITT in that they do not determine which organ(s) may be insulin sensitive or insulin resistant. This limitation is important because insulin resistance may develop in selective organs (e.g., skeletal muscle, liver) during the prediabetic stage but compensatory hyperinsulinemia may increase glucose metabolism in adipose tissue *(10)*. Additionally, the euglycemic clamp is capable of detecting a small change in insulin sensitivity that would not be possible with GTT/ITT and therefore has important advantages as a tool to measure insulin sensitivity in individual organs.

In principle, the hyperinsulinemic-euglycemic clamp raises and maintains circulating insulin levels by intravenously infusing insulin at a constant rate *(11)*. Insulin may be primed with a bolus injection at the start of euglycemic clamp to rapidly raise systemic insulin levels. Insulin is constantly infused at a rate of 2.5 mU/kg/min during the 2-h clamp to raise circulating insulin levels three-to four-fold over basal (target concentration of 300-400 pM). However, insulin infusion rate and therefore target insulin levels may be adjusted for various reasons (*see* **Notes 1** and **2**). During the hyperinsulinemic condition, glucose is intravenously infused at variable rates to maintain euglycemia (approximately 7 mM). This task is particularly challenging for euglycemic clamps involving mice since volume and frequency of blood sampling are greatly limited. In euglycemic clamps without blood transfusion, blood sampling and monitoring of plasma glucose levels are performed at 10–20 min intervals from the tail vessels. Plasma glucose concentrations are rapidly measured using a clinical glucose analyzer, and this information (ambient glucose levels) is used to adjust the variable rates of glucose infusion needed to maintain euglycemia during the euglycemic clamp.

Plasma glucose concentrations measured during the final 30 min of the clamp (steady-state) are used to calculate the specific activity and glucose turnover rates (*see* **Note 3**). Intravenous infusion of insulin (constant) and glucose (variable) uses a microdialysis pump, which performs the delivery with a high degree of accuracy (*see* **Note 4**).

Since glucose is intravenously infused at variable rates to maintain euglycemia, the glucose infusion rate during the steady state represents a crude index of insulin sensitivity. High rates of glucose infusion are required to maintain euglycemia in insulin-sensitive subjects since glucose is rapidly utilized and taken up by tissues during the hyperinsulinemic condition. In contrast, low rates of glucose infusion are required to maintain euglycemia in insulin resistant subjects since glucose utilization and clearance are impaired in these subjects. Additionally, the glucose infusion rates from the euglycemic clamp studies were shown to correlate with commonly used, simple surrogate indices of insulin sensitivity, such as QUICKI (quantitative insulin sensitivity check index) and HOMA (homeostasis model assessment) *(12)*. Thus, hyperinsulinemic-euglycemic clamps can be used to determine insulin sensitivity in various animal models *(12)*.

Prior to the start of euglycemic clamp experiments, [3-^{3}H] glucose is intravenously infused for 2 h to measure the basal rate of whole body glucose turnover. A blood sample is taken at the end of the 2-h infusion to measure basal concentrations of glucose and insulin, specific activity, and rates of glucose turnover. At basal state, HGP is the only source of glucose introduced into the system and therefore equilibrates with peripheral glucose disposal at steady state. Thus, the basal rate of whole body glucose turnover represents the basal rate of HGP. During the euglycemic clamp, [^{3}H] glucose is continuously infused to measure insulin-stimulated rates of whole body glucose turnover. Since [^{3}H] glucose is constantly infused, as is insulin, one infusate solution is concocted with a body weight-adjusted concentration of insulin and a fixed concentration of [^{3}H] glucose. [^{3}H] glucose is primed at the start of the experiment to rapidly raise systemic [^{3}H] glucose levels. Blood samples are taken during the final 30 min of the clamp (steady-state) to measure plasma [^{3}H] glucose concentrations, specific activity, and insulin-stimulated whole body glucose turnover. During the insulin-stimulated condition (hyperinsulinemic-euglycemic clamps), HGP (endogenous glucose production) and exogenous glucose infusion are introduced into the system and equilibrate with peripheral glucose disposal. HGP in the insulin-stimulated state will be calculated as the difference between whole body glucose turnover and glucose infusion rate. Thus, [^{3}H] glucose is used during the euglycemic clamp to measure insulin sensitivity in liver and peripheral organs.

To assess the rates of glucose metabolism in individual organs (e.g., skeletal muscle, adipose tissue), 2-deoxy-D-[1-^{14}C]glucose (2-[^{14}C] DG), a non-metabolizable glucose analogue, is injected as a bolus at 75 min after the start of the 2-h euglycemic clamp. The timing of the 2-[^{14}C] DG injection depends on the assumptions that steady state is achieved by 75 min of the euglycemic clamp and that most of the 2-[^{14}C] DG is cleared from the system during the final 45 min. Blood samples are taken during the final 45 min to measure plasma concentrations of 2-[^{14}C] DG. At the end of the experiment, mice are anesthetized using sodium pentobarbital injection, and tissues (e.g., skeletal muscle, adipose tissue, liver, and heart) are rapidly taken for biochemical and molecular analysis.

2. Materials

2.1. Survival Surgery for Intravenous Catheterization

1. HelixMark Standard Silicone Tubing (0.012″ ID/0.025″ OD; Helix Medical, Inc.) is used as an implantable catheter for intravenous infusion of solutions during the euglycemic clamp.
2. A combined solution of KetaVed ketamine HCl Inj., USP (100 mg/ml) and TranquiVed xylazine Inj. (20 mg/ml) is used for general anesthesia during surgery.

2.2. Hyperinsulinemic-Euglycemic Clamp in Conscious Mouse

1. Radioactive-labeled glucose: [3-^{3}H] glucose (18 μCi per mouse) is used to measure whole body insulin sensitivity. 2-deoxy-D-[1-^{14}C] glucose (10 μCi per mouse) is used to measure glucose uptake in individual organs.
2. Microdialysis pumps (CMA/Microdialysis, North Chelmsford, MA) are used to infuse intravenous solutions (insulin, glucose, [3-^{3}H] glucose) at a constant rate.
3. Beckman Glucose Analyzer 2 (Beckman, Fullerton, CA) or Analox GM7 Micro-stat Rapid Multiassay Analyser (Analox Instruments Ltd., London, UK) are used for a rapid and accurate measurement of plasma glucose levels using a small blood volume (20 μl).
4. Humulin regular insulin human Inj. USP (100 U/ml, #U100; Novo Nordisk) is intravenously infused to raise circulating insulin levels during the euglycemic clamp.
5. Twenty percent dextrose solution is intravenously infused at variable rates to maintain euglycemia during the clamp.
6. Sodium chloride (0.9%) is used to suspend and prepare infusion solutions.

7. One milliliter tuberculin syringes are used to set up an infusion line.
8. Microhematocrit capillary tubes are used to collect blood samples from tail vessels.
9. Heparin-coated blue polyethylene open-top tubes (400 μl) are used to transfer blood samples from capillary tubes for centrifugation and collection of plasma samples.
10. Microcentrifuge tubes (1.5 ml) are used to collect plasma samples to be stored for biochemical analysis.

2.3. Biochemical Assay: Whole Body Glucose Metabolism

1. Barium hydroxide monohydrate (0.3 N) is used to deproteinize plasma samples to measure whole body glucose metabolism.
2. Zinc sulfate heptahydrate (0.3 N) is used to deproteinize plasma samples to measure whole body glucose metabolism.
3. Scintillation cocktail is used to measure radioactivity in serum and tissue samples.
4. Liquid scintillation counter with dual channels for the separation of ^{3}H and ^{14}C is used to measure radioactivity in all samples.

2.4. Biochemical Assay: Glucose Uptake in Individual Organs

1. Poly-prep columns prefilled with AG 1-X8 resin (Bio-Rad) are used in anion-exchange chromatography to separate 2-[^{14}C] DG-6-phosphate from 2-[^{14}C] DG to measure glucose uptake in individual organs.
2. A solution containing 0.2 M formic acid and 0.5 M ammonium acetate is used for anion-exchange chromatography: Prepare 900 ml dH_2O in a graduate cylinder and add 7.69 ml formic acid. Add 38.54 g ammonium acetate (kept refrigerated), and adjust the solution pH to 4.9 ± 0.05 using dH_2O. Add dH_2O to make the final volume of solution of 1 L.

2.5. Biochemical Assay: Glycogen Synthesis in Individual Organs

1. 30% potassium hydroxide: 16.4 g KOH is added to 40 ml dH_2O and stirred until the solute is completely dissolved.
2. 95% ethanol: 190 ml 100% ethanol is added to 10 ml dH_2O and kept in the freezer.

2.6. Biochemical Assay: Plasma Metabolite Profiles

1. Beckman or Analox glucose reagent kits are used to measure plasma glucose concentrations using Beckman or Analox glucose analyzer.
2. Both regular and ultrasensitive mouse insulin ELISA kits or Luminex (Bio-Rad) are used to measure plasma insulin concentrations.

3. Methods

There are a few important topics to address when designing a study involving the euglycemic clamp in mice.

1. Gender: Male mice are preferred since the metabolic phenotypes of female mice may be affected by hormonal and menstrual cycles. Exceptions can be made for studies involving gender-specific phenotypes.
2. Background strain: It is important to be consistent on the background strain. It is well known that different genetic strains of mice have different levels of insulin sensitivity *(13)*. It is also well established that the metabolic effects of obesity (e.g., high-fat diet) or diabetes (e.g., streptozotocin) intervention differ based on the genetic strain of mice. Thus, all study groups should have the same background genetic strain and an equal number of generations of back-crosses. For obesity studies, C57BL/6 mice are commonly chosen since these mice are sensitive to obesity and diet intervention. The C57BL/6 background is also the most commonly used background strain of transgenic mouse models of obesity, diabetes, and its complications. The number of back-crosses should be considered since too little or too many may affect the genetic composition of the study mice. Typically, more than four and less than ten back-crossed generations are recommended.
3. Appropriate controls: It is important to study an appropriate control group to which the data comparison will be performed. This is often a group of mice with the same background genetic strain as the experimental mice. The use of littermates as controls is highly recommended since it minimizes potential effects of genetic manipulation and environment. The control group should be gender- and age-matched.
4. Age: The age of the animal has a profound effect on glucose metabolism. Young mice are preferred since the metabolic effects of aging are evident as early as 6 months of age. For standard insulin sensitivity measurements, mice at 3–4 months of age are preferred for their optimal size and maturity. Exceptions can be made for studies involving age-associated phenotypes. It is essential to study control mice that are closely age-matched.
5. Housing and acclimatization: If mice are obtained from a commercial vendor or different institution, they should be studied after 1-2 weeks of acclimatization in the new environment. Mice are typically housed under controlled temperature (23°C) and lighting with free access to water and standard mouse chow. It is important to consider the composition of

the standard chow diet, which differs in fat composition between institutional animal care facilities. In some mouse models, small differences in fat composition may affect insulin sensitivity.

6. Minimizing stress: Stress significantly affects glucose metabolism, and all efforts are needed to minimize stress in mice. Study animals should be brought to the laboratory where the euglycemic clamps are to be performed at least 1 day before the experiments. Transportation causes a stress to the animals and may exert unwanted metabolic effects. Housing of animals in the laboratory for 1 day before the experiment also acclimates the mice to the new environment.

3.1. Survival Surgery for Intravenous Catheterization

To measure insulin sensitivity in the physiological state, the euglycemic clamp is performed in the conscious mouse. Mice are placed in an oversized restrainer to minimize stress during experiments. The mouse is tail-restrained using tape to obtain blood samples from the tail vessels. This setup is performed at least 2 h before the start of the euglycemic clamp in order for the mouse to acclimatize. It is very important that the mouse is minimally stressed since stress affects glucose homeostasis. Some laboratories perform the euglycemic clamp in anesthetized mice, but anesthesia is known to affect glucose homeostasis. Thus, it is most physiological to perform the clamp in a conscious mouse.

Survival surgery, to place an indwelling intravenous catheter, is performed at 4–5 days before euglycemic clamps. This is important since mice are anesthetized, and show reduced food intake 24–48 h following surgery. By 4–5 days after surgery, mice fully recuperate, as evidenced by a regaining of body weight.

1. Mice are anesthetized with an intraperitoneal injection of ketamine (100 mg/kg body weight) and xylazine (10 mg/kg body weight), and the level of general anesthesia is confirmed using a pinch stimulus of the tail and/or foot.
2. A transverse incision (~0.5 cm) is made over the trachea, and the right jugular vein is isolated.
3. A silastic catheter (PE 10) is inserted into the vessel. The catheter is filled with a saline solution containing heparin (10 U/ml) and plugged.
4. The catheter is then tunneled to the back of the neck, and placed under the back skin to prevent its accessibility to the mouse.
5. A suture is tied to the catheter, and a small opening is made at the back of the neck. This silk, which is partially exposed, is used/pulled on the day of the euglycemic clamp to expose the catheter.

The catheter requires no other care until the day of the euglycemic clamp when it is flushed with a heparinized saline solution to reopen. This surgery requires approximately 15 min to complete. All surgical procedures are performed using standardized aseptic techniques. All surgical tools are autoclaved following the surgery. For each day of surgery, the tools are sterilized using a heat-sterilizer for the use on five mice at a time and cooled to room temperature before use.

3.1.1. Postoperative Care

In order to prevent hypothermia, a heating pad is used during the surgery, while a heating lamp and/or heating pad is used during the postoperative recovery period. After surgery, the mice are monitored closely in a postoperative cage with gauze bedding. Mice are monitored until they are awake and ambulatory (usually within 1-2 h). Mice are then housed in individual cages and monitored for postoperative recovery and weight gain on a daily basis for 48 h for evidence of catheter infection. If this occurs, the mice are euthanized as appropriate. In order to minimize pain, Ibuprofen (30 mg/kg body weight/day) is administered via the drinking water for 48 h.

3.2. Hyperinsulinemic-Euglycemic Clamp in Conscious Mice

The euglycemic clamp may be performed following an overnight fast (~15 h) or in the fed state, as insulin sensitivity was shown to be minimally different between either state *(14)*. It is important to be consistent with one metabolic state for the entire study. If the euglycemic clamps are performed in a fed state, it is important to remove the food in the morning and start the clamp at least 5 h after food removal. This approach ensures null or minimal effects of gastrointestinal absorption of nutrients at the start of the clamp.

The following euglycemic clamp procedure is performed in conscious mice **(Fig. 2)**.

1. On the day of the euglycemic clamp experiment, place a mouse in a rat-size restrainer with its tail tape-tethered at one end. This approach minimizes stress during the experiments **(Fig. 3)**.
2. Expose the intravenous catheter and connect to the infusion pump. This procedure is applied for 2 h before the start of the euglycemic clamp for mice to acclimatize to this partially restrained state and recover from the initial stressful handling.
3. To obtain blood samples from the tail vessels during the experiments, cut less than 0.5 cm of tail end and tape to prevent bleeding. All blood samples are taken from the tail vessels after removing the tape and using tail massage. After blood sampling, retape the tail end to prevent bleeding, and repeat during the clamp.

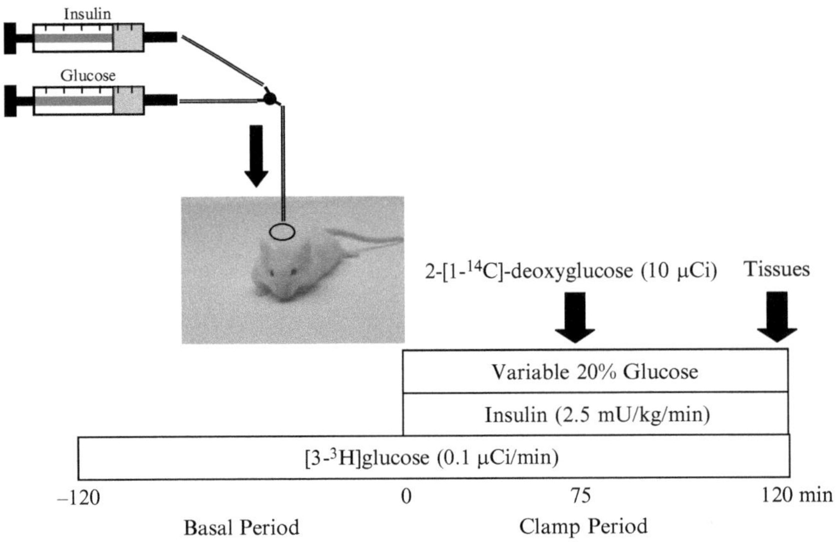

Fig. 2. A 2-h hyperinsulinemic-euglycemic clamp to assess insulin sensitivity and glucose metabolism in individual organs.

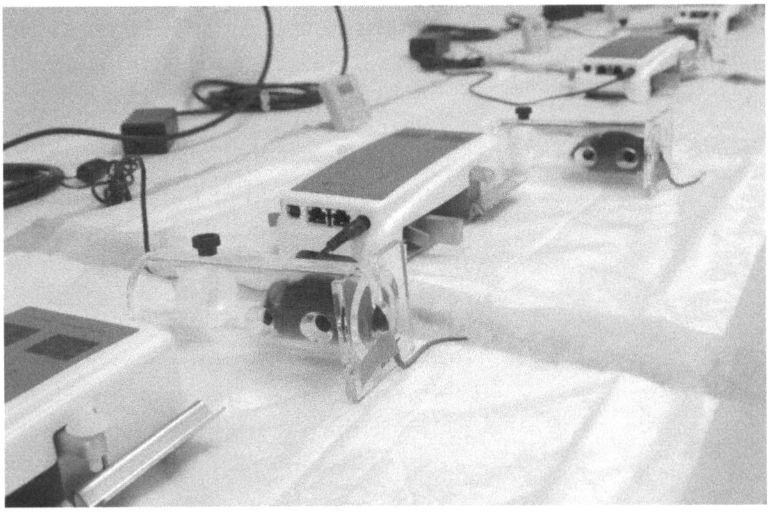

Fig. 3. This picture illustrates the hyperinsulinemic-euglycemic clamp. A conscious mouse is placed in the oversized restrainer with the tail tape tethered to one end of the restrainer to allow access for blood sampling during the euglycemic clamp. This partial restraint is applied at least 2 h prior to the start of the euglycemic clamp for acclimatization.

4. During this 2-h acclimation period, infuse D-[3-^{3}H] glucose (0.05 μCi/min) using a microdialysis pump to assess the basal rate of whole body glucose turnover.
5. Collect a blood sample (60 μl) at the end for the measurement of plasma glucose, insulin, and [^{3}H] glucose concentrations (basal parameters).

6. Following the basal period, conduct a 2-h hyperinsulinemic-euglycemic clamp with a primed (150 mU/kg body weight) and continuous infusion (2.5 mU/kg/min) of human insulin to raise plasma insulin within a physiological range (approximately 300 pM) *(11)*.
7. Collect blood samples (20 μl) at 10–20 min intervals for the immediate measurement of plasma glucose concentrations using a clinical glucose analyzer.
8. Infuse 20% glucose at variable rates to maintain plasma glucose at basal concentrations (~6 mM) during the euglycemic clamp.
9. Insulin-stimulated whole body glucose turnover can be estimated with a continuous infusion of [3-^{3}H] glucose throughout the clamp (0.1 μCi/min).
10. To estimate insulin-stimulated glucose uptake in individual organs, administer a bolus of 2-deoxy-D-[1-^{14}C] glucose (2-[^{14}C]DG) (10 μCi) 75 min after the start of the clamp *(11)*.
11. Take blood samples (20 μl) at 80, 85, 90, 100, 110, and 120 min for the measurement of plasma [^{3}H] glucose, $^{3}H_2O$, and 2-[^{14}C] DG concentrations. Take a final blood sample (20 μl) at the end of the clamp to measure plasma insulin concentrations.
12. At the end of the euglycemic clamp, anesthetize the mice, and dissect out skeletal muscles (gastrocnemius, tibialis anterior, and quadriceps) from both hindlimbs, white and brown adipose tissues, liver, and heart. Rapidly freeze the tissues in liquid N_2, and store the samples in a –80°C freezer for biochemical/molecular analysis *(11)*.

3.3. Biochemical Assay: Plasma Metabolite Profiles

1. Measure glucose concentrations during the clamp with 5-10 μl plasma using a Beckman Glucose Analyzer 2 or Analox GM7 Micro-stat Rapid Multiassay Analyser.
2. Measure plasma insulin concentrations by ELISA or Luminex.

3.4. Biochemical Assay: Whole Body Glucose Metabolism

Plasma concentrations of [3-^{3}H] glucose, 2-[^{14}C]DG, and $^{3}H_2O$ are determined following deproteinization of plasma samples (10 μl plasma suspended in 20 μl dH_2O) as follows:

1. Add 25 μl of $Ba(OH)_2$ to the plasma samples and vortex for 10 s.
2. Add 25 μl of $ZnSO_4$ to the plasma samples and vortex for 10 s.
3. Centrifuge the samples at 17,000 × *g* for 5 min.
4. Prepare two sets of scintillation vials (dry and non-dry samples) for each sample.

For dry samples (in order to eliminate ^3H_2O from the samples):

5. Add 25 μl of the supernatant obtained from **step 3** to dry sample vials.
6. Place the dry sample vials into a vacuum oven and dry overnight. This drying step must not use any heat, and the vacuum oven should be set at room temperature.
7. On the next day, add 100 μl of dH_2O to the dry sample vials and vortex for 30 s.
8. Add 3 ml of scintillation cocktail and vortex for 10 s.
9. Count the radioactivity using a liquid scintillation counter on dual channels for the separation of ^3H and ^{14}C.

For nondry samples:

10. Add 75 μl of dH_2O to the non-dry sample vials.
11. Add 25 μl of the supernatant obtained from **step 3** to the non-dry sample vials.
12. Add 3 ml of scintillation cocktail and vortex for 30 s.
13. Count the radioactivity using a liquid scintillation counter on dual channels for the separation of ^3H and ^{14}C.

At the end of the euglycemic clamp, basal and clamp infusate samples containing [3-^3H] glucose will be saved, and the infusate concentrations of [3-^3H] glucose will be determined using the same procedure as described. Plasma concentrations of ^3H_2O will be calculated as the difference in ^3H counts between dry and non-dry samples and will be used to calculate the rate of whole body glycolysis.

3.5. Biochemical Assay: Glucose Uptake in Individual Organs

The rate of insulin-stimulated glucose uptake in individual organs is determined using 2-[^{14}C] DG. 2-[^{14}C] DG is taken up by cells, phosphorylated by glucokinase to become 2-[^{14}C] DG-6-P, and not further metabolized. Thus, organ-specific accumulation and level of 2-[^{14}C] DG-6-P during the clamp reflect insulin-stimulated glucose uptake in individual organs. Intracellular concentrations of 2-[^{14}C] DG-6-P are determined as follows:

1. Prepare a heat block set to ~100°C.
2. Prepare anion-exchange columns by washing with 5 ml of dH_2O.
3. Homogenize 50–100 mg of frozen tissue samples by adding ten times the volume of dH_2O (50 mg of tissue in 500 μl of dH_2O) in glass tubes using a tissue homogenizer.
4. Following homogenization, place the glass tubes in the heat block for 10 min, vortex for 2 s, and then cool to room temperature.
5. Transfer the homogenized samples to microcentrifuge tubes using transfer pipettes and centrifuge at 16,000 × *g* for 5 min.

6. Add 33 μl of homogenate (supernatant) to 467 μl dH_2O in a scintillation vial labeled "total" sample. Add 5 ml of scintillation cocktail, vortex, and count the samples for ^{14}C using a liquid scintillation counter (total ^{14}C samples).
7. Transfer 333 μl of homogenate (supernatant) to the anion-exchange columns for the separation of 2-[^{14}C] DG-6-P from 2-[^{14}C] DG.
8. Wash the columns with 2 ml of dH_2O three times and collect the samples into a scintillation vial labeled "wash" sample.
9. Vortex the "wash" samples, and transfer 500 μl of "wash" samples to another set of scintillation vials to be counted for ^{14}C using a liquid scintillation counter (wash samples containing 2-[^{14}C] DG).
10. Elute the columns with 2 ml of 0.2 M formic acid/0.5 M ammonium acetate three times, and collect the samples into a scintillation vial labeled "eluate" sample.
11. Vortex the "eluate" samples, and transfer 500 μl of "eluate" samples to another set of scintillation vials to be counted for ^{14}C using a liquid scintillation counter (eluate samples containing 2-[^{14}C] DG-6-P).

3.6. Biochemical Assay: Glycogen Synthesis in Individual Organs

The rate of insulin-stimulated glycogen synthesis is determined using [3-^3H] glucose, which is taken up by cells and metabolized via glycolysis and glycogen synthesis. In adipose tissue, [3-^3H] glucose is also metabolized via lipogenesis.

1. Prepare a heat block set to ~100°C.
2. Add 500 μl of 30% KOH to the glass tubes.
3. Add approximately 50 mg of tissue samples to the KOH, and homogenize using a tissue homogenizer.
4. Following homogenization, place the glass tubes in the heat block for 15 min, vortex for 2 s, and cool to room temperature.
5. Add 3 ml of ice-cold 95% ethanol to the homogenate samples, parafilm, and incubate in a freezer for 1 h.
6. Following incubation, centrifuge the samples at 400 × *g* at 4°C for 15 min.
7. Discard the ethanol supernatants using a transfer pipette.
8. Add 3 ml of ice-cold 95% ethanol for the second and third washes and repeat the process.
9. Following the third wash, dry the glycogen pellets by placing the glass tubes in the heat block set at 100°C for 1–2 min.
10. Add 0.6 ml of dH_2O to the glycogen pellet, and completely dissolve by vortexing.

11. Transfer 500 μl of the samples to scintillation vials, and add 3 ml of scintillation cocktail to count for ^{3}H-glycogen using a liquid scintillation counter.

3.7. Calculations

Basal HGP or basal glucose turnover is calculated as the ratio of the basal [^{3}H] glucose infusion rate (dpm/min) to the specific activity of plasma glucose (dpm/μmol) at the end of the basal period **(Fig. 4)**. Insulin-stimulated whole body glucose turnover is calculated as the ratio of the clamp [^{3}H] glucose infusion rate (dpm/min) to the specific activity of plasma glucose (dpm/μmol) during the final 30 min of the euglycemic clamp **(Fig. 5)**. Insulin-stimulated HGP (during the euglycemic clamp) is calculated by subtracting the glucose infusion rate from the whole body glucose turnover rate. Whole body glycolysis is calculated from the rate of increase in plasma ^3H_2O concentrations, as determined by linear regression of the measurements at 80, 85, 90, 100, 110, and 120 min **(Fig. 6)**. Whole body glycogen plus lipid synthesis are estimated by subtracting whole body glycolysis from whole body glucose turnover.

Since 2-deoxyglucose is a non-metabolizable glucose analogue, insulin-stimulated glucose uptake in individual organs is estimated by determining the organ-specific level of 2-[^{14}C] DG-6-P. To this end, organ-specific glucose uptake is calculated from the plasma 2-[^{14}C] DG decay profile, which is fitted with a

$$\text{Rd} = \frac{\text{basal } [^3\text{H}]\text{-glucose infusion rate}}{\text{specific activity of glucose}}$$

$$= \text{basal hepatic glucose production}$$

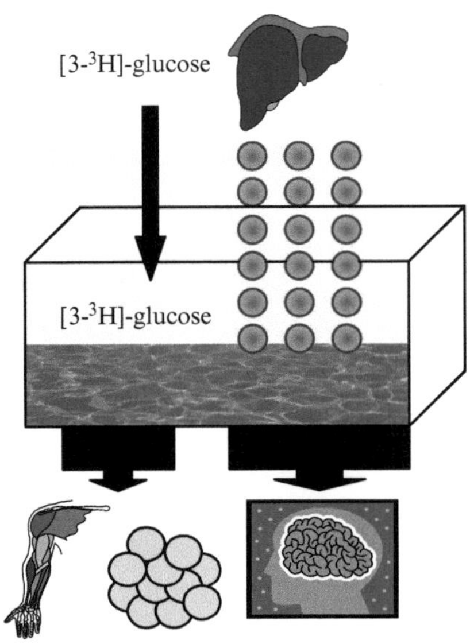

Fig. 4. This picture illustrates the maintenance of glucose homeostasis by hepatic glucose production (*HGP*) and glucose utilization in peripheral organs (e.g., skeletal muscle, adipose tissue, and brain) in the basal state. Basal whole body glucose turnover (Rd) is calculated as the ratio of basal [^{3}H] glucose infusion rate and specific activity of glucose at the end of the basal period.

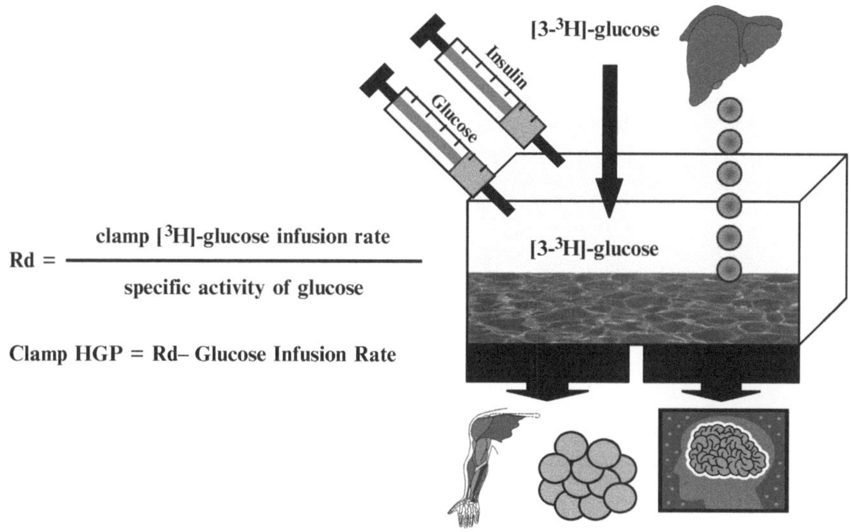

Fig. 5. This picture illustrates the introduction of insulin and exogenous glucose during the euglycemic clamp. Insulin maintains glucose homeostasis by suppressing hepatic glucose production (*HGP*) and increasing glucose utilization in peripheral organs. Insulin-stimulated whole body glucose turnover (Rd) is calculated as the ratio of clamp [^{3}H] glucose infusion rate and specific activity of glucose during the last 30 min of the clamp. Insulin-stimulated HGP is calculated as the difference between whole body glucose turnover and glucose infusion rate.

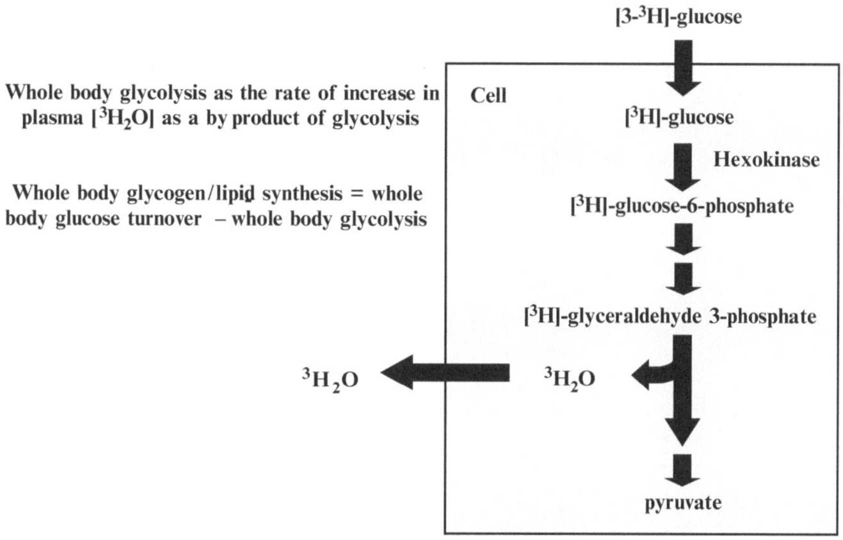

Fig. 6. This picture illustrates the estimation of whole body glycolysis using [3-^{3}H] glucose infusion and the rate of increase in plasma [3 (supernatant) H_2O] during the euglycemic clamp. Whole body glycogen plus lipid synthesis is calculated as the difference between whole body glucose turnover and glycolysis.

double exponential or linear curve, and intracellular 2-[^{14}C] DG-6-P content (**Fig. 7**)*(11)*. The equation for tissue glucose uptake (R'_g) is as follows: $R'_g = C_p C_m / \int_{t=0}^{45} C_p(t)dt$, where C_p is the plasma glucose concentration at steady state, C_m is the tissue concentration of 2-[14C] DG-6-P, and $C_p(t)$ is the plasma 2-[14C] DG concentration t minutes after 2-[14C] DG injection. Tissue-specific glycogen synthesis is calculated from ^3H incorporation into tissue glycogen **(Fig. 8)**. Tissue glycolysis is estimated as the difference between glucose uptake and glycogen synthesis in individual organs.

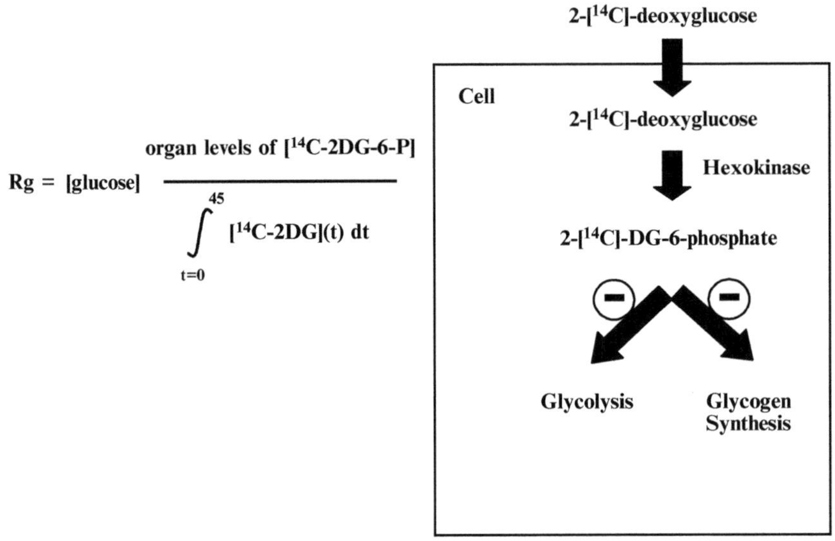

Fig. 7. This picture illustrates the estimation of organ-specific glucose uptake using 2-[14C]-deoxyglucose (14C-2DG) injection during the euglycemic clamp. 2-DG is a non-metabolizable glucose analogue, and tissue glucose uptake rate (R_g) is based on organ-specific accumulation of 14C-2DG-6-P and the plasma decay profile of 14C-2DG.

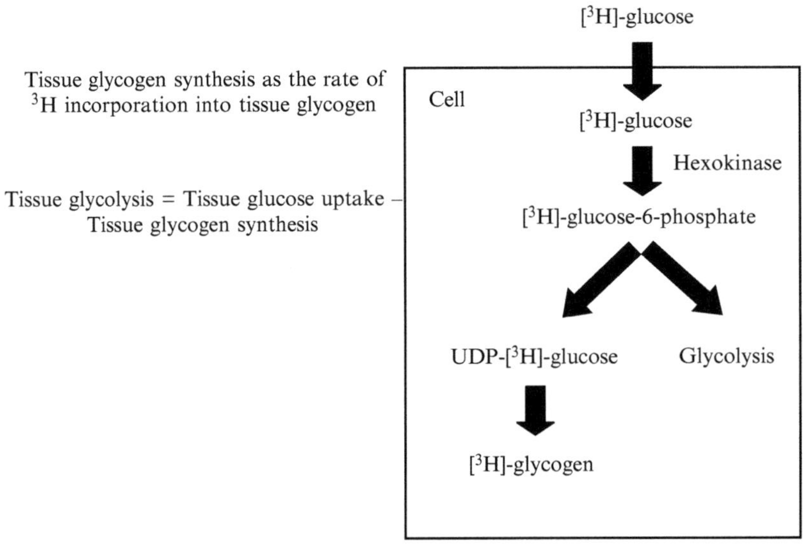

Fig. 8. This picture illustrates the estimation of organ-specific glycogen synthesis using [3H]-glucose infusion and 3H incorporation into tissue glycogen. Organ-specific glycolysis is calculated as the difference between glucose uptake and glycogen synthesis.

4. Notes

1. An insulin infusion rate of 2.5 mU/kg/min causes a maximal suppression of HGP in some genetic strains, and such effects make it difficult to assess the changes in hepatic insulin sensitivity in response to diet or genetic manipulations. In this case, a lower insulin infusion rate of 1.25 mU/kg/min, which causes a submaximal suppression of HGP in most genetic strains, may be used to assess insulin sensitivity in liver. This is exemplified in the metabolic characterization of SHP-1-deficient *Ptpn6*$^{me-v/me-v}$ mice, which showed increased insulin sensitivity in the liver **(Fig. 9)** *(15)*.
2. In severely insulin resistant and diabetic animals, such as leptin-deficient Lep^{ob} mice, the standard insulin infusion rate of 2.5 mU/kg/min is not sufficient to overcome insulin resistance, and the mice remain hyperglycemic during the euglycemic clamp. In this case, a higher insulin infusion rate of 4 mU/kg/min may be used to elicit an insulin response during the euglycemic clamp, thereby making insulin sensitivity assessment possible.
3. The accuracy of measuring the plasma glucose concentration is highly important. Some laboratories use a portable glucometer to measure blood glucose concentrations. Although such an approach is acceptable to monitor blood glucose levels and maintain euglycemia during euglycemic clamps, it is strongly discouraged for the calculation of specific activity and glucose turnover rates. This is due to the fact that any differences between blood versus plasma glucose concentrations

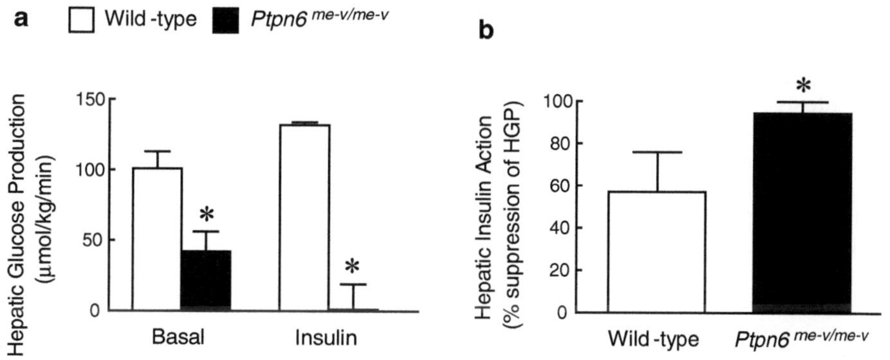

Fig. 9. Hepatic insulin sensitivity was measured using hyperinsulinemic-euglycemic clamps with a low-insulin dose in conscious mice. *Ptpn6*$^{me-v/me-v}$ mice showed lower hepatic glucose production (*HGP*) during the insulin-stimulated state (clamp), and hepatic insulin action, calculated as percent suppression of basal HGP, was increased in *Ptpn6*$^{me-v/me-v}$ mice as compared with wild-type littermates. *$p < 0.05$ versus wild-type mice.

will result in over- or underestimation of specific activity (ratio of [^{3}H] glucose concentrations and circulating glucose concentrations) and glucose turnover rates.

4. A routine test to confirm its accuracy is highly recommended.

Acknowledgments

This work was supported by grants from the US Public Health Service (U24 DK-59635 and R01 DK-80756), the American Diabetes Association (1-04-RA-47 and 7-07-RA-80), the American Heart Association (0855492D), and the Pennsylvania State Department of Health. I thank Prof. Gerald Shulman for technical advice.

References

1. Kahn, C.R. (1994). Insulin action, diabetogenes, and the cause of type II diabetes. *Diabetes* **43**, 1066–1084
2. Reaven, G.M. (1988). Role of insulin resistance in human disease. *Diabetes* **37**, 1595–1607
3. DeFronzo, R.A. (1988). The triumvirate: beta-cell, muscle, liver. A collusion responsible for NIDDM. *Diabetes* **37**, 667–687
4. Haldane, J.B.S., Wigglesworth, V.B., Woodcow, C.E. (1924). Effects of reaction changes on human carbohydrate and oxygen metabolism. *Proc Roy Soc Lond, Ser B* **96**, 15–32
5. Shen, S.-W., Reaven, G.M., Farquhar, J.W. (1970). Comparison of impedance to insulin-mediated glucose uptake in normal subjects and in subjects with latent diabetes. *J Clin Invest* **49**, 2151–2160
6. DeFronzo, R.A., Beckles, A.D. (1979). Glucose intolerance following chronic metabolic acidosis in man. *Am J Physiol* **236**, E328–E334
7. White, M.F., Kahn, C.R. (1994). The insulin signaling system. *J Biol Chem* **269**, 1–4
8. Shepherd, P.R., Kahn, B.B. (1999). Glucose transporters and insulin action - implications for insulin resistance and diabetes melitus. *N Engl J Med* **341**, 248–257
9. Bruning, J.C. (1998). A muscle-specific insulin receptor knockout exhibits features of the metabolic syndrome of NIDDM without altering glucose tolerance. *Mol Cell* **2**, 559–569
10. Kim, J.K., Michael, M.D., Previs, S.F., Peroni, O.D., Mauvais-Jarvis, F., Neschen, S., Kahn, B.B., Kahn, C.R., Shulman, G.I. (2000). Redistribution of substrates to adipose tissue in mice with selective insulin resistance in muscle promotes obesity. *J Clin Invest* **105**, 1791–1797
11. Kim, H.J., Higashimori, T., Park, S.Y., Choi, H., Dong, J., Kim, Y.J., Noh, H.L., Cho, Y.R., Cline, G., Kim, Y.B., Kim, J.K. (2004). Differential effects of interleukin-6 and -10 on skeletal muscle and liver insulin action in vivo. *Diabetes* **53**, 1060–1067
12. Lee, S., Muniyappa, R., Yan, X., Chen, H., Yue, L.Q., Hong, E-G., Kim, J.K., Quon, M.J. (2008). Comparison between surrogate indexes of insulin sensitivity and resistance and hyperinsulinemic euglycemic clamp estimates in mice. *Am J Physiol* **294**, E261–E270
13. Haluzik, M., Columbo, C., Gavrilova, O., Chua, S., Wolf, N., Chen, M., Stannard, B., Dietz, K.R., Le Roith, D., Reitman, M.L. (2004). Genetic background (C57BL/6J versus FVB/N) strongly influences the severity of diabetes and insulin resistance in ob/ob mice. *Endocrinology* **145**, 3258–3264
14. Ayala, J.E., Bracy, D.P., McGuinness, O.P., Wasserman, D.H. (2006). Considerations in the design of hyperinsulinemic-euglycemic clamps in the conscious mouse. *Diabetes* **55**, 390–397
15. Dubois, M.-J., Bergeron, S., Kim, H.-J., Dombrowski, L., Perreault, M., Fournes, B., Faure, R., Olivier, M., Beauchemin, N., Shulman, G.I., Siminovitch, K.A., Kim, J.K., Marette, A. (2006). The SHP-1 protein tyrosine phosphatase negatively modulates glucose homeostasis. *Nat Med* **12**, 549–556

Chapter 16

Gene Expression Analysis in Diabetes Research

Peter White and Klaus H. Kaestner

Summary

Global gene expression profiling through the use of microarray technology is among the most powerful molecular biological techniques available to diabetes researchers today. In this chapter, we outline how to appropriately perform a microarray experiment using pancreatic islets or total pancreas, based upon over a decade of experience in our laboratory. Through the utilization of careful experimental designs, large numbers of biological replicates, production of high-quality starting material, optimized protocols for hybridization, and sophisticated tools for data processing and statistical analysis, the full potential of high-quality expression profiling can be realized.

Key words: Microarray, RNA extraction, Gene expression profiling, Diabetes, Islet, β-Cell

1. Introduction

The incidence of both type I and II diabetes continues to increase globally and the effectiveness of pharmaceutical treatments for the disease remains limited. A significant proportion of basic research into the disease has focused on understanding the transcriptional programs that regulate the development and function of the endocrine pancreas. Of the numerous research tools and approaches that have been utilized to address these fundamental questions of development, global gene expression profiling has become one of the most powerful techniques employed to date. The use of microarray technology opened the door for researchers to rapidly assess the transcriptional profile for thousands of genes. Through the application of these techniques, we have gained significant insights into the transcriptional programs and

C. Stocker (ed.), *Type 2 Diabetes,* Methods in Molecular Biology, vol. 560
DOI 10.1007/978-1-59745-448-3_16, © Humana Press, a part of Springer Science+Business Media, LLC 2009

signaling mechanisms that control the differentiation of endocrine precursors to mature hormone-expressing endocrine cells of the islet (reviewed in *(1–5)*).

Over the last decade, the methodology involved in expression profiling has become more standardized and the technical variation within the assay has significantly diminished, resulting in highly reproducible gene expression measurements across multiple platforms *(6)*. However, with the power of microarray techniques come significant pitfalls. Initially, the high cost of arrays resulted in inappropriate application of the technology, with studies being conducted and conclusions being drawn from the use of only one or two biological replicates. Even though the price of commercial arrays has now fallen to under $200, this inappropriate practice is still commonplace, resulting in the production of low-quality data sets and consequently wasting time and resources following up on potentially wrong hypotheses. In our hands, the use of four or more true biological replicates per experiment has resulted in the production of numerous high-quality data sets *(3, 7–11)*.

One of the biggest challenges in conducting genomics research in the diabetes field is the production of high-quality RNA. Microarray analysis is exquisitely sensitive to RNA quality, and requires RNA of very high integrity. The pancreas is the major source of ribonucleases (RNase) in the body and therefore it is very difficult to isolate RNA from this tissue. Furthermore, expression profiling using the whole pancreas may be inappropriate if the aim is to investigate gene expression profiles at the level of the endocrine islet. With islets accoun-ting for less than 5% of total pancreas mass, expression profiling using RNA from the whole pancreas will predominantly provide information on the exocrine pancreas and a small subset of the most highly expressed endocrine genes. To overcome this limitation, islets must first be purified from the pancreas using collagenase digestion in Hanks buffer, followed by separation of islets from exocrine tissue in a Ficoll gradient *(12)*. Finally, once islets have been purified, they must be purity matched before microarray analysis can begin. We have developed a method of purity matching using quantitative real-time reverse transcription polymerase chain reaction (qRT-PCR) which allows the investigator to hybridize islet samples of similar purity by determining the ratio of exocrine and endocrine markers *(3)*. This additional step of purity matching allows the investigator to remove the confounding factors contributed by even slight differences in purity between islet preparations.

Having designed the experiment and carefully prepared the samples, the next step is to label and hybridize. Numerous commercial kits are available for this purpose, but in this chapter, we focus on an indirect labeling method that we have significantly optimized and in our hands consistently produces better results than the commercial kits we have tested *(13)*. A choice must be made at this point between using a single- or dual-color approach. In the one-color procedure, a single sample is fluorescently labeled and hybridized to each array, whereas in a two-color approach, samples are labeled in pairs (e.g., test and control) with different fluorophores and hybridized together on a single microarray. There are advantages and disadvantages to both approaches, but we have found that the two-color procedure, which allows for direct comparisons of test and control samples, reduces variability and results in greater sensitivity and accuracy in determining differential gene expression. There are many different array-based platforms for assessing transcript abundance including spotted cDNA arrays (e.g., the PancChips *(14)*), spotted long oligo arrays, in-situ synthesized short (e.g., Affymetrix GeneChips) or long (e.g., Agilent Technologies Whole Genome Arrays) oligo arrays, and long oligo bead arrays (e.g., Illumina BeadChips). The mouse and human PancChip microarrays developed by the NIDDK-funded Beta Cell Biology Consortium have proved to be invaluable tools for diabetes research and will be the array platform of choice for this chapter. The content of these arrays was chosen based upon transcripts known to play important roles in pathways relating to pancreatic development and glucose homeostasis and for their expression in various stages of pancreatic development. These arrays contain many novel and rare transcripts known to be expressed in the pancreas and yet not available on many commercial platforms. Moreover, these arrays provide a low-cost alternative to commercial platforms and are distributed at cost through the Beta Cell Biology Consortium (http://www.betacell.org/microarrays).

The final stumbling blocks for many researchers performing gene expression profiling experiments lie in the data analysis and interpretation steps. Numerous commercial and public domain applications exist for the purpose of data preprocessing and normalization [for detailed reviews see *(15, 16)*]. Although we provide some recommendations regarding the informatics tools that can be employed, for best results it is our recommendation that you consult a qualified bioinformatics expert for assistance. Once the data has been processed and statistical analyses have been conducted, interpretation of the data remains the final step. There are many resources available for this purpose, and in the following chapter, Dr. Dunbar provides a review of several of these tools. Finally, once a hypothesis has been drawn, it is back to the bench for experimental validation and verification of the results, leading ultimately to discovery and publication of the new findings.

2. Materials

2.1. Sample Collection

1. Collect samples for expression analysis based upon the optimal experimental design to answer the biological question of interest.

2.2. Preparation of High-Quality RNA

1. Choose the most appripriate kit for your sample. Consult the Qiagen web site for more specifics, or call Qiagen technical support (1 (800) 362-7737):
   (a) Qiagen RNeasy® Mini Kit *(12)*: Qiagen (Cat. No. 74104). Yields <100 μg RNA from 0.5 to 30 mg tissue or 1×10^5–1×10^7 cells.
   (b) Qiagen RNeasy® Midi Kit *(12)*: Qiagen (Cat. No. 75142). Yields <1 mg RNA from 20 to 250 mg tissue or 5×10^6–1×10^8 cells.
   (c) Qiagen RNeasy® Maxi Kit *(12)*: Qiagen (Cat. No. 75162). Yields <6 mg RNA from 150 mg to 1 g of tissue or 5×10^7–5×10^8 cells.
2. TRIzol® Reagent (a ready-to-use mixture of phenol, guanidine isothiocyanate, red dye, and proprietary components): Invitrogen (Cat. No. 15596-026).
3. TRIzol® LS Reagent (recommended for liquid samples, e.g., FACS sorted cells): Invitrogen (Cat. No. 10296-010).
4. Chloroform.
5. RNaseZap® RNase Decontamination Solution, 250 ml: Ambion (Cat. No. 9780).
6. Nuclease-free water.
7. 100% (200 proof) ethanol.
8. 70% Ethanol in RNase-free H_2O.
9. Agilent 2100 bioanalyzer: (Agilent Technologies, Cat. No. G2940CA).
10. Agilent RNA 6000 Nano Kit: (Agilent Technologies, Cat. No. 5067-1511). For RNA in the concentration range of 25–500 ng μl^{-1}.
11. Agilent RNA 6000 Pico Kit: (Agilent Technologies, Cat. No. 5067-1513). For RNA in the concentration range of 50–5,000 pg μl^{-1}.
12. MessageAmp™ II aRNA Amplification Kit (Ambion, Cat. No. AM1751). Required for samples where RNA yield is limited.

2.3. Sample Labeling and Hybridization

1. Mouse PancChip 6 (Functional Genomics Core, University of Pennsylvania). Contains approximately 13,000 mouse cDNAs chosen for their expression in various stages of pancreatic development.

2. Human PancChip 1 (Functional Genomics Core, University of Pennsylvania). Contains over 12,000 cDNAs known to be expressed in the human pancreas and islets.
3. Anchored Oligo $dT_{20}VN$ Primer. 1 μg μl^{-1}. Stored at –20°C.
4. $pd(N)_6$ Random Hexamer. 500 ng μl^{-1}. Stored at –20°C.
5. 25× aa dNTP Mix: dATP, dGTP, dCTP, and dTTP. 5-(3-aminoallyl)-dUTP (Ambion, Cat. No. AM8439). Prepare as detailed in **Table 1** and aliquot into five tubes of 100 μl each and store at –80°C. A working stock can be kept at -20°C and is stable for a month, with several freeze/thaw cycles.
6. SuperScript III RT: (Invitrogen, Cat. No. 18080044). 10,000 Units. Supplied with 5× First Strand Buffer and 0.1 M DTT. Stored at –20°C.
7. RNasin® Plus RNase Inhibitor: (Promega, Cat. No. PR-N2615). 10,000 Units @ 40 U μl^{-1}. Stored at -20°C.
8. Sodium hydroxide (NaOH; 1 N Solution). Stored at room temperature.
9. Hydrochloric acid (HCl; 1 N Solution). Stored at room temperature.
10. 3 M Sodium acetate, pH 5.5. Stored at room temperature.
11. MinElute Reaction Cleanup Kit (50): (Qiagen, Cat. No. 74104). For cleanup of up to 5 μg DNA (70 bp to 4 Kb) from enzymatic reactions.
12. Sodium bicarbonate, pH 8.6-9.0. Dissolve 0.84 g in 100 ml nuclease-free water to make 100 mM stock, having adjusted the pH with NaOH. Aliquot in 500 μl aliquots and store at –20°C.

Table 1
25× aa-dNTP mix

Component	Initial (mM)	Volume (ul)	25× Stock (mM)	Final (mM)
dATP	100	62.5	12.5	0.5
dGTP	100	62.5	12.5	0.5
dCTP	100	62.5	12.5	0.5
dTTP	100	37.5	7.5	0.3
Aminoallyl-dUTP	50	75	7.5	0.3
H_2O	–	200	–	–

13. Amersham CyDye Post-Labeling Reactive Dye Packs: (GE Healthcare, Cat. No. RPN5661). 12 vials Cyanine (Cy3) *N*-hydroxysuccinimide (NHS) ester, 12 vials Cy5 NHS ester. Use 3 μl of DMSO to resuspend the dye and then add it to the cDNA eluted in 100 mM sodium bicarbonate, pH 9.0. Stored at –20°C.
14. DMSO. Stored at room temperature.
15. Shandon Complete Staining Assembly: (Thermo Scientific, Cat. No. 121). Includes staining rack for up to 30 slides and staining dish with lid holding up to 350 ml of solution.
16. Prehybridization buffer: 1% BSA, 5× SSC, 0.1% SDS; 500 ml. Dissolve 5 g BSA (Sigma, Cat. No. A9418-100G) in 372.5 ml nuclease-free H_2O. Add 125 ml 20× SSC and 2.5 ml 20% SDS. Stored at 4°C. Can be reused up to five times.
17. Formamide: (Sigma, Cat. No. F9073-100ML). (100 ml deionized, nuclease free). Stored at 4°C.
18. 2× Hybridization buffer: 50% Formamide, 10× SSC, 0.2% SDS; 10 ml. Combine 5 ml of formamide, 5 ml 20×SSC and 100 μl 20% SDS. Aliquot in 20 × 500 μl and store at –20°C. Stable for 1–3 months.
19. Mouse Cot-1 DNA: (Invitrogen, Cat. No. 18440016). 1 mg ml^{-1}. Stored at –20°C.
20. LifterSlips™: (Erie Scientific Company, Cat. No. 22x60I-2-4861). 22 × 60 mm. Clean LifterSlips with clean water followed by 100% EtOH rinse. Dry LifterSlips with a clean compressed air supply.
21. Corning Microarray Hybridization Chambers: (Corning Life Sciences, Cat. No. 2551).
22. 20× SSC. Stored at room temperature.
23. 20% SDS. Stored at room temperature.
24. Wash buffer 1: 2× SSC, 0.1% SDS; 5 L. Combine 500 ml of 20 × SSC, 25 ml of 20% SDS, and 4,475 ml of nuclease-free H_2O.
25. Wash buffer 2: 0.2× SSC, 0.1% SDS; 5 L. Combine 50 ml of 20 × SSC, 25 ml of 20% SDS, and 4,925 ml of nuclease-free H_2O.
26. Wash buffer 3: 0.2× SSC; 5 L. Combine 50 ml of 20 × SSC and 4,950 ml of nuclease-free H_2O.

3. Methods

When designing a microarray experiment with a local core facility, it is important to consult with the core's Technical Director before beginning the study. This consultation is essential to the success of your experiment. Not only will it ensure that the experiment is designed correctly, but it will help the investigator to avoid the many traps that hamper the success of microarray analysis. That being said, the following protocols are designed for those who do not have access to a core facility and for core facility personnel, conducting expression profiling experiments for investigators in the diabetes research field (*see* **Fig. 1** for overview).

3.1. Experimental Design

Choosing a design for gene expression profiling experiments requires care and time if issues are to be avoided at the stages of data analysis and beyond. The design of the experiment should be as simple as possible, with the preferred method being a direct two-state comparison. Especially in a first attempt at microarray analysis, multiple conditions or time points should be avoided. Rather, if it is possible, just compare two conditions (e.g., treated vs untreated or KO vs WT) or focus on the single time point that would likely answer the most interesting question. The more complex the experimental design, the greater is the potential for being overwhelmed with the data output produced. When a single direct comparison is not possible, a common control reference design should always be used over a loop design. Our preferred method of analysis is the utilization of a two-color approach, which requires the following special considerations.

3.1.1. Direct Comparison Design

This is the simplest and often most sensitive and accurate approach for a given gene expression profiling experiment. In this design, a test sample is typically labeled with Cy5 (red) and a control sample with Cy3 (green) and the two are hybridized competitively on a single array. The resulting ratio between red and green signal allows for the determination of differential expression between the test and control samples (*see* **Note 1**).

3.1.2. Reference Design

When investigating gene profiles over multiple time points or in multiple treatment groups, a direct comparison design is not possible and a common control or reference design must be used. In this scenario, test conditions are compared against a common reference condition. The reference sample should be matched to the experimental samples as closely as possible, for example, a pool of the different test conditions. When evaluating RNA samples taken from different tissue types, a Universal Reference RNA might be an appropriate control.

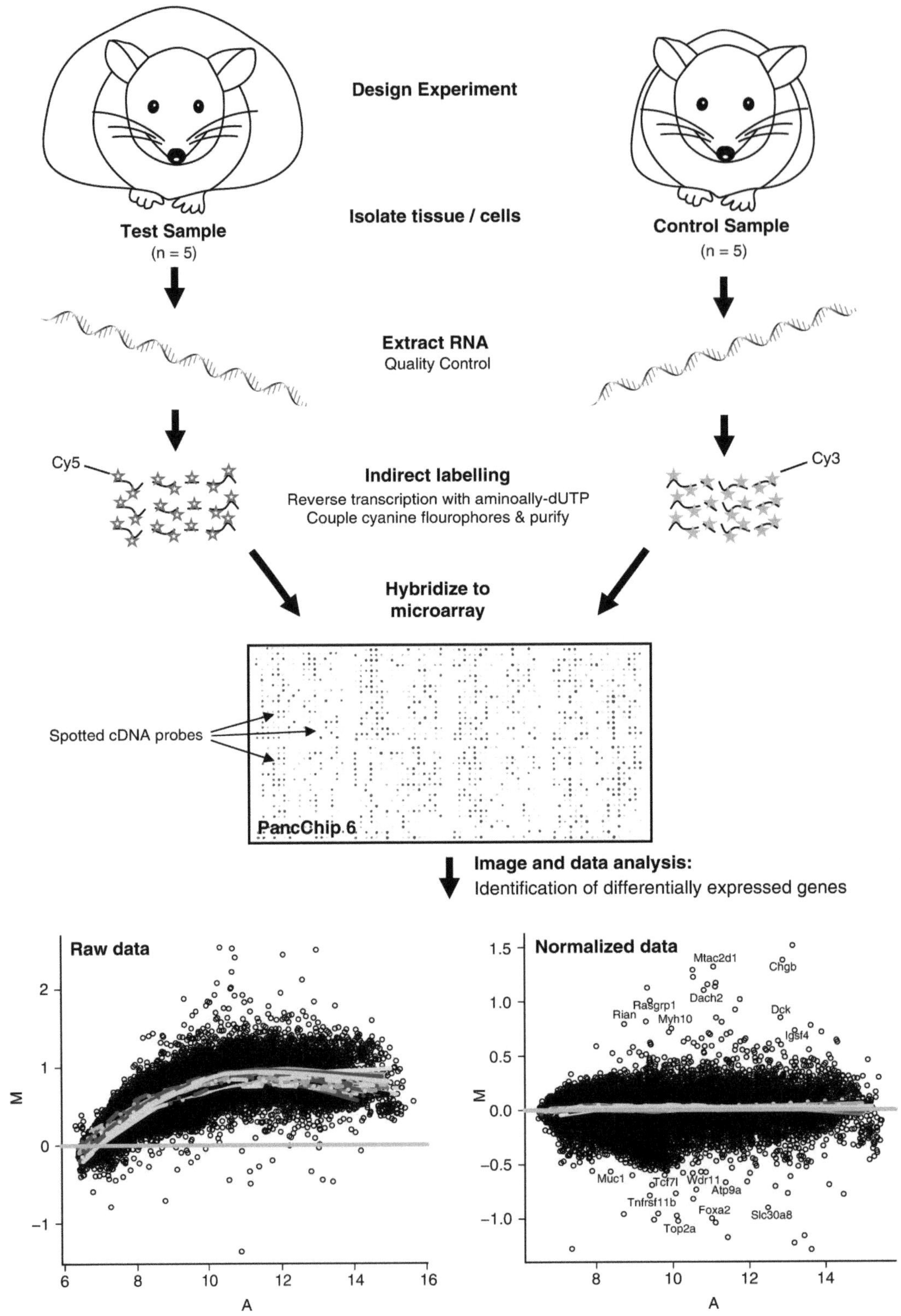

Fig. 1. Overview of gene expression profiling. The figure highlights the key steps in performing gene expression profiling from designing an experiment to data analysis. The data used to generate the MvA plots have been deposited at Array Express with the accession number E-CBIL-39 *(7)*.

3.1.3. Replicates

The number of biological replicates (a technical replicate is not the same as a true biological replicate) used in any given study is directly proportional to the confidence with which one can call any given gene on the array as being differentially expressed. For experiments conducted using congenic mouse strains or cell cultures, we recommend five or more biological replicates, with an absolute minimum of four biological replicates. In human studies where genetic variation is dramatically increased, the number of replicates needs to be significantly higher if one is to observe changes related to a particular disease condition rather than normal population variation.

3.1.4. Avoiding Confounding Factors

When designing the experiment, care should also be taken to minimize and if possible eliminate potential confounding factors. Such factors include isolating samples for a given test condition on one day and then the control samples on another, extracting RNA using different methods, or processing samples differently. Where possible always use age- and sex-matched samples. Hybridizations should not be conducted over multiple days, as hybridization date is well known to be a significant confounding factor for microarrays.

3.2. Preparation of High-Quality RNA for Expression Analysis

The protocol outlined in this section is an enhancement of the Qiagen RNeasy protocol. In essence, the lysis steps using Buffer RLT in the kit have been replaced with the TRIzol® Reagent, a ready to use mixture of phenol and guanidine isothiocyanate (Invitrogen). When preparing RNA from small samples, such as islets, higher yields and better quality of RNA can be achieved, as lysis of the sample and inhibition of RNase is more efficient with TRIzol than with Buffer RLT. After phase separation, the Qiagen protocol is then followed, as the selective binding properties of the silica-gel-based membrane provided in the kit confers significant advantages over traditional ethanol precipitation methods. The RNeasy procedure enriches mRNA since most small RNAs (such as 5.8S rRNA, 5S rRNA, and tRNAs, which together comprise 15-20% of total RNA) are selectively excluded by the purification column which isolates all RNA molecules longer than 200 nucleotides.

3.2.1. Sample Preparation and Homogenization

There are two key prerequisites for successfully preparing RNA: use of RNase-free technique (*see* **Note 2**) and speed. When isolating RNA from mammalian tissue, it is essential that the RNA be stabilized by homogenization and lysis of the tissue or cells in at least ten volumes of a denaturing buffer that will inhibit RNase. Our preference is that the tissue be immediately homogenized or if this is not possible, snap frozen in liquid nitrogen (*see* **Note 3** if using pancreas). Once homogenized, the lysate can be snap frozen and stored at –80°C until all samples have been collected and are ready for completing the RNA isolation procedure (*see* **Note 4**). The following guidelines should be followed dependant upon the tissue of interest:

1. *Islets.* Prepare the islets according to standard protocols, working quickly, and at the last step, remove any residual wash buffer. Resuspend the islet pellet (no more than 500 mouse islets) in a 2.0 ml microcentrifuge tube in 1 ml TRIzol and vortex well to ensure complete lysis.
2. *Cells.* To a pellet of cells (<1 × 10^7 cells), add 1 ml TRIzol or for direct lysis of cells grown in a monolayer, add 1 ml TRIzol (<10 cm diameter dish) and collect cell lysate with a rubber policeman, transferring to a 2.0 ml microcentrifuge tube.
3. *Sorted Cells.* The issue with extracting RNA from sorted cells is the volume of cells after sorting must not dilute the denaturing agent beyond its ability to denature RNase. As such we recommend the use of TRIzol LS which remains active when diluted up to 1:3. If possible, sort cells directly into 750 µl of TRIzol LS (sample volume must not exceed 250 µl - if this is a problem, use more reagents and adjust the protocol accordingly).
4. *Tissue.* This protocol should only be followed with small amounts of tissue (<30 mg); if using larger amounts of tissue follow the protocols provided with larger RNeasy Midi or Maxi kits. The volume of lysis reagent should be at least tenfold greater than the volume of tissue, to ensure complete inhibition of endogenous RNase. Thus, for <30 mg of tissue, use 1 ml TRIzol. The tissue must be completely disrupted by homogenization, using a homogenizer probe that is appropriate for small sample volume in a 2 ml microcentrifuge tube (*see* **Note 5**). Clean the homogenizer probe by running it at maximum speed in the probe wash tubes (15 ml conical tubes) as follows:

RNaseZAP®	30 s
DEPC water	30 s
100% ethanol	30 s
DEPC water	30 s

Immediately, homogenize the tissue using a conventional rotor–stator homogenizer for at least 45 s at maximum speed until the sample is uniformly homogeneous. Place homogenate on ice and when all samples are complete, proceed immediately to the steps in **Subheading 3.2.2**. Alternatively, snap freeze the homogenate in liquid nitrogen and store at -80°C for future RNA extraction. Wash the homogenizer probe as above for each sample and when finished, ensure that the probe is thoroughly cleaned.

3.2.2. RNA Isolation Using Qiagen RNeasy® Mini Columns

1. Ensure that the sample is completely lysed in TRIzol: if working with cells or islets vortex well, or if working with tissue ensure complete homogenization.
2. Incubate sample/TRIzol lysate for 5 min at room temperature.
3. Add 0.2 ml of chloroform for every 1 ml of TRIzol used. Shake vigorously for 15 s and incubate at room temperature for 2–3 min.
4. Centrifuge samples 5 min at 12,000 × g at 4°C (*see* **Note 6**).
5. Transfer the aqueous phase to a fresh microcentrifuge tube (*see* **Note 7**). Proceed immediately to the next step.
6. Add 1 volume (usually 600 μl) of 70% ethanol to the cleared lysate, and mix immediately by pipetting. Do not centrifuge. Continue without delay to the next step.
7. Apply up to 700 μl aliquots of the sample successively, including any precipitate that may have formed, to an RNeasy mini column placed in a 2 ml collection tube (supplied). Close the tube gently, and centrifuge for 15 s at ≥8,000 × g (≥10,000 rpm). Discard the flow-through, but not the collection tube, after each centrifugation step until it has all been passed over the column.
8. Add 700 μl Buffer RW1 to the RNeasy column. Close the tube gently and centrifuge for 15 s at ≥8,000 × g (≥10,000 rpm) to wash the column. Discard the flow-through and collection tube.
9. Transfer the RNeasy column into a new 2 ml collection tube (supplied). Pipet 500 μl Buffer RPE onto the RNeasy column (*see* **Note 8**). Close the tube gently, and centrifuge for 15 s at ≥8,000 × g (≥10,000 rpm) to wash the column. Discard the flow-through, but not the collection tube.
10. Add another 500 μl Buffer RPE to the RNeasy column. Close the tube gently, and centrifuge for 2 min at ≥8,000 × g (≥10,000 rpm) to dry the RNeasy silica-gel membrane (*see* **Note 9**).
11. To elute, transfer the RNeasy column to a new 1.5 ml collection tube (supplied). Pipet 30-50 μl RNase-free water directly onto the RNeasy silica-gel membrane. Close the tube gently, wait 1 min, and centrifuge for 1 min at ≥8,000 × g (≥10,000 rpm) to elute (*see* **Note 10**).
12. Keep eluted RNA on ice at all times and store at -80°C (*see* **Note 11**).

3.2.3. Determination of RNA Quantity and Quality

Quantitation of RNA

The concentration of RNA should be determined by measuring the absorbance at 260 nm (A260) in a spectrophotometer (*see* **Note 12**). If using a standard spectrophotometer, with a 1 cm path length, readings should be greater than 0.15 to ensure accuracy. An absorbance of 1 unit at 260 nm corresponds to 40 μg of RNA per ml, for measurements in water (concentration = A260 × 40 × dilution factor). The ratio of the readings at 260 and 280 nm (A260/A280) provides an estimate of the purity of RNA with respect to contaminants that absorb in the UV, such as protein and phenol (*see* **Note 13**). Pure RNA has an A260/A280 ratio of 1.9-2.1 in 10 mM Tris-Cl, pH 7.5. If there is contamination with protein or phenol, the A260/A280 will be significantly less than the values given above, and accurate quantitation of the amount of RNA will not be possible.

Determination of RNA Integrity

Microarray analysis requires RNA of very high integrity. As a standard practice, all samples to be used for array analysis must be analyzed for integrity using an Agilent bioanalyzer, to confirm that the ratio of 18S:28S ribosomal subunit RNA is close to the theoretical maximum of 2.5 (*see* **Note 14**). The bioanalyzer provides a complete RNA profile and can quickly reveal sample degradation. If prepared correctly, RNA samples prepared from animal tissues should resemble the high-quality RNA trace in **Fig. 2a**. However, with some tissues that have a high RNase content, such as adult pancreas, a trace similar to that of the partially degraded RNA sample might be expected **(Fig. 2b)**. Degraded RNA should never be used **(Fig. 2c)**. If a bioanalyzer is not available, sample integrity can be determined by denaturing gel electrophoresis (*see* **Note 15**).

3.3. Probe Preparation for Expression Array Analysis

To obtain appropriate signal strength on the microarray, 10-20 μg of total RNA is required for this labeling procedure. However, RNA isolated from small amounts of tissue, such as islets, is often available in considerably lower quantities. If you have less than 10 μg of total RNA, or if your sample is very precious, then it must be first amplified. A number of commercial kits exist for this, and for the purposes of this chapter, we will assume that you either have enough total RNA or have amplified your sample to produce amplified RNA (aRNA, *see* **Note 16**). In outline, the indirect labeling procedure involves reverse transcribing the mRNA in the sample in the presence of 5-(3-aminoallyl)-dUTP. This modified dUTP is readily incorporated by reverse transcriptase and provides a reactive group enabling downstream labeling of the cDNA with Cy amine-reactive NHS esters. Once labeled, the test and control samples need to be paired for hybridization and subsequent analysis (if working with islets, *see* **Fig. 3** and **Note 17**).

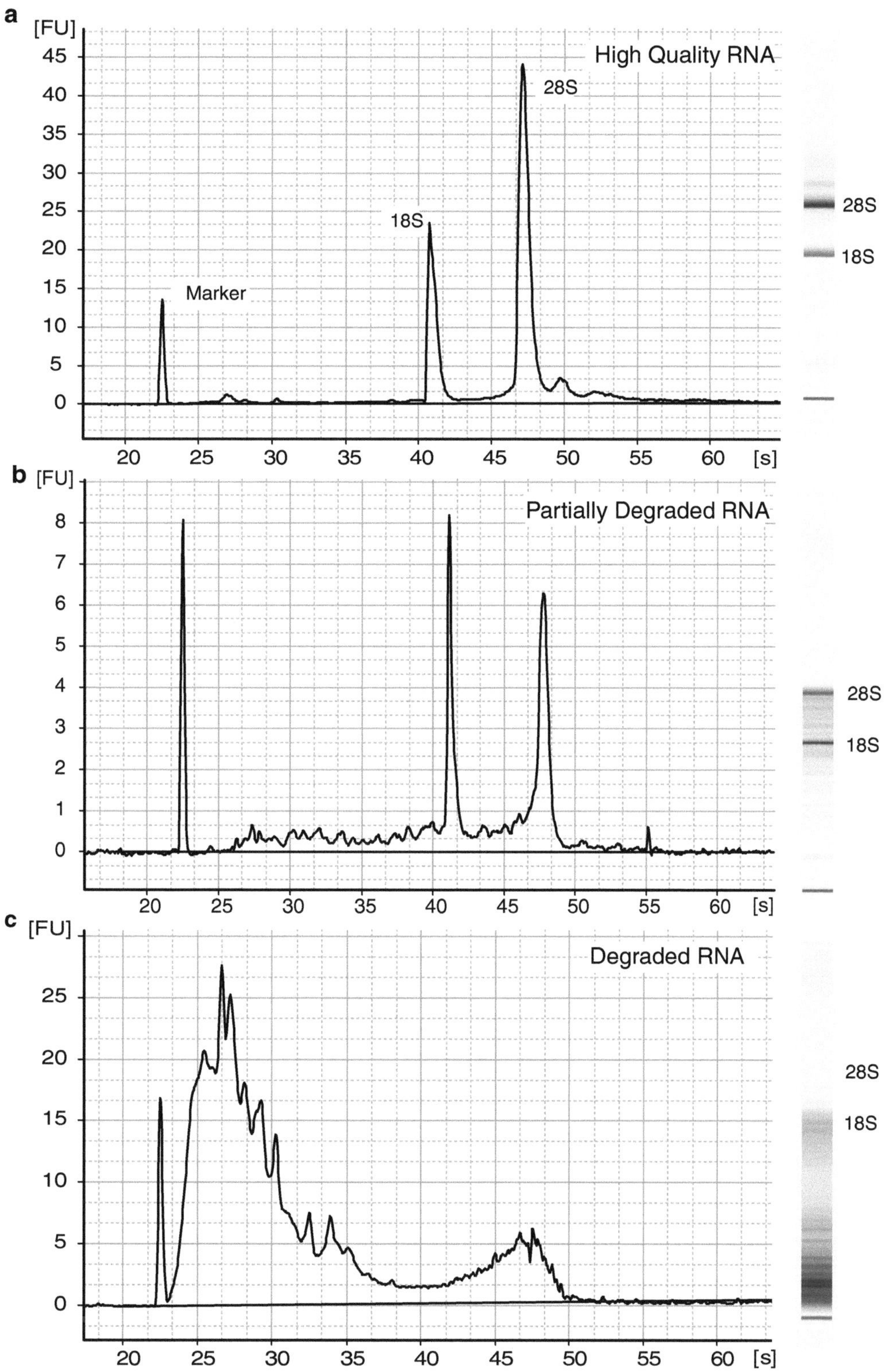

Fig. 2. RNA quality control using the Agilent Bioanlyzer. The electropherograms (*left*) and gel-traces (*right*) show total RNA samples with decreasing quality in terms of integrity. RNA should have integrity somewhere between the intact RNA trace (**a**) and the partially degraded trace (**b**). RNA prepared from total pancreas should resemble the center partially degraded trace (**b**). The 18S and 28S ribosomal RNA peaks are no longer detected in the degraded RNA sample (**c**).

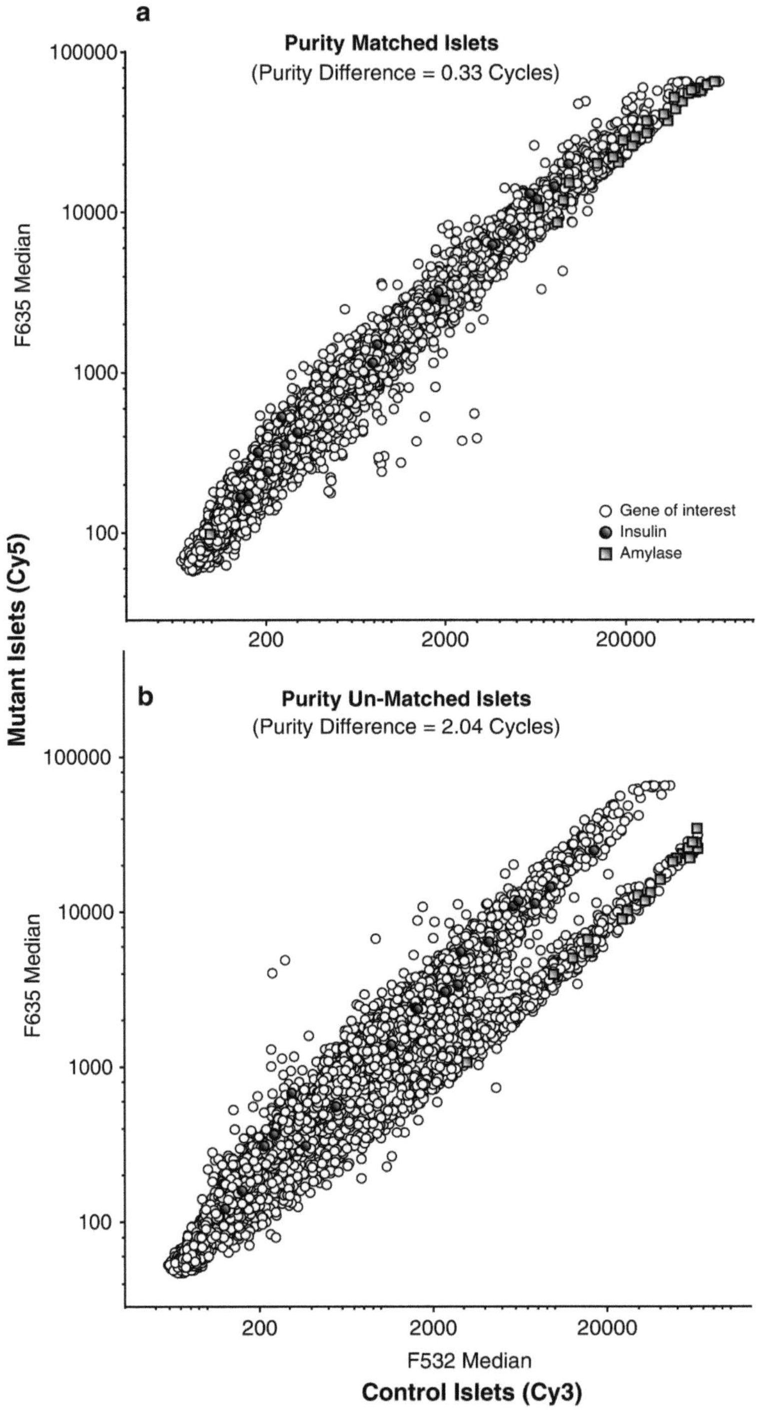

Fig. 3. Islet purity matching is critical for the success of microarray analysis performed using isolated islets. In outline, qRT-PCR is used to determine the relative levels of endocrine (Insulin) and exocrine (Amylase) gene expression levels in each sample. This then allows hybridization of samples that are well matched for purity in terms of the amount of exocrine contamination found in every islet preparation. In this way, differential gene expression as a result of the islet preparation technique can be minimized (**a**), allowing the investigator to accurately determine islet gene expression profiles. In poorly matched samples, the results will be confounded by significant differential expression of contaminating exocrine genes (**b**).

3.3.1. cDNA Synthesis

1. Aliquot 10 μg total RNA or 2 μg aRNA per reaction into separate microtubes - maximum volume of sample is 28 μl.
2. Add 2.5 μl anchored Oligo dT primer (1 μg μl^{-1}) to total RNA sample or 2.5 μl Random Hexamers (500 ng μl^{-1}) to aRNA sample.
3. Add nuclease-free H_2O to 30.5 μl total volume.
4. Heat tube at 70°C for 5 min – cool on ice for at least 1 min.
5. Prepare a Master Mix sufficient for the number of reactions plus one extra reaction to ensure sufficient volume:
   10 μl 5× first strand buffer.
   2 μl 25× aa-dNTP mix.
   5 μl 0.1 M DTT.
   0.5 μl RNAsin (40 U μl^{-1}).
   2 μl Superscript III RT (200 U μl^{-1}).
6. Keep Master Mix at room temperature and add 19.5 μl of Master Mix. Mix gently and spin down.
7. Incubate at 46°C for 2 h.
8. Add 20 μl 1 N NaOH. Heat 70°C for 10 min.
9. Spin down briefly and add 20 μl of 1 N HCl.
10. Add 10 μl 3 M sodium acetate, pH 5.2 (*Note*: MinElute reaction volume must not exceed 100 μl).
11. Add 300 μl Qiagen Buffer ERC and follow Qiagen MinElute Reaction Cleanup protocol:
    (a) Place a MinElute column (stored at 4°C) in a 2 ml collection tube in a suitable rack.
    (b) To bind cDNA, apply the entire sample to the MinElute column and centrifuge for 1 min.
    (c) Discard the flow-through and place the MinElute column back into the same tube.
    (d) To wash, add 750 μl 80% ethanol (do not use PE) to the MinElute column and centrifuge for 1 min.
    (e) Discard the flow-through and place the MinElute column back in the same tube.
    (f) Centrifuge the column for an additional 1 min at maximum speed.
    (g) Place the MinElute column in a clean 1.5 ml microcentrifuge tube.
    (h) Elute in 10 μl of 100 mM sodium bicarbonate buffer pH 9.0, prewarmed to 50°C. Make sure that buffer is added precisely to the center of the column matrix.
    (i) Let stand for 2 min, centrifuge the column for 2 min at maximum speed.

12. Proceed immediately to the coupling step. If necessary, purified cDNA samples may be stored at –20°C.

3.3.2. Fluorescent Dye Coupling and Purification

1. Resuspend Cy dye pellet in 3 μl DMSO.
2. Transfer 3 μl dye solution to 10 μl cDNA sample. Mix well (do not vortex), pulse spin, and place the tube at room temperature in the dark or wrapped in aluminum foil.
3. Incubate at room temperature for 1 h (*see* **Note 18**).
4. Combine Cy5-labeled sample with the Cy3-labeled sample (~26 μl) and add 2 μl 3 M sodium acetate, pH 5.2.
5. Add 300 μl Qiagen Buffer ERC to combined labeled probe and follow Qiagen MinElute Reaction Cleanup protocol (*see* **Note 19**), washing twice with Buffer PE (*see* **Subheading 3.3.1** steps 11a–g).
6. Add 24 μl of Elution Buffer (prewarmed to 50°C) to the column, let stand for 2 min.
7. Centrifuge the column for 2 min at maximum speed.

3.4. Array Preparation and Hybridization

3.4.1 Prehybridization

Following printing of the PancChip, DNA has been immobilized on the array by baking at 80°C for 2 h and then UV cross-linking at 250 mJ. Immediately before hybridization, the unused surface of the slides should be blocked by prehybridization with BSA and washed to remove loosely bound reporter DNA. Use array immediately after prehybridization (within 1 h) after blocking.

1. Warm prehybridization solution to 42°C.
2. Incubate 45–60 min in prehybridization buffer (5× SSC, containing 0.1% SDS and 10 mg ml^{-1} BSA) at 42°C, with gently agitation if possible.
3. Wash 2 × 5 min in 350 ml of 0.1% SSC on an orbital shaker.
4. Wash the arrays in two dH_2O washes and one isopropanol wash by plunging the rack of arrays up and down ten times.
5. Dry the arrays by centrifugation (~70-100 × g) to avoid any water stains on the slide surface.

3.4.2. Array Hybridization

1. Warm 2× hybridization buffer (50% formamide, 10× SSC, and 0.2% SDS) to 42°C.
2. Take the eluted sample of fluorescently labeled cDNA probe (from **Subheading 3.3.2**) and add 3 μl Cotl DNA (1 mg ml^{-1}) and 3 μl oligo-dT (1 mg ml^{-1}).
3. Add 30 μl of 2× hybridization buffer, flick to mix, and pulse spin (final volume of 60 μl).
4. Denature probe 95°C for 5 min Spin down quickly and keep at 42°C until applied to slide.

5. Set up Corning Hybridization Chambers with the slides to be used and place 10 μl H_2O at either end of the chamber (this is critical or the slide will dry out).
6. Place a cleaned LifterSlip over the printed area with white rails facing down.
7. Slowly pipette the denatured probe from one corner of the LifterSlip – the pipette should be as close as possible to the LifterSlip/Array junction – but not touching. As the probe is expelled from the pipette tip, it will spread under the LifterSlip via capillary action.
8. Carefully seal hybridization chamber, while maintaining the chamber in a horizontal plane, and gently submerge in a 42°C water bath. Allow hybridization to proceed overnight.
9. Preheat wash buffer 2 at 42°C in preparation for the next day.

3.4.3. Washing and Scanning the Arrays

The aim here is to remove excess and unbound probe from the arrays so that they may be scanned and signal intensity of the reporter elements on the array can be determined (*see* **Note 20**).

1. Prepare slide jars with 300 ml of each of the three wash buffers:

Wash buffer 1	2× SSC; 0.1% SDS	Room temperature
Wash buffer 2	0.2× SSC; 0.1% SDS	42°C
Wash buffer 3	0.2× SSC	Room temperature

2. Remove LifterSlip by gently dipping the slide into 500 ml of low stringency Wash buffer 1 until it falls off. Once LifterSlip is removed, store the slide in a separate container of Wash buffer 1 until all LifterSlips have been removed (never allow the slide to dry).
3. Place into high stringency Wash buffer 2 and gently agitate for 5 min.
4. Place the slide into Wash buffer 3 and gently agitate for 5 min.
5. Centrifuge the slide for 5 min at ~72 × g (600 rpm) in a swinging bucket rotor.
6. Scan immediately (*see* **Note 21**).

3.5. Data Processing

After completion of the experimental work, computational analysis of the data must follow. A series of steps are required to take the image files generated by the hybridization and process them into final data for downstream analysis. Having generated TIFF images of the hybridized arrays, the first step of data processing is to derive quantified intensity values for all of the arrayed elements. Several commercial and freeware applications exist for this feature extraction process [for a review, *see* *(17)*] (*see* **Note 22**).

Post feature extraction, the subsequent data processing steps are performed using R, a free software environment for statistical computing and graphics (http://www.r-project.org). At this point, seeking help from a qualified bioinformatics expert is strongly recommended (*see* **Note 23**). In outline, the median foreground intensities obtained for each spot are imported into R, which is subsequently used for all data input, diagnostic plots, normalization, and quality checking steps of the analysis process using scripts we have developed in-house. The ratio of expression for each element on the array is calculated in terms of M (log2(Red/Green)) and A ((log2(Red) + log2(Green))/2)). The data set is filtered to remove positive control elements (Cy3 anchors and spike-in control elements) and any elements that had been manually flagged. The M values are then normalized by the print-tip loess method using the BioConductor limma package *(18)*. Normalization is an essential step for all microarray data sets and is required to remove systematic sources of variation that can be introduced at various stages during the entire sample preparation, labeling, and hybridization procedures *(19)*.

3.6. Generation of Differentially Expressed Gene Lists

The ultimate aim of the gene expression profiling procedures described in this chapter is to generate a list of genes that demonstrate differential expression as a result of the biological model in question. Because microarrays measure the expression of thousands of genes simultaneously, identification of changes in gene expression between different biological states requires methods to determine the significance of these changes while accounting for the enormous number of genes tested. Numerous statistical analysis tools exist for this purpose, including significance analysis of microarrays (SAM) *(20)*, Extraction and analysis of differential gene expression (EDGE) *(21)*, linear models for microarrays (limma) *(18)*, and patterns of gene expression (PaGE) *(22)*. Of these tools, SAM has proved to be particularly accurate in our hands for identifying differentially expressed genes in a given data set. SAM uses the false discovery rate (FDR) to measure the expected proportion of false positives in the set of all differential expression calls. Typically we have used an FDR or 10-20% to maximize sensitivity without significantly impacting accuracy of the analysis.

The final step is to take the list of significantly differentially expressed genes and apply a fold change filter (*see* **Note 24**). Typically only those genes whose fold change is greater than 50% (1.5-fold) are considered differentially expressed (*see* **Note 25**). There are a number of tools available to help investigators move forward with their gene list, including tools to discover biologically relevant pathways (*see* **Note 26**), functional annotation enrichment analysis, and literature mining [for examples of the application of these tools, see *(7, 11)*]. These tools and others are described in more detail in Chapter 17.

4. Notes

1. It is possible to hybridize each pair of samples twice, in what is known as a dye-swap. In this scenario, the samples are labeled as test (Cy5) and control (Cy3) and then technically replicated by swapping the channels, such that control (Cy5) and test (Cy3) are also hybridized. After image analysis, the reciprocal is taken for these dye-swapped arrays and the data from the two technical replicates is averaged. This approach does reduce technical variation within the assay, but it doubles the cost and is not strictly necessary. We have found that equally good results can be achieved by labeling half of the biological replicates one way and the remaining half the other: test1 (Cy5), test2 (Cy5), test3 (Cy3), and test4 (Cy3) versus control1 (Cy3), control2 (Cy3), control3 (Cy5), and control4 (Cy5). In this way, variations introduced by any dye bias can be eliminated at the experimental level.
2. If you are not experienced with RNA isolation, please read the literature and tips found on Ambion's website: http://www.ambion.com/techlib/basics/rnaisol/index.html
3. If working with the pancreas, the animal should be anesthetized and the pancreas removed while the animal is still living and homogenized in the appropriate volume of TRIzol immediately (an additional pair of hands will help here). Never snap freeze adult murine pancreas for later homogenization - the RNA will be severely degraded **(Fig. 2c)**.
4. We do not recommend the use of the RNAlater RNA stabilization reagent (this should not be confused with Buffer RLT). Direct disruption of the tissue or cells in TRIzol or Buffer RLT yields the best results in our experience. If the tissue has been stored in RNAlater, the tissue must first be removed and placed into Buffer RLT and immediately disrupted.
5. We use the Model PT 1200 E Kinematica® Polytron Ergonomic Handheld Homogenizer with a 5 mm EasyCare generator (Brinkmann).
6. The 4°C spins are essential for phase separation. Room temperature spins may result in variable phase separation, thus resulting in variable RNA yields.

7. The aqueous phase is the colorless upper phase that corresponds to ~60% of the volume of TRIzol used. The interphase should be fairly well-defined. Take care not to touch the interphase - it is better to loose some of the recoverable sample volume than to contaminate it.
8. Buffer RPE is supplied as a concentrate. Ensure that ethanol is added to Buffer RPE before use.
9. Following the centrifugation, remove the RNeasy mini column from the collection tube carefully, so the column does not contact the flow-through as this will result in carryover of ethanol.
10. Never elute with less than 30 µl water. If the expected RNA yield is >30 µg, repeat the elution step with a second volume of RNase-free water. Elute into the same collection tube.
11. The RNeasy kits allow for treatment of the sample with DNase directly on the column. However, we do not recommend DNase treatment of RNA samples for microarray analysis.
12. We recommend use of the ND-1000 Spectrophotometer (NanoDrop Technologies) which allows direct measurement of the sample in as little as 1.5 µl. See http://www.nanodrop.com for details
13. The OD 260/280 ratio is a measure of purity not integrity. It is common for researchers to erroneously assume that their RNA is intact based upon this ratio, yet completely degraded RNA can have a good OD 260/280 ratio.
14. It is very important that there is consistency in the quality of your RNA samples within an experiment, and samples that produce a high-quality trace should never be compared with a sample that showed partial degradation.
15. If a Bioanalyzer is not available, the integrity and size distribution of isolated total RNA should be confirmed by denaturing agarose gel electrophoresis and ethidium bromide staining, prior to submitting samples. The respective ribosomal bands should appear as sharp bands on the stained gel. 28S ribosomal RNA bands should be present with an intensity approximately twice that of the 18S RNA band. If the ribosomal bands in a given lane are not sharp, but appear as a smear of smaller sized RNAs, it is likely that the RNA sample suffered major degradation during preparation. Mouse 18S = 1.9 Kb, 28S = 4.7 Kb. Human 18S = 1.9 Kb, 28S = 5.0 Kb.
16. The MessageAmp™ II aRNA Amplification Kit (Ambion) has worked very well for us, and is based on the RNA amplification protocol developed in the Eberwine laboratory.

17. Our extensive experience in working with islet samples has enabled us to develop an Islet Purity Matching assay that we have found to be essential for the production of high-quality microarray analysis from islets. In outline, qRT-PCR is used to determine the relative levels of endocrine (insulin and prohormone convertase) and exocrine (amylase and chymotrypsin) gene expression levels in each sample. This then allows us to only hybridize samples that are well matched for purity in terms of the amount of exocrine contamination found in every islet preparation. In this way, differential gene expression as a result of the islet preparation technique can be minimized, allowing the investigator to accurately determine islet gene expression profiles (**Fig. 3**).
18. Coupling time can be extended to 2 h and occasional mixing may result in a modest increase in coupling efficiency.
19. Use the MinElute Reaction or PCR Cleanup Kit protocol to purify labeled cDNA fragments of 100 bp to 10 Kb from salts and unincorporated dye.
20. It is essential to work carefully and quickly when preparing microarrays to be scanned. Under no circumstances should coverslips be pulled off of the slide as this will result in scratching the array surface. Cy5 is very sensitive to humidity and ambient ozone levels, with as little as 5 ppb O_3 resulting in rapid degradation of the signal. Avoid performing experiments on summer days when high heat and humidity can result in soaring ozone levels. If this is not possible then there are ways in which ozone can be eliminated from the laboratory. See http://cmgm.stanford.edu/pbrown/ and http://www.genomics.princeton.edu/dunham/ozone.html
21. If arrays cannot be scanned immediately, they may be stored in the dark in a vacuum or under N_2 for a short period. There are a number of microarray scanners available to scan the arrays. We have had very good results with the Agilent DNA Microarray Scanner (http://www.chem.agilent.com/Scripts/PDS.asp?lPage = 398). A lower cost alternative is the Molecular Devices GenePix 4000B (http://www.moleculardevices.com/pages/instruments/gn_genepix 4000.html).
22. For image analysis, we use GenePix Pro http://www.moleculardevices.com/pages/software/gn_genepix_pro.html. Care should be taken during this process to manually inspect the images and flag any features that have been scratched or otherwise compromised.
23. For analysis of two-color microarray, use of the BioConductor package limma has proved to be an extremely powerful

tool. A graphical user interface (GUI), limmaGUI, which simplifies use of this package can be downloaded from the Bioinformatics group at the Walter & Elizer Hall Institute of Medical Research, Melbourne, Australia (http://bioinf.wehi.edu.au/limmaGUI/).

24. A fold change cutoff must always be used in conjunction with an associated statistical test. With the PancChip arrays, we have been able to successfully confirm differential expression of genes called with fold changes as low as 30%, although a minimum change of 50% leads to fewer false positives.
25. It should be noted that microarrays typically underestimate fold changes due to sensitivity limits of the assay. qRT-PCR is considerably more sensitive, and having determined that a gene is differentially expressed with the microarray, if it is desired to more accurately determine or confirm this change then qRT-PCR should be used.
26. Discovery of biologically relevant pathways in a given gene list can be aided through the use of Ingenuity Pathways Analysis, a commercial web-delivered application (http://www.ingenuity.com/) that enables the visualization and analysis of biologically relevant networks to discover, visualize, and explore therapeutically relevant networks.

References

1. Edlund H. (2002). Pancreatic organogenesis - developmental mechanisms and implications for therapy. *Nat. Rev. Genet.* **3**, 524–532
2. Habener J. F., Kemp D. M., and Thomas M. K. (2005). Minireview: transcriptional regulation in pancreatic development. *Endocrinology* **146**, 1025–1034
3. Lantz K. A. and Kaestner K. H. (2005). Winged-helix transcription factors and pancreatic development. *Clin. Sci.* **108**, 195–204
4. Wilson M. E., Scheel D., and German M. S. (2003). Gene expression cascades in pancreatic development. *Mech. Dev.* **120**, 65–80
5. Jensen J. (2004). Gene regulatory factors in pancreatic development. *Dev. Dyn.* **229**, 176–200
6. Shi L. and Consortium T. M. (2006). The MicroArray Quality Control (MAQC) project shows inter- and intraplatform reproducibility of gene expression measurements. *Nat. Biotechnol.* **24**, 1151–1161
7. Gao N., White P., Doliba N., Golson M. L., Matschinsky F. M., and Kaestner K. H. (2007). Foxa2 controls vesicle docking and insulin secretion in mature beta cells. *Cell Metab.* **6**, 267–279
8. Gupta R. K., Gao N., Gorski R. K., White P., Hardy O. T., Rafiq K., Brestelli J. E., Chen G., Stoeckert C. J., Jr., and Kaestner K. H. (2007). Expansion of adult beta-cell mass in response to increased metabolic demand is dependent on HNF-4alpha. *Genes Dev.* **21**, 756–769
9. Hardy O. T., Hohmeier H. E., Becker T. C., Manduchi E., Doliba N. M., Gupta R. K., White P., Stoeckert C. J., Jr., Matschinsky F. M., Newgard C. B., and Kaestner K. H. (2007). Functional genomics of the beta-cell: short-chain 3-hydroxyacyl-coenzyme A dehydrogenase regulates insulin secretion independent of K+ currents. *Mol. Endocrinol.* **21**, 765–773
10. Mazzarelli J. M., White P., Gorski R., Brestelli J., Pinney D. F., Arsenlis A., Katokhin A., Belova O., Bogdanova V., Elisafenko E., Gubina M., Nizolenko L., Perelman P., Puzakov M., Shilov A., Trifonoff V., Vorobjeva N., Kolchanov N., Kaestner K. H., and Stoeckert C. J., Jr. (2006). Novel genes identified

by manual annotation and microarray expression analysis in the pancreas. *Genomics* **88**, 752–761

11. White P., Brestelli J. E., Kaestner K. H., and Greenbaum L. E. (2005). Identification of transcriptional networks during liver regeneration. *J. Biol. Chem.* **280**, 3715–3722
12. Vatamaniuk M. Z., Gupta R. K., Lantz K. A., Doliba N. M., Matschinsky F. M., and Kaestner K. H. (2006). Foxa1-deficient mice exhibit impaired insulin secretion due to uncoupled oxidative phosphorylation. *Diabetes* **55**, 2730–2736
13. Manduchi E., Scearce L. M., Brestelli J. E., Grant G. R., Kaestner K. H., and Stoeckert C. J., Jr. (2002). Comparison of different labeling methods for two-channel high-density microarray experiments. *Physiol. Genomics* **10**, 169–179
14. Scearce L. M., Brestelli J. E., McWeeney S. K., Lee C. S., Mazzarelli J., Pinney D. F., Pizarro A., Stoeckert C. J., Jr., Clifton S. W., Permutt M. A., Brown J., Melton D. A., and Kaestner K. H. (2002). Functional genomics of the endocrine pancreas: the pancreas clone set and PancChip, new resources for diabetes research. *Diabetes* **51**, 1997–2004
15. Allison D. B., Cui X., Page G. P., and Sabripour M. (2006). Microarray data analysis: from disarray to consolidation and consensus. *Nat. Rev. Genet.* 7, 55–65
16. Grant G. R., Manduchi E., and Stoeckert C. J., Jr. (2007). Analysis and management of microarray gene expression data. In: Current Protocols in Molecular Biology (Ausubel F. M., Brent R., Kingston R. E., Moore D. D., Seidman J. G., Smith J. A., Struhl K., Eds.), John Wiley & Sons, Inc., Hoboken, NJ, pp. **19**.16.11-19.16.30
17. Yang Y. H., Buckley M. J., and Speed T. P. (2001). Analysis of cDNA microarray images. *Brief Bioinform* **2**, 341–349
18. Smyth G. K., Michaud J., and Scott H. S. (2005). Use of within-array replicate spots for assessing differential expression in microarray experiments. *Bioinformatics* **21**, 2067–2075
19. Smyth G. K. and Speed T. (2003). Normalization of cDNA microarray data. *Methods* **31**, 265–273
20. Tusher V. G., Tibshirani R., and Chu G. (2001). Significance analysis of microarrays applied to the ionizing radiation response. *Proc. Natl. Acad. Sci. U.S.A.* **98**, 5116–5121
21. Leek J. T., Monsen E., Dabney A. R., and Storey J. D. (2006). EDGE: extraction and analysis of differential gene expression. *Bioinformatics* **22**, 507–508
22. Grant G. R., Liu J., and Stoeckert C. J., Jr. (2005). A practical false discovery rate approach to identifying patterns of differential expression in microarray data. *Bioinformatics* **21**, 2684–2690

Chapter 17

Gene Expression Mining in Type 2 Diabetes Research

Donald R. Dunbar

Summary

Microarray analysis has become a core part of biomedical research and its value can be seen in thousands of research papers. A successful microarray experiment needs to be augmented by specialized data mining techniques if the data are to be fully exploited. Here, tools that concentrate on three areas – gene enrichment analysis, literature mining, and transcription factor binding site analysis – are described for the novice user of microarray technology. The focus of this chapter is on free, publicly available, web-based tools.

Key words: Bioinformatics, Microarray, Gene expression, Data mining, Gene enrichment, Literature mining, Transcription factor binding site

1. Introduction

The methods and utility of microarray gene expression studies have been described in Chap. 16 by Drs. White and Kaestner. For biologists, the main limiting step in the process from experiment design to publication of results is usually the interpretation of the data. Modern microarrays measure gene expression on a genome-wide level, and depending on the experimental system being studied, routinely identify from tens to thousands of genes that are differentially expressed. This creates a problem for the biologist. The biological annotation for a handful of genes is relatively easy to collate and any strong themes within the data will be simple to spot. However, when presented with a list of a hundred

C. Stocker (ed.), *Type 2 Diabetes,* Methods in Molecular Biology, vol. 560
DOI 10.1007/978-1-59745-448-3_17, © Humana Press, a part of Springer Science+Business Media, LLC 2009

or more genes, interpretation of the biological changes underlying the data becomes an enormous challenge. High-throughput methods that help the biologist make sense of their microarray data have been developed over the last few years, and the purpose of this chapter is to guide the inexperienced user of microarrays through a selection of them. The selection includes tools to identify overrepresented biological functions and processes associated with the gene list, mine the biomedical literature for associations between genes and biological terms of interest, and identify transcription factor binding sites (TFBSs) in the gene sequences. The focus of this chapter will be on free, publicly available, web-based tools.

The protocol section of this chapter is split into five short sections (one method for preparing gene lists and four web-based tools). Each describes one method or tool that helps the biologist to gain some insight into the biology behind their data. The aim is to give enough information to allow the novice user of microarrays, with little or no bioinformatics support, to use each tool. Each of the tools has additional functionality (and usually adequate online help pages), and indeed there are many other similar tools available in addition to those described here.

1.1. Gene Enrichment Analysis

Gene enrichment analysis uses statistical procedures to discover overrepresented features within a dataset. Given a gene list and some biological information, these tools can identify categories (e.g., biological processes and molecular functions from the Gene Ontology consortium or molecular pathways from KEGG) that appear more often in the gene set that they would be by chance in a random gene set of the same size. If a category is overrepresented, then this might have biological significance and point to that part of biology being perturbed in the experiment *(1)*. Gene enrichment analysis with the online tool DAVID (Database for Annotation, Visualization, and Integrated Discovery) will be described *(2)*.

1.2. Literature Mining

Literature mining probes the huge body of information available to biomedical scientists, for example, in the Medline database *(3)*. If two or more genes or proteins occur in the same paper, it is possible that they have some sort of association. Biologist faces two main problems when mining the literature however. First, because there are often hundreds of genes of interest, looking for pairwise associations using manual web-based searching (e.g., through the Pubmed web interface) is unfeasible. Computationally, however, these searches are trivial. The Pubmatrix text mining tool will be described *(4)*. Second, genes often have multiple synonyms that are used in the literature. For example, the human gene transcription factor 7-like 2 (T-cell specific, HMG-box) (official gene symbol, TCF7L2) has several synonyms: HMG box transcription factor 4, hTCF-4, T-cell-specific transcription factor 4, TCF4, TCF-4, transcription factor 7-like 2. Many of these are used in scientific publications and this makes exact text matching difficult unless a complicated query string is built for each gene. The Information Hyperlinked over Proteins (iHOP) tool makes good use of synonym information and offers several useful features, and its use will be described here *(5)*. These text mining tools give the biologist a good entry to mining the literature. Further tools that include more advanced information extraction and retrieval, entity recognition, and natural language processing will be available to the biologists over time.

1.3. TFBS Analysis

TFBS analysis can identify binding sites that are statistically overrepresented in the sequences of a gene list. Finding such enriched sites can give an idea of the factors that are driving gene expression locally at the cellular level in the experimental model. TFBSs often bind to several similar sequences, and computational tools that access TFBS databases can use sequence models to predict binding sites in gene sequences *(6)*. In addition, if a binding site is conserved between species, it is more likely to be functionally important. Whole Genome RVista allows identification of conserved (between pairs of species) statistically overrepresented TFBSs in specified regions (e.g., 5 kb upstream) of groups of genes *(7)*.

2. Materials

The description of protocols for downstream analysis of microarray data is strongly aimed at the inexperienced user of microarray technology with little or no bioinformatics support. As such, the reader only needs access to the processed, statistically analysed data (*see* Chap. 16) and a computer with web access, spreadsheet (e.g., Microsoft Excel or OpenOffice) software, and text file editing software.

3. Protocols

The following protocols require the user to have a list of selected genes. These have been generated by a statistical tool (e.g., Affymetrix GCOS), and genes will be included or excluded based on a threshold score for some statistics of the gene expression (e.g., *p*-value or fold change). These protocols require that the user can copy a list of gene identifiers (e.g., Affymetrix Probeset IDs or Entrez Gene IDs for protocols 3.2 "Gene Enrichment Analysis with DAVID" and 3.5 "TFBS Analysis with Whole Genome RVista," and gene symbols and names for protocol 3.3 "Literature Mining with Pubmatrix") for further use. Data should be available to the user in the form of a spreadsheet or a tab-delimited text file.

3.1. Gene List Preparation

1. Open the file containing gene expression data with spreadsheet software.
2. Copy the gene identifiers.
3. Paste into a new spreadsheet.
4. Sort the identifiers.
5. Remove duplicate entries (*see* **Note 1**).
6. Save as a plain text file with appropriate name, for example, "exp1_up_2fold_AffyIDs.txt."

3.2. Gene Enrichment Analysis with DAVID

1. Open the gene list text file (*see* **Note 2**).
2. Copy the identifiers, noting their type (e.g., Affymetrix ID, Entrez Gene IDs).
3. Go to the DAVID Web site: http://david.abcc.ncifcrf.gov/
4. Click "Start Analysis" in the menu bar.
5. Paste the gene list into "Step 1: Enter Gene List" box.
6. Select the type of identifier (e.g., AFFY_ID) in "Step 2: Select Identifier."
7. Select "Gene List" from "Step 3: List Type."
8. Submit list (this will take the reader to the analysis wizard).
9. Click "Rename," rename the list in the dialog box, and click "OK."
10. The "Current Background" will be automatically selected (*see* **Note 3**).
11. If your data are Affymetrix IDs, click "Background" in the navigation bar.
12. Click the "+" beside "Affymetrix." Choose the appropriate GeneChip.
13. Click "Functional Annotation Tool" in the analysis wizard.
14. Click "Functional Annotation Chart."
15. Click the "+" for "Options." Check "Fold Enrichment" then "Rerun Using Options."
16. Explore the results (*see* **Note 4**).

3.3. Literature Mining with Pubmatrix

1. Go to the Pubmatrix site (http://pubmatrix.grc.nia.nih.gov/) and register for an account, and then log in to the "authenticated site."
2. Prepare a list of gene names and symbols up to a maximum of 100 (*see* **Note 5**).
3. Prepare a list of relevant words to analyse alongside the genes (e.g., diabetes, obesity, insulin, diet, glucose, metformin, regulate, and expression).
4. Give the "Search Terms" and "Modifier Terms" appropriate names (e.g., "upregulated genes experiment 2," "T2D terms 1-10").
5. Copy the gene list into the "Search Terms" list.
6. Copy the word list into the "Modifier Terms" list.
7. Submit to Pubmatrix (*see* **Note 6**).
8. On the following day, go to the Pubmatrix site and click "Your past results." Check the status of your search, and if completed, click the link.
9. Explore your results. In the matrix displayed, each combination of Search Term (gene) and Modifier Term (extra word) has a number indicating how many abstracts were found. Click one.
10. This takes you to a Pubmed search for the titles and abstracts that contain both the search and modifier terms (*see* **Note 7**).

3.4. Literature Mining with iHOP

1. Go to the iHOP Web site: http://www.ihop-net.org
2. Enter a gene name, symbol, or ID in the first box.
3. Select the appropriate fields to search (leaving "all fields" is usually fine, if it is a gene ID, select "NCBI Gene"). Select a species if required.
4. Click the "SEARCH" link.
5. Explore your results.
6. If successful, the search gives one or more rows. Click any of the links in the row that matches your gene (all the links in a row are to the same page).
7. This page is the current iHOP page for that gene (highlighted red). Sentences from Pubmed abstracts are displayed and other genes and annotation are highlighted and hyperlinked (*see* **Note 8**).
8. Click a link for another gene mentioned in the sentence along with your gene of interest and you will be taken to the iHOP page for that gene.
9. Use some of the other functions available in iHOP page (*see* **Note 9**).

3.5. TFBS Analysis with Whole Genome RVista

1. Go to the Whole Genome RVista site: http://genome-test.lbl.gov/cgi-bin/WGRVistaInputCommon.pl
2. Choose a genome alignment to use (e.g., TFBS in Mouse May 2004 assembly conserved in the alignment with the Human May 2004 assembly) and "GO."
3. Select the length of upstream sequence you would like to analyse (5 kb default).
4. Open the file with the Entrez Gene IDs. Copy the IDs into the box and select "I am submitting locus link IDs" (*see* **Note 10**), and click on Submit.
5. Explore your results. The results table shows overrepresented (statistically significant) conserved TFBSs, ordered by $-\log_{10}p$-value (0.005 gives 2.3). Click one of the buttons on the right, marked with a TFBS symbol. This then shows the genes in your list that have this sequence at least once in the region searched (*see* **Note 11**).
6. Go back to the main results page and scroll down to the second table. Click on one of the "show" links in the "Summary of all conserved TFBS upstream of this gene" column. This will then show a table of conserved TFBSs upstream of the gene with those overrepresented in the input gene list, marked in green.

4. Notes

1. Often lists of genes that are differentially expressed will have two or more entries for the same gene. This can cause problems in further analysis, especially where statistics require no redundancy. If a gene (e.g., its Entrez Gene ID) is present two or more times in a list, then it will be counted twice in the analyses used, for example, by DAVID (protocol 3.2) and RVista (protocol 3.5). When working with tools that accept chip identifiers (such as Affymetrix Probeset IDs), redundancy is not usually a problem as the chip identifiers will normally be unique. Although many tools deal with this redundancy at the gene level, it is safer to remove it at source. Paste the IDs into a worksheet, sort, and then remove duplicate items.
2. Many tools allow identifiers or sequences to be input either by pasting text or directly form a file. If the file is in the appropriate format, then these methods are equivalent. Choose the method that suits you.
3. Enrichment analysis requires a "benchmark" to test against. A background gene set is used for this and can be the

complement of genes on a microarray, or in the whole genome. (The "Current Background" in DAVID defaults to complete knowledgebase gene set for the input species.) If, for example, 10 genes in your gene list of 200 (5%) belong to (or map to) one Gene Ontology term (GO term), this might sound exciting. However, if 5% of the genes on the microarray also belong to that GO term, then your finding is no different from chance. But if only 1% of the genes on the microarray map to the GO term, then it is likely that your result is a real enrichment. You can then proceed to investigate the biological significance of the result.

4. The DAVID functional annotation chart is a table displaying those terms that are statistically enriched in your gene list. The "term" column gives a hyperlinked name of the enriched term. The hyperlink goes to the database outlined in the "category" column: for example, GOTERM_ goes to QuickGO at EBI, SP_ goes to Uniprot, and KEGG_ and BIOCARTA_ go to those pathway databases that are stored within DAVID. The links are not all ideal as they can be to text searches rather than direct links to database entries using the ID of the term: these text searches using the term name can often match more than the term of interest. Further information about the term can be obtained from the "RT" column, which gives a hyperlink to related terms for each term, ranked by relatedness based on overlap of gene lists. This can be useful to get a wider view of the biology around the enriched term. There is usually a lot of redundancy in this list: mainly due to the hierarchical nature of the GO database (e.g., genes in GOTERM_BP_5 are a subset of genes in GOTERM_BP_4). The table is ordered by the *p*-value for the statistical test (Fisher Exact) used to determine enrichment. In addition, there is a column "Benjamini" that lists the *p*-value corrected for multiple testing. The "count" tells us the number of genes from our list that were mapped to the term, and "%" gives the number as a percentage of the full list of genes mapped to that term. The "fold enrichment" column gives a ratio for the enrichment. Clicking on the blue bar in the "Genes" column will show the genes in the list that map to the term and useful links to the database entry for each gene and a set of related genes.

5. Pubmatrix does not map the gene's ID onto its name or symbol, so it is essential to prepare a gene name and symbol list. These, of course, can be used separately, but can also be used as a query together, separated by "OR." Copy and paste name and symbol from your gene list into a worksheet. Insert a column between them and add the word "OR" to each cell in the column by filling down, so that we have gene name in column 1, "OR" in column 2 and

gene symbol in column 3. Now, in the column 4, add the following function: =CONCATENATE(A1," ",B2," ",C1), and fill or copy it down the column. This will give terms like "aquaporin 4 OR Aqp4." These can then be stored in a text file with an appropriate name and can be used in a Pubmatrix search.

6. Because of the restrictions placed on using Pubmed servers at NCBI, Pubmatrix will only run searches from 5 pm to 8 am Eastern Standard Time. Jobs will, however, go into the queue if submitted outside this window and are almost always completed by the next day.
7. Pubmatrix searches are fairly crude and as with other text searches of Pubmed, are sensitive to false positives and negatives. False negatives usually happen because none of the gene's synonyms were used in the search. False positives are frequently the fault of gene symbols having alternative meaning in the literature. Symbols that are also short words or abbreviations are often the culprits. Adding extra synonyms where appropriate and removing problematic symbols can help. Just resubmit the new list to Pubmatrix.
8. The main advantage of using iHOP is its use of synonym data to search the literature and link genes/proteins. This means that searching with one synonym will also find publications that cite other synonyms or symbols for the gene or protein. iHOP makes extensive use of links and markup. Each iHOP page has links to the pages for other genes: this is the essence of iHOP. "Marking up" abstracts means that it is immediately obvious where in the abstract the current and other genes are. In addition, informative verbs such as associated, interacts, biding, complexed, affect, inhibits, suppresses, activates etc.; MESH (Medical Subject Headings) terms; and chemical compounds are also marked up and have additional links. Links on the right of the screen will take you to abstracts at Pubmed.
9. An extremely useful feature of iHOP is the "show overview" link. This link takes you to a list of genes that are associated with the gene of interest, ordered by the number of sentences in the literature that cocite the two genes and whether there is any interaction evidence in several databases including IntAct. This immediately guides you to genes that are highly cocited with the gene of interest. Click a gene link to see both the original and linked genes that are marked up in the sentences. Enhanced Pubmed and Google searches (using all synonyms, symbols, and additional terms) are useful for further searching, and genes can be added to a useful "Gene Model" that shows interactions visually.

10. Locus link was the predecessor of the Entrez Gene database. Locus link IDs map exactly to Entrez Gene IDs.

11. In the Whole Genome RVista output, the "number of hits in the submitted regions" column tells us the total number of hits rather than the number of genes that contain the conserved TFBS sequence. This is compared with the "total number of hits on genome" to generate the statistic. Clicking the "show genes where..." buttons will then show the genes that have the TFBS.

References

1. Curtis, R. K., et al. (2005). Pathways to the analysis of microarray data. *Trends Biotechnol* **23**, 429–435
2. Dennis, G., Jr., et al. (2003). DAVID: Database for Annotation, Visualization, and Integrated Discovery. *Genome Biol* **4**, P3
3. Jensen, L. J., et al. (2006). Literature mining for the biologist: from information retrieval to biological discovery. *Nat Rev Genet* 7, 119–129
4. Becker, K. G., et al. (2003). PubMatrix: a tool for multiplex literature mining. *BMC Bioinformatics* **4**, 61
5. Hoffmann, R., et al. (2004). A gene network for navigating the literature. *Nat Genet* **36**, 664
6. Elnitski, L., et al. (2006). Locating mammalian transcription factor binding sites: a survey of computational and experi mental techniques. *Genome Res.* **16**, 1455–1464
7. Loots, G. G., et al. (2002). RVista for comparative sequence-based discovery of functional transcription factor binding sites. *Genome Res* **12**, 832–839

INDEX

Q

R

S

T

V

Z

MIX
Papier aus verantwortungsvollen Quellen
Paper from responsible sources
FSC® C105338

If you have any concerns about our products,
you can contact us on
ProductSafety@springernature.com

In case Publisher is established outside the EU,
the EU authorized representative is:
Springer Nature Customer Service Center GmbH
Europaplatz 3, 69115 Heidelberg, Germany

Printed by Libri Plureos GmbH
in Hamburg, Germany